The human future depends on a spreading awakening to a spiritual reality that Western cultures have been prone to deny. Salmon and Maslow bring together ancient Eastern spiritual teachings with the most advanced of Western science to help us penetrate the illusions of culture, helping us not only to understand the nature of spirituality, but even more, to experience it. A profoundly important book.

—David C. Korten, Ph.D., board chair *YES!* Magazine;
author, *The Great Turning: From Empire to Earth Community*

Developing a global consensus about the nature and evolution of consciousness provides a major challenge for 21st Century thought. Nothing could be more important for an understanding of human nature. Drawing largely on the integral yoga philosophy and psychology of Sri Aurobindo, the authors provide an in-depth account that sheds a very different light on the view currently prevalent in the West. Fascinating and provocative.

—Max Velmans, Ph.D., cognitive psychologist; author,
Understanding Consciousness; science editor, *The Blackwell Companion to Consciousness*

Don Salmon and Jan Maslow liberate us from the limited prison of ego psychology and awaken us to the realm of real consciousness, the true consciousness that lies at the root of all of life. Here is a map to help us escape the confines of our contemporary culture, a way to understand what it really means to be fully alive to our infinite nature. Here are signposts for individual and collective transformation: read them!

—Llewellyn Vaughan-Lee, Sufi teacher;
author, *Awakening the World: A Global Dimension to Spiritual Life*

As a neuroscientist, a long-time practitioner of Theravada Buddhist meditation, and a budding Christian theologian, I find the ideas presented by Salmon and Maslow wonderfully complementary to my own perspective, particularly with respect to the nature of the self. Those interested in how the wisdom of ancient India can help shed light on the nature of consciousness in both traditional Christian and classical Buddhist contexts would be well advised to study this text closely. It is a high quality, authentically serious effort, and very nicely written.

—Jeffrey M. Schwartz, MD, research psychiatrist, UCLA;
author, *The Mind & The Brain*

This book builds a bridge between science and spirituality in order to perceive Reality in an integral way. The authors have distilled a common vocabulary, experiences, practices, diagrams and concepts from various writings to show that Reality and science can only be encompassed by an ever-growing understanding and experience of spirituality. Such an understanding can lead to a holistic change in the perception of Reality, which in turn induces deep transformative powers to formulate new solutions to address complex challenges within and outside us. In all, here's a truly well-researched book for those of us who want to attempt to sense Reality.

—Arnab B. Chowdhury, founder, Nināad Consultancy Services

The authors range widely through contemporary thinking in consciousness studies, philosophy of science and psi research, providing provocative challenges to traditional thinking at every step.

—William A. Adams, Ph.D., psychologist;
author, *What Does It All Mean? A Humanistic Account of Human Experience*

This book tackles in an elegant yet incisive manner one of the necessities of our time —the synthesis of science and spirituality. Bringing to bear the insights of Indian philosopher-sage Aurobindo Ghose, it helps us understand our experiences from a spiritual perspective. It offers optimism about our world's future which is needed in this time of transformation. Read it.

—Elmer Green, Ph.D., psychophysicist and biofeedback pioneer

The book is excellent—informative, easy to read, well-researched and organized, and most of all it has a wonderful spiritual atmosphere. I can feel the breath of Infinity behind every page.

—Michael Miovic, M.D., attending psychiatrist,
Dana Farber Cancer Institute, Boston

YOGA PSYCHOLOGY AND THE TRANSFORMATION OF CONSCIOUSNESS

YOGA PSYCHOLOGY AND THE TRANSFORMATION OF CONSCIOUSNESS

SEEING THROUGH THE EYES OF INFINITY

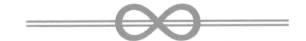

Don Salmon   Jan Maslow

First Edition 2007

Published in the United States by
Paragon House
1925 Oakcrest Avenue, Suite 7
St. Paul, MN 55113

Library of Congress Cataloging-in-Publication Data

Salmon, Don, 1952-
  Yoga psychology and the transformation of consciousness : seeing through the
    eyes of infinity / Don Salmon, Jan Maslow. -- 1st ed.
    p. cm.
  Includes bibliographical references and index.
  ISBN 1-55778-835-9 (pbk. : alk. paper) 1. Consciousness. 2.
Transpersonal psychology. 3. Yoga--Psychological aspects. 4. Ghose, Aurobindo,
    1872-1950. I. Maslow, Jan, 1950- II. Title.
  BF311.S333 2007
  150.19'8--dc22
                                    2006035188

Manufactured in the United States of America
10 9 8 7 6 5 4 3 2 1

The paper used in this publication meets the minimum requirements of American National Standard for Information Sciences—Permanence of Paper for Printed Library Materials, ANSIZ39.48-1984.

For current information on all releases from Paragon House
visit the website at: www.paragonhouse.com

ACKNOWLEDGMENTS

We have each, in our own way, spent more than twenty-five years studying and meditating on various facets of yoga psychology. During this time there have been many who influenced and inspired us. We are grateful to our parents, our families, and our friends who have supported and encouraged us in so many ways over the years. For guidance in our spiritual practice, we offer our deep gratitude to Sri Aurobindo and Mirra Alfassa, Swami Ramananda, Roy Eugene Davis, Kumar S. Kumar, Llewellyn Vaughan-Lee, and Morton Klausen.

Though we have both studied psychology, we've also learned much that was relevant to our understanding of yoga psychology from other experiences. Don would especially like to thank the dancers, choreographers, and dance teachers with whom he worked. He feels that learning to create music to match the rhythmic flow of dance taught him a great deal about the play of various colors and textures of consciousness. Jan is grateful to Gene Maslow and others in the arts who helped her gain an appreciation for the relationship between yoga psychology and the creative process. She is also grateful to all those with whom she worked and studied in the course of helping to create a collaborative workplace; an endeavor that gave her a richer understanding of different aspects of consciousness as they play out in human nature.

We are grateful for the online Integral Psychology forum that provided the opportunity for an in-depth exploration of Sri Aurobindo's synthesis of yoga psychology. We thank all the participants for their support, encouragement, and penetrating insight—and equally for their incisive criticism, which helped us see how much we had to learn and clarify in our own understanding.

We are grateful for the generous support of the Infinity Foundation as well as to Rajiv Malhotra, its founder and president. The book is a different book as a result of what we learned from Rajiv's formulation of the issues involved in presenting yoga psychology in a contemporary context. Thanks also to the Foundation for World Education for their support.

We would like to express our appreciation to all those who have helped us to better understand yoga psychology as well as those who've given us invaluable feedback as we struggled to put our understanding into words, including Bill Adams, Anne-Marie, Imants Baruss, Soumitra Basu, Jonathan Bricklin, Sitansu Chakravarti, Jim Chamberlain, Janis Coker, Brant Cortwright, Brad Coupe, Lynn Crawford, Luke Crouse, Don Cruse, Dr. Dalal, Bhavana Dee, Deshpande, Larry Dossey, Astrid Fitzgerald, Charles Flores, Bob Forman, Richard Geldard, Neil Gore, Rod Hemsell, Mark Henry, Alan Herbert, Neeltje Huppes, Liz Inglis, Ben Irvin, Gary Jacobs, Cleo Kearns, Barbara Kimmel, Pete Kimmel, Amal Kiran, Lorna Kohler, Maggi Lidchi, Martha Miller, Ulrich Moerher, Jennifer Morgan, Jugal Mukherjee, Aster Patel, Dean Radin, Arthur Reber, Ananda Reddy, Kitty Reddy, Lakshman Sehgal, Larry Seidlitz, Kosha Shah, Jonathan Shear, Bahman Shirazi, Shraddavan, Andy Smith, Charles Tart, Georges Van Vrekhem, Vladimir, Julie Weinberg, Daniel Winstel, Klaus Witz, and Mark Woodhouse.

We offer special thanks to those who devoted extra time to carefully reviewing the entire manuscript: Bob Salmon, Stephanie Golden, Will Moss, Michael Miovic, Matthijs Cornelissen, Rhianon Allen, Rich Carlson, and Neil Gore.

We want to thank Rosemary Yokoi at Paragon House, whose kindness, patience, and unfailing good humor were a great balm all along the way, and especially at critical moments just before our deadline(s!). Thanks to John White, the editor of the Omega Series, for shepherding us from the proposal stage up to publication. We are grateful to Tommy Wyche for the beautiful photograph that served as the basis for the cover of the book. We deeply appreciate the dedication, time, and talent of Carolyn Vaughan for her work on the cover, the charts, and diagrams.

We are deeply grateful for the opportunity of collaborating with each other in the writing of the book. We have been sharing our interest and passion for yoga psychology since we met in 1993, talking about it together, and—to whatever extent possible—trying to live it as well. Don began working on the book while we were still living in

New York City. Not long after moving (in the wake of 9/11) to the Nature's Spirit community in South Carolina, circumstances changed such that we were able to begin working on the book together. It has been very gratifying to give shape to something that has been so central to both our lives. We hope that in some small way our efforts will contribute to a fuller realization of what we believe to be the potential transformative power inherent in yoga psychology.

Contents

BOOK I
THE STORIES

BOOK II
PREPARATION FOR THE JOURNEY

BOOK III
THE JOURNEY

PART I
THE VIEW FROM INFINITY

PART II
THE EVOLUTION OF THE FIELD

PART III
THE KNOWER OF THE FIELD

APPENDIX D

Table of Contemplative Practices

List of Tables and Figures

...to the seeing eye each finite carries in it its own revelation of the infinite.[1]

—Sri Aurobindo, *Essays on the Gita*

FOREWORD

Skillful yoga practice restores the practitioner's awareness to its original, pure wholeness. Three effective ways of allowing this process to be experienced are by: 1) removing attention and awareness from objective phenomena and modified states of mind and consciousness; 2) using discriminative intelligence to discern the difference between what is observed and one's self as the detached observer; 3) skillful meditation practice that calms the wave—like movements and changes in the mind that keep awareness confined. When awareness is clarified, the reality of one's pure essence of being is said to be self-shining.

The meditative way is described in Patanjali's yoga-sutra's (1:2): "Yoga [unification] is realized when movements and changes in the individual field of awareness are turned back to their origin. The enlightened or fully awake state of consciousness is naturally experienced when identification of awareness with modified states of mind and consciousness ceases. Spiritual enlightenment is spontaneously realized when obstacles to its emergence are removed.

It was from my teacher Paramahansa Yogananda that I learned the fundamentals of yoga and with his personal guidance and encouragement was soon able to proficiently apply them. Having experienced the positive results of dedicated practice, I can wholeheartedly attest to its practical usefulness.

For the reader who is sincerely interested in knowing about the positive, transformative changes and states of consciousness that are possible to be experienced by right personal endeavor, this book will be extremely helpful.

Roy Eugene Davis
Director, Center For Spiritual Awareness
Author of *The Eternal Way: The Inner Meaning of the Bhagavad Gita*
and *The Science of Self-Realization:*
A Guide to Spiritual Practice in the Kriya Yoga Tradition

PREFACE

In recent decades Yoga has crossed into the popular culture in the West and is dramatically growing on the American scene. Unfortunately the depth and transformative power of genuine Yoga Science and Philosophy often gets lost in "translation" across cultures. It is well known in Eastern meditative traditions that Yoga focuses on the awakening transformation of the Self and the dilation of consciousness beyond the ego-based psyche and egocentric patterns of consciousness. And yet this vital essence often gets lost and is not sufficiently brought front and center. Don Salmon and Jan Maslow in their beautifully presented book break new ground in daring to suggest and remind us that we humans are meant to come into direct encounter with the Primal Infinite Force and Presence that permeates us all and surrounds us in every moment of our daily lives.

Their innovative and transformative narrative builds on the great advances in Yoga Philosophy developed by the eminent Indian sage Sri Aurobindo in the 20th Century. Aurobindo brings this amazing and evolving classical tradition of Yoga Science into the modern world in showing that this Infinite Presence (called *Aum* and *Brahman* in the Indian tradition) is proactive in the evolution of the cosmos and culture, and is itself in boundlessly dynamic process and evolution. In this light Aurobindo shows that Nature, Matter, and Body, as expressions of Brahman, are sacred and integral to spiritual life and human flourishing.

Indeed, as we enter a new and unprecedented global age and rise to a more inclusive global perspective it becomes clear that this Infinite Presence, by whatever name we use—*Tao, Yahweh, Aum, Allah, Christ, Brahman, Logos, Energy*—infinitely situates and surrounds us in every pulse of life, and across all our cultural, religious and disciplinary boundaries. And the bottom line in this wondrous perennial and global wisdom is that we humans suffer and perish when we are cut off from direct connectivity with this global Infinite Presence, and we thrive and flourish in Well-being and boundless Life when we awaken into communion with this Infinite Presiding Force-field. This is the more advanced and mature way to understand and process our psychic and spiritual development, indeed, every aspect of our daily cultural lives.

In this spirit Don and Jan in their highly readable book lead the reader in a meditative and mind-expanding way ever deeper into this evolutionary awakening of consciousness and the maturation of the human psyche. They demonstrate a solid inner grasp of the Science and Philosophy of Yoga and beautifully bring this vital teaching into our contemporary cultural lives as we face the challenges of the 21st Century. This important book speaks deeply to all emerging global citizens, to all persons who are on the awakening path and who seek wholeness, well-being, and inner peace. The narrative dares to recognize and open the lens to the encounter with Infinite Presence, and to seeing through the eyes of Infinity. This book is an accessible manual for rising into this higher life for all humans living in the 21st Century.

Ashok Gangadean
Professor and Chair of Philosophy, Haverford College
Founder-Director of the Global Dialogue Institute
Co-Convenor of the World Commission on
Global Consciousness and Spirituality
Author of *The Awakening of the Global Mind*

INTRODUCTION

The day-to-day life of our distant ancestors remained essentially unchanged for more than a hundred thousand years. In the past hundred years, we have experienced a dizzying acceleration in the pace of change fueled by a seemingly never-ending cascade of new technologies—from the airplane and the automobile to the cell phone and the Internet.

Advances in transportation and communication have woven the world together. While the increased contact with cultures in far-flung parts of the world has been enriching, the clash of differing world-views has challenged the core of our identity. To the extent our identities have been wrapped up in the rapidly receding past, our sense of ourselves has been fractured.

Having depended on age-old cultural norms to tell us what is good and what is bad, many feel lost in a world that seems to make no sense. Adrift in a sea of growing numbers of meaningless things, we are bombarded with information and have no yardstick with which to measure the value of one thing relative to another.

Psychologists who study animal intelligence tell us that the capacity to stand back and reflect on ourselves and our world is a uniquely human capacity. Caught up in the whirlwind of change, flooded with meaningless bits of information, we lose touch with this ability and react blindly to passing circumstance. Without consciously setting out to do so, we produce a world that makes no sense. We create air that is not fit to breathe, water that is not fit to drink, and in the midst of plenty, millions go hungry. In just the past twenty-four hours, over forty-five thousand people have died of starvation—more than a dozen times the number of people who died in the World Trade Center on September 11, 2001. In the same twenty-four-hour period, we have poured another 13 million tons of toxic chemicals into our environment.[1]

SLOWING DOWN, TURNING EAST

This increasing tension has compelled many to look for a way out, for a way to insert a pause in the frenzied pace of life. Looking for something that has not been infected by the rush and meaninglessness of modern life, many have turned to the spiritual traditions of India.

India is for many a land of contradictions that conjures images of the majestic Taj Mahal, crowds of impoverished children begging for money, ascetic yogis meditating in Himalayan caves, and wealthy businessmen negotiating high-tech deals. Whatever truth may lie behind these clashing images, it is a place that has held a fascination for the West for centuries. This has been the case at least since Christopher Columbus set sail in search of a faster trade route to India, then one of the wealthiest countries in the world.

What began centuries ago as a desire for exotic material goods soon grew into a quest for the subtler treasures of the spirit. In the early 1800s, German philosophers and poets looked to ancient Indian writings for inspiration. As a result of the British colonization of India, knowledge of yogic practices began to filter back to England. In response to the Industrial Revolution then under way, some were drawn to these practices as a way to keep their balance in the face of widespread social upheaval and an increasingly mechanized way of life.

While greater peace of mind was the goal for some, others sought greater understanding. In the early twentieth century, physicist Erwin Schrodinger turned to Indian spiritual texts to help him solve the mysteries raised by the new discoveries of quantum physics.[2] During the same period, William James announced to his psychology class at Harvard that the Buddhist understanding of the mind, rooted in Indian teachings more than two thousand years old, would one day provide the foundation for modern psychology.[3]

Schrodinger and James looked to the wisdom of the ancient yogic tradition in search of something outside their familiar framework that might illumine it in a new way. William James in particular understood the potential of the psychological and spiritual aspects of yoga to revolutionize our basic understanding of reality. Many decades later, in the 1960s and '70s, scientists like biofeedback pioneer Elmer

Green and mindfulness meditation teacher Jon Kabat-Zinn initiated research programs with the goal of explaining these practices in modern scientific terms.

Recognizing that the culture of the time would not have been receptive to the psychospiritual roots of the yoga tradition, they presented the practices in a way that did not challenge the prevailing materialistic view. By using acceptable scientific language—for example, defining meditation as an attitude of "attentional manipulation"—they were able to bypass the foreign cultural and spiritual context from which they had borrowed the yogic techniques.[4] Their cautious terminology was effective in gaining respectability within the mainstream scientific culture for what were essentially yogic practices in disguise.

One of the more skillful bridge-builders between science and yoga has been Dr. Herbert Benson. An associate professor of medicine at Harvard Medical School and chief of behavioral medicine at Beth Israel Deaconess Medical Center in Boston, Benson has become one of the foremost pioneers in the field of mind-body medicine and the integration of spirituality and healing. Looking back, he admits that it was with great "trepidation and footdragging" that he initially came to engage in mind-body research. As a young cardiologist in the 1960s, he recognized there was a real possibility that he could be severely criticized, if not ostracized, by his colleagues for exploring topics that were at the time considered taboo.

Benson was first persuaded to take up his research in mind-body medicine in 1968, when some practitioners of Transcendental Meditation approached him with the claim they could induce physiological changes through the practice of meditation. Benson turned down their initial request, but their persistence and enthusiasm eventually persuaded him to embark on what was soon to become a vital part of his life's work.

After studying the effects of Transcendental Meditation for several years, Benson extracted from it the components that he believed were essential to its effectiveness. Patients were thus taught to sit or lie quietly and repeat a sound or phrase such as the word "one." This practice was found to result in a significant reduction of physiological and psychological stress. In order to avoid association with the yoga tradition, Benson referred to the effects of this practice simply as "the relaxation response."

Other researchers, including Jon Kabat-Zinn, Richard Davidson, and John Teasdale, have since discovered that meditative practices have psychophysical effects beyond those that Benson attributes to the relaxation response.[5] In recent years millions of people have become involved in meditative practices, and many as a result have developed a new sense of joy and inner peace. Meditation and other practices based on the yoga tradition have been adapted for a wide variety of uses, from the rehabilitation of longtime convicts to the training of Olympic athletes. Biologists, cellists, CEOs and even priests, among many others, have found that these practices have helped them be more effective in what they do and find deeper satisfaction in their lives.

The initial motivation for taking up yogic practices is often the desire to bring about a change in one's health or performance—perhaps a reduction in pain or stress, an improvement in athletic abilities, or an increased effectiveness in the workplace. However, after some time, as the body learns to relax and the mind becomes calmer, some begin to have glimpses of a deeper experience. Accompanying these glimpses, there may be a vague sense that something still more is possible. Benson himself found, after years of cautiously presenting his technique in secular terms, that patients occasionally would share with him spiritual experiences that arose spontaneously while experiencing the relaxation response. Reflecting his recognition that bringing a spiritual context to the practice makes it richer and more powerful, Benson began to speak openly of the importance of the "faith factor"—that is, a "faith in an eternal or life-transcending force."[6]

Like Benson and others, we had initially felt the need to present meditative practices in a "safe" secular form. Don conducted research on the effectiveness of Buddhist meditation in reducing pain and applied his findings to his clinical work. Inspired by the yogic underpinnings of Peter Senge's work with learning organizations,[a] Jan developed a program to help create a more collaborative atmosphere in her workplace—one based on learning and a deeper sense of purpose.

---

a. For more information on learning organizations, see Peter Senge's book *The Fifth Discipline*.

These early attempts were limited in their effectiveness. Part of this was due to our inexperience, but we also felt it was a result of having taken these practices out of their deeper spiritual context. In recent years we've integrated some of that larger context, and to the extent we've done so, the work has been more effective. Still, we continued to feel that something was needed to counter the influence of a culture that in so many ways is opposed to a spiritual sense of things.

While this may have been difficult to do even ten years ago, it seems the time may now be ripe for a fuller presentation of the essence of the Indian spiritual tradition. The fact that a small but growing group of eminent scientists is beginning to challenge the prevailing materialistic perspective suggests an increased receptivity to an alternative view. Nobel Prize–winning physicist Brian Josephson,[7] biologist Mae Wan-Ho, and psychiatrist Jeffrey Schwartz, for example, are saying, respectively, that the laws of nature, the process of evolution, and the workings of the brain cannot be explained without taking some form of conscious intelligence into account. Articles in leading scientific journals have explicitly called for a spiritual, or non-material, understanding of consciousness, an understanding that is fundamental to the yoga tradition.

The presentation of yoga and meditation separated from its spiritual roots may have been a wise and necessary accommodation at the time. And thanks to the work of pioneering spirits like Dr. Benson, Jon Kabat-Zinn, and others, it has now become possible to present the deeper view underlying the yoga tradition.

THE METHOD AND FORMAT OF THE BOOK

Intimations of Infinity

One of our major aims in this book is to both describe and evoke this deeper view that sees everything in the universe as the expression of an infinite consciousness. Some of what we describe may seem at first to be remote from everyday life. But if there is any validity to the yogic idea that everything is an expression of an infinite reality, then that reality must be an intimate part of our most ordinary experience.

Many spiritual writings point to intimations of the pervasive presence of an infinite reality in our lives. The Sufis speak of a longing we sometimes feel, a longing that is an intimation of the presence of something deep within us, some "place" of harmony, a source of profound contentment. The Buddhists speak of the "sky of mind" to refer to a feeling of spaciousness, that is an intimation of that greater reality beyond all time and space which holds the entire universe in its embrace. Both use familiar experiences—the sense of longing or the simple perception of space—to point to a deeper spiritual reality. Throughout the book, we use such familiar experiences to show how this greater reality is reflected in our everyday lives.

One way we do this is through the presentation of Sharon's story, which is based on events in the lives of several army veterans, some of whom served in the Vietnam War. For example, the awareness of "something strange yet familiar" that came to her while sitting in the backyard of her father's house is an intimation of a greater presence in the depths of her being. Her story is offered as an invitation to readers to examine similar intimations in their own experience.

The Basis of the Book

What is yoga psychology? Psychology refers to the study of the mind. Yoga—literally to yoke or unite—is a means of helping us to recognize the connection between our individual consciousness and an infinite, all-pervading consciousness. Thus, yoga psychology is the study of the mind in light of its inherent connection to an infinite Reality.

We base our presentation of yoga psychology, for the most part, on the synthesis of the yoga tradition presented by twentieth-century Indian philosopher-sage Sri Aurobindo. However, we use the term "yoga psychology" in a generic sense to mean an intuitive, experiential study of our conscious experience in light of an infinite Reality. We also at times use it to refer to the large body of psychospiritual knowledge accumulated over thousands of years by those who have engaged in this kind of intuitive study.

To underscore our understanding that "yoga psychology" is ultimately about a way of looking that transcends any particular perspective, we draw from a number of sources besides Sri Aurobindo, including Hindu, Buddhist, Sufi, and Christian sacred texts, as well as the writings of William Blake, Sri Krishna Prem, and other "yoga psychologists."

We understand, however, that there are some real differences among different branches of the yoga tradition. Whenever we write "according to yoga psychology" or "from the yogic perspective," it means we believe the idea we're presenting is in harmony with the yogic tradition as a whole. When an idea represents something about which there may be different perspectives, we will specify the source, as in "according to Sri Aurobindo," "according to Sri Krishna Prem," and so on.

Potentially, the most troublesome aspect of our usage of the term "yoga psychology" is the implication of a common perspective between Buddhists and Hindus. In this, we are following the lead of Robert Thurman, a prominent authority on Tibetan Buddhism, who in recent years has used the phrase "yoga psychology" to refer to themes common to the whole Indo-Tibetan tradition.[8]

The Format of the Book

The book is organized around the theme of the evolution of consciousness. Book One gives an overview of what scientists have discovered to date regarding the emergence and development of consciousness in the universe. Book Three gives the yogic understanding of the evolution of consciousness. Because the yogic view is so profoundly different from the way we ordinarily see the world, we examine in Book Two the assumptions which shape that ordinary view. We devote two chapters to the examination of these assumptions because, to the extent we are unaware of them, they will make it more difficult to consider those aspects of yoga psychology that are most at variance with our conventional way of seeing things. We also develop the idea in these chapters that there is no inherent conflict between the vision of yoga psychology and the findings of science—at least, not when those findings are distinguished from the materialistic philosophy sometimes assumed to be inseparable from them.

Yoga Psychology: Fact or Fantasy?

Since the vision of yoga psychology is so much at variance with the conventional view of things, by what authority do we claim it to be valid? Perhaps yogis are mistaken in their views; perhaps Sri Aurobindo's understanding is mistaken; and we're certain that our own understanding of yoga psychology is limited.

The main aim of this book is not so much to present the "truth" of "how things are" but rather to present a way of looking. Our descriptions of various aspects of yoga psychology are offered as a series of what might be thought of as intuitive hypotheses. We have developed these hypotheses based on our intimations of what Sri Aurobindo refers to as the essential "movements of consciousness" underlying the processes of biological and human evolution.

We hope that, in the future, others who are more knowledgeable in these various fields will be inspired to come up with their own intuitive hypotheses, and that all such hypotheses will be tested and confirmed or discomfirmed by appropriately trained contemplative scientists.[a] We believe this way of seeing—what we are calling the "view from infinity"—can be of immense practical value. In addition to contributing to the development of a new science of consciousness, it can provide the foundation for personal and societal transformation.

YOGA PSYCHOLOGY AND THE TRANSFORMATION OF SOCIETY

The issues crying out for attention are all around us. At the national level, we face ailing health care systems, unemployment, violence in the schools; at the planetary level, weapons of mass destruction, global

---

a. A method for developing this way of looking is described in the section on intuition in the last chapter of the book. There is a description of how it might be used for the development of a yogic science of consciousness in Appendix A. Alan Wallace's "Samatha Project," described in chapter 17, is an excellent example of a rigorous training program designed to produce expert contemplatives capable of serving as consultants in scientific research.

warming, and the possibility that the flow of oil will run dry before the end of this century. If we grant that some level of societal transformation is in order, we might wish to consider what would be required to bring it about.

Generally, our initial tendency when faced with social and economic problems is to look for some kind of external solution. Some look to institutions, private or governmental. Others look to technological innovations—alternative energy sources, new medicines, or new machines to increase productivity. It does seem likely that far-reaching technological, economic, and political reform will, in fact, be needed as part of any truly fundamental transformation.

But will such structural reforms be long-lasting? What evidence is there from the recent past that gives us reason to believe continued reliance on external change will solve our problems?

What if the essential problem is not insufficient energy, failed institutions, or inadequate technology? What if the core of our problem is an inadequate view? The view underlying our predominant institutions is one that sees the world as made up of essentially separate competing individuals, countries, and ideologies, fated to be forever in conflict. So long as we are subject to this view, we will feel compelled to do whatever is required to support and defend ourselves, our country, and our "way of life" against those we perceive to be a threat. All actions flowing from that view will only continue to create conflict and disharmony.

But is it really possible that changing something as intangible as a "view" could bring about the magnitude of change that is needed in the world at this time?

Extensive psychological research has shown that when an individual's view of himself changes, problems with anxiety, depression, hopelessness and despair diminish, leading to a life of greater happiness, satisfaction, and fulfillment.[9] Perhaps it is not too great a leap to imagine then, that a radical transformation of society might come about if there were a fundamental change in the view that currently shapes the minds, hearts and actions of human beings. If this is true, what kind of view is needed?

Theologian-ecologist Thomas Berry and physicist Brian Swimme, among others, propose what they refer to as a "New Story," based on the inspiring findings of modern science regarding the origin and evolution of the physical universe.[10] Focusing on the sense of beauty and aliveness conveyed in astronomers' descriptions of the birth and evolution of stars, and biologists' portrayal of the birth and evolution of life, they use this story to evoke a feeling of awe and a greater awareness that each of us is an essential part of a greater creative process occurring throughout the universe. While Berry and Swimme succeed in imbuing this story with a sense of wonder, they refrain from challenging the basis of the materialistic perspective underlying the scientific view.

It just may be that there is a "new" New Story that is, in a way, a very old story, one with a very different basis from that of modern science. We believe that the "story" of the universe at the foundation of yoga psychology, taken in its full spiritual context, has the power to get to the very roots of our modern malaise. If these roots were to be addressed, a transformation in the structure and function of business, government, and other institutions might be a natural result.

Is this an overly utopian vision? Or is it possible that even a partial beginning to such a radical transformation is already under way? A number of individuals who have conducted extensive research on this question suggest that something along these lines is definitely happening.

Over the past several decades, sociologist Paul Ray has interviewed more than ten thousand people.[11] He found that an increasing number—from less than 1 percent of the American population in the 1970s to more than 25 percent at present—feel that something is lacking in the prevailing materialistic view. Similar numbers have been found in other countries as well. These individuals are looking for a view that brings together mind, body, and spirit, one that can inform everything from the way they eat and work to their choices about how they might contribute to cultural and political transformation. Philosopher Robert Forman spent several years in the 1990s interviewing leaders in the fields of business, education, and medicine.[12] His results, published in "The Grassroots Spirituality Project," suggest that high-level people in hospitals, universities, and other major institutions are looking for ways to integrate a nondogmatic, nonsectarian spirituality into all aspects of their respective organizations.

In 1969, Dr. Herbert Benson felt he had to conduct his research on meditation after-hours in order to conceal his work from the potential disapproval of his colleagues. More than thirty years later, he now reports that the desire for a spiritual approach to health care has become so great, he cannot train meditation teachers fast enough to meet the demand.[13] According to Dr. Larry Dossey, a longtime leader in the movement to integrate spirituality and medicine, a majority of the medical schools in the United States have developed courses in alternative/complementary medicine, and nearly two-thirds offer "courses on religious and spiritual issues."[14]

If such a change is actually under way, is there some way of understanding what is happening that can help us discern a larger purpose and align ourselves with it? Tibetan Buddhist scholar Robert Thurman suggests that we are on the verge of a second Renaissance.[15] Thurman believes that, just as the first Renaissance five hundred years ago brought about major changes in European civilization through the reexamination of ancient Roman and Greek culture, similarly a worldwide Renaissance may be sparked by a reexamination of the yogic culture of India. Sociologists David Loye and Riane Eisler suggest another perspective on change—that we are approaching the end of the five thousand-year "age of empire," leading to a new era of global collaboration.[16] And a few, like Eckhart Tolle and Sri Aurobindo, go still further, proposing that what is happening now may be a shift in consciousness as great as that which began 5 million years ago, resulting ultimately in the emergence of a new species—*Homo sapiens*.[17] Perhaps, to some extent, all three are correct.

Whatever the ultimate nature of the change, what we see depends on how we look. What might we see if we were to look through the eyes of infinity?

BOOK I

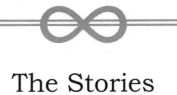

The Stories

OVERVIEW

We present in this section an overview of what scientists have discovered to date regarding the emergence and evolution of consciousness in the universe. This unfolding of consciousness is not something remote from our daily experience, taking place only millions of years ago. It occurs on a smaller scale over the course of our lives, and on an even smaller scale over the course of a few minutes or even fractions of a second. In one sense, the whole process of the evolution of consciousness is reflected in each moment of our lives, in all that we are. Even just sitting reading a book, our capacity to see and hear, to feel, move, and understand is the result of billions of years of evolution.

Throughout the book, to help establish this connection between the larger evolutionary unfolding of consciousness and our own lives, we describe several incidents in the life of Sharon Jefferson Price, showing how different grades of consciousness are at play in her experience. Here, in Book I, we introduce Sharon at a critical moment in her life, providing some background information about the hopes and aspirations as well as the fears and conflicts that brought her to that moment.

Chapter 1

Sharon's Story: A Reason to Live

Sharon had nearly given up trying to make sense of her life. She saw no reason to go on living. It had been more than a quarter century since she had returned from tending wounded soldiers in Vietnam. Now forty-seven years old, she felt it was unlikely she would ever understand what had happened during the war to so completely undo her sense of who she was and what her life was about. She couldn't imagine anything else she could do to resolve the persistent feelings of futility. Her childhood faith—which had been a source of comfort for her growing up amidst the violence and poverty of the inner city—no longer offered any solace. And none of her achievements—neither setting up her own successful business, nor being elected the first African-American councilwoman in her district—seemed to make any difference.

After walking away from her job as councilwoman, Sharon went to stay with her father for a time. She spent her days sitting by the pond in his backyard, trying to gain some perspective on the mounting tension she'd been experiencing in recent years. One day, several weeks after she arrived at her father's house, watching a leaf fall from a tree overhanging the pond, she began to feel a warm, embracing Presence.

~~~~~~~~~~

Whether or not we've experienced a personal trauma, for many of us the world has become so complex that, like Sharon, we find it hard to make sense of things. In the modern world, an increasing number of people find that religious faiths that had their origin in a very different time do not speak to the need for meaning in their lives. Turning to science, we find a wealth of truly amazing facts about the birth of the universe, the process of evolution, and the intricate workings of the brain. These facts by default have come to represent the story of our world and who we are. However, the facts in themselves offer us no way of understanding why we are here or what we need to be doing.

There are different ways of understanding the scientific facts about the universe, each of which carries with it very different implications for our lives. Perhaps the facts with most relevance to our search for meaning are those that relate to the nature of our consciousness—how it has evolved and how it works. After reviewing the details of what scientists now understand about the evolution of consciousness in the universe, we'll explore two contrasting ways of viewing them.

But before embarking on this journey of exploration, we'll first go back and look more closely at Sharon's state of mind when she first arrived at her father's house. In subsequent chapters, we'll look at what happened in the intervening weeks that led Sharon to the experience that began to resolve her suffering, and gave her a reason to live.

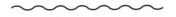

Caught up in a reverie of disjointed memories, Sharon hadn't noticed the sound of the truck idling on the street behind her father's house until the engine was turned off. She cringes as the sound of the truck door brings her back to the medical compound in Vietnam. She imagines she hears the sound of soldiers unloading the dead bodies from the back of the truck parked on the dirt road just outside the compound. She remembers the smell of the jungle air thick with death and a feeling of nausea sweeps over her. Closing her eyes, she sees the faces of the dying soldiers for whom she had provided comfort in the final moments of their lives. She feels her hand grasping the metal cup half filled with water as she prepares to lift it to the parched lips of one of these men. Startled, Sharon opens her eyes and glances down, seeing not a metal cup but the bottle of pills she is holding in her hand. Attempting to reorient herself, she quickly looks up and surveys her surroundings.

Her eye is caught by the light reflecting off the rippled surface of the pond in front of her. Several bright orange goldfish with long flowing tails swim to the surface for a moment, then dart away. A cardinal on one of the higher branches of the oak tree to her left is singing.

It had been only a few weeks since she arrived at her father's house in this quiet residential area, a world away from the noisy urban neighborhood where she had served as councilwoman for the past ten years. Leaving her job at the peak of success, she thought that spending some time with her family might help her make sense of her life. Her mother had died several years before, but her brother Willie lived down the street, and her sister Clarissa frequently drove there from her home two hours away in the mountains.

Thinking about the senseless killing of Bobby Thompson, Sharon recalls the flashbacks that began not long after she'd heard about his death. She can hardly believe, sitting here in this quiet place, that the crime-filled neighborhood where she spent her childhood is only a few miles away. She is so lucky to have had such a loving, close-knit family, her parents instilling in her a sense of endless possibility, and so carefully nurturing her passion to make a difference in her community. How had things come to this? Neither the drug addicts nor gang members who populated her childhood neighborhood had distracted her from actively pursuing her ideals—organizing youth groups, marching for civil rights, running successfully for student council president. Her path had seemed so clear—she would study nursing, go to Vietnam to help tend wounded soldiers, come back to study medicine, and work toward establishing health clinics in her community.

She recalls how after Vietnam, none of this seemed to matter. She had lost all interest in becoming a doctor and tried working briefly as a nurse, but could no longer bear being around illness and pain. She recalls her family's futile efforts to comfort her, their inability to understand why she was unable to continue on the path she had set out for herself. Somehow their cheerful faith in her had left her feeling even more despondent.

She half smiles thinking of her next move—relocating to a distant city, hoping to find some new way to live out her ideals, imagining that might help resolve her uneasiness, help her lessen the sense of burden she was carrying. She set up the boutique soon after meeting Nicole, and it wasn't long before they had become successful enough to donate a significant portion of their profits to help fund community projects. But the unease and restlessness continued to grow, and when Martin suggested she run for office, she was happy to move on. Though she turned out to be a good politician, she didn't like some of what she saw in herself during that period—the ambition, the ease with which she got drawn into questionable deal-making, the determination to win even at the expense of others. But still, she had done good things. Even before the end of her first year in office, her proposal for creating an agency to help women get started in small businesses was already off the ground.

But it seemed that with every new success, the sense of burden and meaninglessness only grew deeper. She had money and respect as well as many opportunities to do good, but she still couldn't shake the feeling that nothing mattered. No amount of success seemed to quell the painful restlessness she felt inside. And the more she was admired, the lonelier she became. She'd never really been able to give herself to the men who pursued her; she only ended up feeling more desperate and alone when she was with them.

In the eyes of others, she had been functioning well enough. But she knew she could not continue what she was doing while sinking further into despair. And now, just a few weeks after leaving her job, she can't imagine there is anything she can do to change the way she feels.

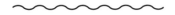

Bearing in mind the questions with which Sharon—and perhaps, in some form, each one of us—is grappling, we'll go on to the story of the evolution of consciousness. We'll then consider different ways of looking at that story to see if there's one that might illumine our pressing questions.

CHAPTER 2

The Story of the Evolution of Consciousness

WHEN DID CONSCIOUSNESS FIRST APPEAR?

Some say consciousness was there at the beginning, and exists throughout the universe. Physicist Freeman Dyson, describing the mysterious discoveries of quantum physics, writes "[a]toms are weird stuff, behaving like active agents rather than inert substances. They make unpredictable choices between alternative possibilities according to the laws of quantum mechanics. It appears that mind, as manifested by the capacity to make choices, is to some extent inherent in every atom."[1] In contrast, others like psychologist Susan Blackmore and philosopher Paul Churchland advise us to be realistic and face the fact that consciousness does not really exist anywhere, that it is nothing more than a word that describes a particular activity of the brain. Apart from these two extremes, most scientists agree that consciousness does in fact exist, but disagree about when it first appeared.[a] In the last decade, as scientists have had access to more sophisticated tools for investigating

---

a. There is a wide range of positions amongst scientists regarding the nature of consciousness. For example, some, like Trewavas and Nakagaki, who see evidence of the workings of intelligence in plants and one-celled organisms, might not see this as evidence that a paramecium or pomegranate has any kind of subjective experience (i.e., feelings). On the other hand, there are some (e.g., psychologist Harry Hunt) who believe there is evidence for subjectivity even in primitive organisms. There are very few who would assert that either intelligence or subjective experience is anything more than a complex working of matter. In this chapter, we're using the word "consciousness" to include both subjective experience and intelligence. For now, the term is intended to be entirely neutral with regard to whether or not consciousness can be explained as a purely material phenomenon.

intelligence, it has become possible to detect intelligent behavior much earlier in the evolutionary chain.

According to Anthony Trewavas, professor of biology at the University of Edinburgh, "plants have senses and can detect a wide variety of external variables, such as light, water, temperature, chemicals, vibrations, gravity, and sounds. They can also react to these factors by changing the way they grow. Plants can forage and compete with one another for resources. When attacked by herbivores, some plants signal for help, releasing chemicals that attract their assailants' predators. Plants can detect distress signals let off by other plant species and take preventive measures. They can assimilate information and respond on the whole-plant level. And they use cell-to-cell communication based on molecular and electrical signals, some of which are remarkably similar to those used by our own neurons. When a plant is damaged, its cells send one another electrical signals just like our own pain messages."[2]

Trewavas does not claim that plants can think or have anything resembling human self-awareness. However, he does consider these facts about plants to be a clear demonstration that they are sentient and respond intelligently to what they sense.

Toshiyuki Nakagaki is an associate professor of biology at Hokkaido University in Sapporo, Japan. In articles such as "Amoeboid Organisms May Be More Clever Than We Had Thought," Nakagaki describes some remarkable abilities in the organism known as the "true slime mold"—a creature formed by the merging together of thousands of amoebae into a single cell. Though it does not have eyes or a nervous system, it is able to "move, navigate and avoid obstacles. [It] can also sense food at a distance and head unerringly toward it."[3]

When researchers place separate pieces of true slime mold into a maze, the pieces rejoin to form a single organism that spreads out into every corridor of the maze, covering all the available space. "[W]hen food is placed at the start and end points of the maze, the slime mold withdraws from the dead-end corridors and shrinks its body to a tube spanning the shortest path between food sources…[and it] solves the maze in this way each time it is tested." Nakagaki and his collaborators conclude "[t]his remarkable process of cellular computation implies that cellular materials can show a primitive intelligence."[4]

Some may be reluctant to consider the possibility that the activity of such primitive organisms reflects any kind of conscious intelligence. If, however, one is willing to concede that a shrub or slime mold possesses some form of intelligence, it seems hard to dispute that it is probably less complex than that of a snowy owl or a South American sea lion. Nevertheless, the idea that consciousness has somehow grown in complexity over the course of evolution continues to be very controversial.

DOES CONSCIOUSNESS BECOME MORE COMPLEX OVER THE COURSE OF EVOLUTION?

Some scientists who dispute the notion of a hierarchy of consciousness suggest that adaptability should be the main measure of intelligence. According to this line of thought, a frog's intelligence is no less than a human's, since a frog's intelligence helps it adapt to its environment equally as well as our human intelligence helps us adapt to ours. Such scientists might suggest, for example, that human beings would be hard-pressed to live on lily-pads and subsist on a diet of whatever flies we could catch with our tongues. But is adaptability the same as intelligence? Neuropsychologist Merlin Donald points out that if we use the criterion of adaptability, one might say "corporate CEOs are no more or less intelligent in an adaptive biological sense than, say, maggots, a conclusion that may have a certain emotional resonance for many, but falls a bit short on the evidence."[5]

There is another, more powerful reason for resistance to the idea that consciousness has become more complex. Many scientists are concerned that even the suggestion of some kind of directionality in evolution might open a door through which religious dogma could enter and distort their objective findings. However, as we see from the work of those like Trewavas and Nakagaki, it is possible to pursue these questions in a rigorous scientific manner.

Some who object to the idea of directionality suggest that if we look at the course of evolution over several thousand or even several million years, it appears as though changes in intelligence have occurred in many directions rather than as a straightforward increase in complexity. However, physicist and theologian Ian Barbour suggests that if we take the long view, "evolutionary history shows an overall trend toward greater complexity, responsiveness and awareness. The capacity of organisms to gather, store and process information has steadily increased."[6]

Recent studies in developmental psychology and cognitive neuroscience have shown that there is a remarkable parallel between the increasing complexity of consciousness over the course of evolution and the way in which it unfolds over shorter time frames. As Harvard neuroscientist J. Allan Hobson describes it, "Consciousness is graded across evolutionary time, over the course of development, and even continuously from moment to moment."[7] Hobson himself has described the emerging complexity of consciousness over the time span of billions of years. Developmental psychologists such as Susan Harter and John Flavell have tracked a similar emergence over the course of a human lifetime. Francisco Varela, Brian Lancaster, and other cognitive neuroscientists suggest that a comparable progression of consciousness unfolds in each moment of human experience.

In the sections that follow, we will describe what science has discovered about the increasing complexity of consciousness as it unfolds over these three different time frames.[a] We will do this in terms of three categories—knowing (cognition), feeling (affect), and willing (volition). Many centuries ago, Aristotle used these categories to encompass the full range of conscious activities. While many ways of describing consciousness have since been developed, cognitive scientists continue to use a framework that is essentially the same as the one used by Aristotle.[8] For the present, we'll define knowing as the

---

a. It is important to keep in mind as we present the scientific evidence of the increasing complexity of consciousness, that it is all based upon speculation derived from observation of external behavior and, in some cases, similarities between human and animal brain structure or function. Scientists have had no direct experience of the consciousness of these creatures (or, if they do, they don't acknowledge it in mainstream academic journals).

capacity for registering and (to a lesser or greater degree) compre-
hending distinctions in the environment; feeling as the largely physiological responses that accompany acts of knowing and willing; and
willing as the active response to what is known and felt.[a]

The Emergence of Consciousness in Animals over the Course of Evolution

As consciousness evolves, the organism becomes capable of distinguishing more of the world. That is, it knows more of the world, has
a wider range of feeling about it, and a wider array of responses to it.
This progression ranges from the slime mold's extremely limited registration of external stimuli to the sea anemone's ability to recognize
distinguishable patterns, the bee's capacity to "understand" some simple relationships between those patterns, the lizard's ability to define
a particular territory, and the crow's capacity to engage in complex
problem-solving within and around its territory.

Whatever the nature of the primitive intelligence Nakagaki identified in a single-celled organism, the way in which it experiences the
world would be unimaginable to us. What kind of consciousness could
one possibly ascribe to such a primitive creature? At best, we might
imagine its experience to be little more than the faintest blur. It has
no sense organs, yet is able in some way to detect the presence of
food, indicating it has a primitive "knowing" of its environment. The
fact that it was able to determine that the substance was desirable is
thought to indicate the presence of a primitive form of "feeling." Its
response to the food—arranging itself to optimally obtain it—reflects
a primitive form of "willing."

What began as a faint glimmer of knowing in the most primitive
creatures was greatly enhanced in early multicellular organisms by the

---

a. These definitions, along with the rest of the information provided in this chapter, are stated in terms that are acceptable within the prevailing scientific perspective. We will give an understanding of knowing, willing, and feeling in terms
of yoga psychology later in the book.

emergence of primitive sense organs. The dim blurry world of the true slime mold became a world of distinguishable patterns. The senses of a sea anemone living in a rock pool, for example, are stimulated by certain patterns in its environment. In response to these patterns, the anemone registers a "feeling"—slightly more differentiated than in the slime mold—that is positive, negative, or neutral depending on whether the pattern is perceived as friendly, unfriendly, or irrelevant to its survival. If the pattern signifies food, in a primitive act of "will" it will grab at it; if it signifies a threat, it will attack or retreat. These responses are even subject to a primitive form of learning known as habituation. For example, if you gently tap a tentacle, the anemone will initially withdraw. If, however, repeated taps prove to be harmless, it will cease to respond.

In multicellular creatures, the specialized sensory cells developed into sense organs. A primitive nervous system emerged that could coordinate the information taken in by the various senses, and a more complex external world of hue and shape began to emerge on the canvas of consciousness. The more complex capacities for knowing, willing, and feeling that accompanied these changes are evident in the "waggle dance" ritual of the honeybee.

In the course of its search for nourishment, when a bee sees a patch of flowers that promises to be a rich source of nutrients, it will retrace its route several times in order to memorize the location. Returning to the hive, it performs a complex series of movements that has come to be known as the "waggle dance." Moving in the form of a figure eight, "its orientation indicates the direction of [the] find relative to the position of the sun. The speed of her movement, the number of times she repeats it, and the fervor of her noisy waggling indicate the richness of the food source."[9] The observing bees assess the intensity of her movements and thus discern the relative value of her find.

In this ritual, the bees demonstrate several acts of knowing that include judgment, memory, and the performance of some fairly complex calculations. Both the ability of the dancing bee to perform her highly detailed movements and the concentration required of her audience indicate a more highly developed capacity for willing than that of either the sea anemone or slime mold. Scientists have not yet developed techniques or technology for distinguishing levels of complexity of feeling between creatures as primitive as the slime mold, sea anemone, and bee. However, assuming that consciousness evolves in an integral fashion, it seems likely that whatever level of feeling is present is to some extent commensurate with the bees' capacity for knowing and willing.

Though impressive, this ritual dance is largely instinctive. The bees' capacity for learning is limited, and their response patterns can be quite inflexible. For example, "if placed in a maze with a glass cover, they perform as well as rats up to the point of reaching the food reward, but they are incapable of turning around and going back to where they have come from. Once bees eat, they are rigidly programmed to fly upward"[10] and will thus remain trapped in the maze.

With the appearance of reptiles, we see a further development of knowing, willing, and feeling. The reptile can process sensory information in more complex ways than either the sea anemone or bee. A lizard, for example, can "understand" the notion of territory and engage in behaviors such as defining, patrolling, and defending that territory against trespassers. The world it experiences is somewhat richer by virtue of the primitive feelings of safety, anger, fear, and competitiveness associated with its knowing of a territory, and its activities related to that knowing. While these behaviors are instinctive and automatic, the lizard's larger repertoire of responses represents a further complexity of will.

With the appearance of mammals and birds, we see the emergence of more complex abilities for learning, memory, and problem-solving. While many may have observed these capacities in such familiar mammals as dogs, cats, or the neighborhood raccoon, it may be surprising to hear the extent to which birds demonstrate them as well. Several newspapers and magazines have recently carried the story of Japanese carrion crows who congregate at traffic intersections waiting for a red light. When the traffic stops, the crows fly down to the road to place walnuts they've gathered in front of the cars. When the light turns green, the cars move forward, cracking open the nuts. When the road is clear, the crows return to enjoy the feast.[11]

Perhaps less well known is the astonishing memory of one particular species of crow, the Clark's nutracker, who can remember as many as thirty-thousand hiding places for the seeds it gathers and buries. After burying the seeds, he then recovers them over the course of the next eleven months, using them as his primary diet during the winter.[12]

With mammals and birds, as opposed to more primitive organisms, it becomes much easier to observe emotional reactions. However, it is quite unusual to find an animal that can verbally articulate its feelings. Alex, an African Grey parrot trained for over twenty years by Dr. Irene Pepperberg, has a vocabulary of more than one hundred words. As familiar as Dr. Pepperberg was with Alex's abilities, even she was startled one day when she dropped him off for an overnight stay at a veterinary hospital to have lung surgery. Apparently upset at being left in a strange place, Alex called to her as she was leaving, "Come here. I love you… Wanna go back."[13]

With primates came the ability to make use of more complex symbols, making possible a simple form of reasoning. For example, a chimp, spotting a banana outside his cage just beyond arm's reach, can conjure up the image of a stick and think about how he might use it to retrieve the banana. This capacity freed primates from adherence to rigid instinctive behaviors, allowing for innovation and a far greater degree of flexibility in coping with new situations. The ability to use symbols also allowed for a new form of communication—that of symbolic language.

While chimpanzees and gorillas may not be able to speak as we do, it is for want of a larynx rather than a deficiency of their brains. The world-renowned and much beloved gorilla Koko was taught the deaf sign language and showed a remarkable ability to use it to communicate.[14] She now has a vocabulary of more than a thousand words and is able to compose simple sentences. Her ability to make use of symbolic language gives her a greater capacity than reptiles and most mammals to comprehend the relationship between herself and the things and creatures of her environment. This makes it possible for Koko to have a more highly developed social life, with more complex familial and other interpersonal ties. These more intimate relationships bring the possibility of deeper, more complex emotional feelings and responses. They also facilitate the passing on of social norms to a new generation, giving birth to the possibility of culture.[15]

With the appearance of human beings, something radically new began to emerge—the sense of an individual self with a past, present, and future, and the capacity to be aware of and reflect upon the nature of that self. We've moved from the blurry inchoate world of the amoeba to a highly differentiated world of multidimensional relationships—between past, present, and future, and between an individual and his environment. With a greatly enhanced capacity for memory, analysis, and strategic planning, human beings can arrive at complex theories for making sense of their world. We've graduated from simple feeling responses of pleasure and pain to the complexities of romantic love, self-sacrifice, compassion, and remorse. And along with the capacity for self-awareness has come the power to change ourselves and reshape our environment.

THE EMERGENCE OF CONSCIOUSNESS OVER THE LIFETIME OF AN INDIVIDUAL

Overview

Whatever scientists have learned about intelligence and sentience in animals has been the result of inference rather than direct experience. Because current scientific methodology offers no way of knowing directly the subjective experience of the slime mold or the crow, the nature of their consciousness has been inferred from careful observation of behavior. When we turn to the study of human consciousness, researchers have the benefit of a self-conscious subject whose consciousness is similar to their own and who can report on their own subjective experience. Even in the study of preverbal children, the researcher has the advantage of having once been a child herself and can bring that tacit knowledge to her interpretation of experimental data. Because of this, there is a richness to the language and content of theories of human development that is not possible in the study of animal consciousness.

Jean Piaget is perhaps the name most widely associated with theories of development. Though many of his ideas have been widely critiqued and in some cases replaced, one of his core principles—that the center of attention shifts over the course of development—has endured as a central idea in developmental theory.[16] To put it simply, the infant's attention is completely absorbed in her sensations and the movements of her body, but she does not know they are *her* sensations or *her* body. "The newborn makes no distinction between inner and outer, between stimuli that come from her own body (for example, hunger) and those that come from outside (light), between your hand passing across her eyes and her own hand passing across her eyes."[17] For the newborn infant, light, hunger, and hands are simply sensations belonging to one undifferentiable world, indistinguishable from herself.

By sometime late in the first year, a momentous change takes place. The infant is no longer wholly identified with these sensations and body movements; she is someone who *has* a body and *experiences* sensations. What has happened? The attention that was wholly absorbed in the body has become at least partially disidentified from it. The growing infant's attention shifts and becomes absorbed in the various desires and impulses that are now growing stronger. Over the course of time, she will once again be able to step back and realize (at least to some extent) that she *has* desires and impulses. Once she does this, rather than being wholly subject to them, she can make these desires and impulses the object of her attention and gradually learn to control them. This process of disidentification continues throughout life as the adolescent learns to detach from her feelings, and the adult from her thoughts and ideas about herself and the world.

While this may sound like a simple, uncomplicated process, development is actually a complex dance of shifting attention in which the growing individual explores new ways of knowing, willing, and feeling. It is true that early development —from birth to about age four or five—is generally considered to be predictable, determined at least to some extent by relatively fixed genetic tendencies. However, as the child grows older, cultural influences as well as the individual's evolving intentions and goals play an increasingly important role, providing for a great degree of unpredictability in the developmental process.

We now look in more detail at several important shifts of attention that take place in the course of development. As we do so, we'll see, as we did with biological evolution, how the processes of knowing, willing, and feeling—the ways in which the individual attends to herself and the world—become more complex.

Infant Development

A human infant at birth cannot willfully direct her attention. She lives in an amorphous world of colors, shapes, and sounds from which she cannot distinguish her "self." Her world is pervaded by simple feeling states such as calm, excitement, or distress. Within the first few months of life, she will acquire the capacity to organize her somewhat chaotic sensations into perceptions, enabling her to recognize more distinct, but still ephemeral shapes and forms that exist, then cease to exist, as they enter or leave her field of vision.

There is an experiment that beautifully illustrates the transition from this early stage of "selflessness"[a] to the emergence of a distinct "self." A researcher gives a ball to a four-month-old baby, who engages with the toy, "...pursuing it with eyes and hands, holding it, bringing it to his mouth." The ball is then covered, and the infant seems not to notice. The experimenter removes the cover and, "the child lights up, vocalizes, reaches again for the object."[18] Psychologist Robert Kegan observes, "It seems not that the child loses interest in the covered object, but that the covered object loses its existence for the child. Between the ages of eight and ten months, the same children begin to make tentative steps to [recover the hidden object]."[19] However, when the experimenter foils this attempt by placing two or more screens between the infant and the object, his "exploration...comes to an early halt."[20]

By the time the child is two years old, he generally has no problem retrieving the hidden ball no matter how well it is hidden. Kegan points out that people hearing of this for the first time think of it as involving two entities—a baby, and a ball. However:

---

a. A "selflessness" that could alternatively be described as "self-embedded-in-world."

> [the experiment] takes on a whole new life if one sees that
> a single dynamic organism, "baby-and-ball," is gradually
> undergoing a process of transformation. Over the period
> roughly from nine to twenty-one months, the baby-and-ball
> begins to be something other than a single entity, but does
> not quite constitute, as yet, two distinct entities. Although
> the hidden object is not immediately given up, its pursuit
> is easily defeated. One has the sense of a differentiation
> so fragile, so tentative, that it can very easily merge back
> into oneness…In the early months [when the experimenter
> takes away the ball and covers it] the child gives it up with-
> out protest of any kind. He does not, it seems clear, have it,
> in the sense of its being something apart from [him].[21]

With age, the child not only refines his physical ability to grasp the ball, but his psychological ability to "grasp" it as well:

> [The experiment] is capturing a motion, the motion of dif-
> ferentiation—which creates the object—and the motion of
> integration—which creates [the baby's relationship with and
> independent existence from] the object.[22]

As his attention is freed from the unity of baby-and-ball, the child becomes capable of knowing the ball as separate from himself, having feelings toward it, and choosing how to engage with it. This momentous shift of attention, giving birth to a new self and a new world, is the crux of all transformational processes.

It is as if the newborn infant is living in a forest, aware only of the blur of shifting colors, shapes, sounds, and movements. Over many months of constant interaction with different facets of her experience, she slowly learns to focus and stabilize her attention, thus beginning to distinguish different aspects of the forest. Here and there, a tree, a leaf, a flower, tentatively emerges out of the general blur—though not yet known as "tree," "leaf," or "flower." With this emergence, she too becomes more distinct. And, over time, an environment separate from herself comes into being.

Early Childhood Development

By the time the child is two or three years old, his sense of self has become more defined and he begins to perceive himself as an entity with various attributes—"my" toys, "my" parents, "my" home. His simple responses of pleasure and pain are elaborated into more complex emotions such as desire and craving, anger and fear, directed toward the things of the now separate world. He comes to understand that words and images can be used as symbols of something else, opening up a world of new possibilities. He can think about his parents after they leave the room, imagine how they look and act in their absence, hear their voices in his mind. He also can begin to hold a mental image of himself—a significant step in the emergence of a self-reflective, conscious self.

However, such a fully conscious self is still many years away. The capacity of a toddler to sustain attention is fragile at best, and both his self and his world are correspondingly fluid and changeable. His attention is easily caught by each passing impulse or desire. Unable to shift attention, the child's desires become imperative, demanding immediate satisfaction. The pain of being so completely subject to one's desires was vividly portrayed in an interaction we witnessed in a city park one afternoon between a four-year-old girl and her mother. As the mother looked on helplessly, the little girl, oblivious to everything around her, tears streaming down her face, stamped her foot repeatedly and screamed, "I WANT IT NOW! I WANT IT NOW!"

It is difficult for anyone to see a child in that kind of pain. However, we can remind ourselves that, if the child's attention were suddenly to be drawn to the sight of a colorful balloon flying overhead, the imperative need to satisfy her previous desire might rapidly dissolve.

Because desires and impulses are so changeable and fleeting, the self caught up in them is similarly transitory. As a new, more stable attentional balance develops, the self and its experienced world grow more stable. Describing the momentous shift of attention that usually takes place somewhere between the ages of five and seven, Kegan writes:

> 1) Children on the early side of the 5 to 7 shift seem to
> need rewards which are fairly immediate, sensual and

communicating of praise; children on the other side seem to be more rewarded by the information that they have been correct. 2) Children who lose a limb or become blind before they are through the shift tend not to have phantom limb responses or memories of sight; children on the other side of the shift do.[23]

The fluid, changeable self of the three or four-year-old child is not stable enough to consistently restrain its impulses, nor is it stable enough to retain the memory of sight or the sensation of a missing limb. By age seven, there is

a more [enduring] self—a self which does its own praising...
A self which can store memories, feelings and perceptions...
so that a feeling arm or a seeing eye lives on in some way.[24]

To return to the forest metaphor, the child is now able to see that the trees are part of a larger category—the forest. His development beyond this point will continue to involve learning to free his attention from its absorption in sensations, impulses, and desires, and it will further involve stepping back from the increasingly complex feelings, thoughts and intentions that later emerge. He will learn to observe the "forest" of his experience with a greater detachment, but at the same time with a greater feeling of connectedness to its various trees, leaves, and flowers. This increased freedom of attention not only brings greater capacities of knowledge and feeling, but also a wider range of action. Eventually, having traversed the length and breadth of the forest, he learns that he can leave the forest, journey to other forests, and even find altogether new landscapes.

Adolescent and Adult Development

In the course of development, attention can get caught in many ways, and by many things. However, for most people, the most troublesome entanglement involves their emotions. Jason is a fifteen-year-old white,

Irish Catholic boy who lives in a large city in northwestern Canada. Among his friends are Muslims, Buddhists, Jews, and Protestants, and he shares their open-minded views toward religion. Shortly after he turns sixteen, his family moves to a small rural town, where all non-Christians are considered heathens destined for hell. Within weeks after beginning school, Jason has adopted the views of his new schoolmates, even to the extent of speaking with scorn of his multifaith city friends. Toward the end of the school year, Yusef, a friend from his hometown who is a devout Muslim, comes to visit.

Viewed externally, one might say Jason was an opportunist or hypocrite, consciously espousing a particular view only for the sake of being accepted by his peers. However, Jason's sense of self was so bound up with his need to be accepted that he was hardly even aware of the conflict between his previous and current views. Yusef's arrival forced that conflict to the forefront of his consciousness, making him painfully aware of the way he betrayed his values in order to fit in.

In order to resolve this developmental conflict, Jason will need to be able to stay with these painful feelings rather than struggling with or trying to deny them. The simple act of being present with his experience would in itself lessen his identification with the desire to be accepted by his peers. He would thus be able to see his behavior and attitude as something he had temporarily taken on, rather than an essential aspect of himself. Once having achieved this degree of disidentification, he might even have some difficulty recognizing himself in the person who was so desperately needing to fit in with his peers.

With increasing globalization, groups with conflicting values and worldviews encounter each other more frequently than ever before. As a consequence, we are all being faced with the same developmental challenge that confronted Jason—the need to step back from our identification with any particular group. The current state of the world might be likened to a giant schoolyard inhabited by various gangs, each demanding the allegiance of its members and, at the same time, providing them with an identity to which they are attached. Because the existence of other views stands to threaten that identity, each gang vigorously, often violently, asserts its own views and ways of doing things as superior, attempting to bully other groups into giving up their "inferior," alien lifestyles in favor of its own.

Learning to step back from the beliefs, customs, and desires with which we identify continues to be the quintessential developmental challenge in adulthood. It seems the global conflict in the world today is calling upon us to free ourselves from identification with our respective groups—be they religious, political, national, or economic—so that we can see and be responsive to the whole of humanity.

THE EMERGENCE OF CONSCIOUSNESS IN EACH MOMENT

The gradual unfoldment of cognitive, emotional, and volitional capacities that took place over the course of terrestrial history is repeated over the course of each individual human lifetime. The emergence of consciousness appears to be similarly graded in every moment of our experience as well.[25]

In each moment there are overlapping strands of experience emerging into conscious awareness. And each one of these strands moves through a continuum: from unconscious to pre-conscious status, to what William James calls "fringe" experience[26] eventually emerging into full consciousness. Each arc of experience bears the imprint of our entire evolutionary past as well as our entire lifetime. Yet, at the same time, according to recent research in cognitive science,[27] each moment contains the possibility of freedom from that past. Whether we repeat the patterns of our personal and ancestral history or shift the course of our development seems to depend—at least to some extent—on what we do with our attention in each moment.

The unconscious[a] processing that precedes a moment[b] of conscious awareness in the human adult resembles the workings of consciousness seen in the earliest stages of evolution and the earliest stage of human infancy:

a. "Unconscious," that is, from the perspective of the prevailing materialistic view.

b. In later chapters we will make further distinctions in the way this process unfolds.

1) initially, there is a simple registration of a sound, light or other vibration by the senses (knowing), accompanied by a primitive feeling tone (feeling) and an initial reaction of attraction or aversion (willing); 2) this simple experience is elaborated, with memories, associations, and beliefs coming into play, further shaping the interpretation of the stimulus, giving it richer meaning; 3) more conscious and complex feelings and intentions gradually come into play; 4) finally, a "self" is constructed in relation to the event, and emerges—in conjunction with the feelings, intentions and interpretation of the event—into conscious awareness.[a]

The "self" is thus not a fixed entity, but is reconstructed in each moment of experience. Similarly, the "world" is constructed anew in each moment as well. The world we experience is not a direct perception of something "out there." It is rather a virtual world, an internal construct updated each moment according to new sensory data, filtered through past conditioning, organized and interpreted by the self, and shaped by that to which its attention is drawn. The entire evolutionary spiral of increasing complexity of consciousness, the whole lifetime journey from fetus to adult, emerges in hardly more than an instant of experience.

To get a sense of experience emerging out of the "unconscious"[b] into conscious awareness, you might notice that just a moment ago, the feel of the surface on which you are sitting was probably in the background, emerging into full awareness only as you read these words and direct your attention to the relevant sensations. Yet the whole time, your brain was processing sensory data regarding the contact of your body with the chair. Similarly, the ticking of a clock, the whirring of a fan, the

---

a. We describe it here in a linear fashion, but it actually takes place as a series of overlapping strands.

b. We use quotations for the word "unconscious" because, as we'll see later—from the perspective of the view from infinity—there is nothing that is wholly "unconscious."

hum of a computer are sounds that often remain in the background of awareness, tending to emerge only in rare moments, most often when they change in some way. Though they seem to emerge suddenly, in retrospect you may be able to recall a partial awareness of such sounds in the moment just before they become fully conscious.

It is possible to refine our attention to the point that we can actually perceive the process by which each moment of awareness is constructed. Cultivating this level of refinement provides us with the means to bring about a radical transformation of our experience.

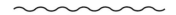

Science has gathered a great deal of information over the past century regarding the unfolding of consciousness in evolution, in human development, and in the course of a single moment. How we view this information, the way in which we understand it, will have a profound impact on our sense of ourselves and the world. Let's look at the view that has come to be associated with these scientific findings—a view that, whether we realize it or not, informs much of the way we think and feel about all that we experience.

BOOK II

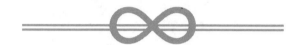

Preparation for the Journey

CHAPTER 3

The View From Nowhere

The core beliefs we hold about the nature of ourselves and the world are powerful forces that shape our behavior, determine our values, and condition the way we feel and think about things. Generally, we are not aware of the underlying view that shapes our experience and, by extension, the society we create. Over the course of time a new view can radically reshape the entire structure of a society.

More than five centuries ago, at the time of the European Renaissance, Galileo helped forge a new method of gaining knowledge, one that would be free from subjection to rigid dogma and superstition. The method Galileo and others developed involved scientists focusing attention exclusively on the objective, measurable aspects of the physical world, temporarily setting aside their personal emotional bias. There were some leaders of the Church who, while they had no objection to this new method, warned scientists to keep in mind that this was only one of many possible ways to view the world.

During the fifteenth and sixteenth centuries, similar developments were occurring in other spheres of society. Artists were developing a method that involved quite literally stepping back from their subject matter to gain a new perspective. People in general were taking a new perspective on their relationship to the rulers of society, questioning absolute authority. What each of these developments had in common was the same shift of attention that a child makes as she moves into adolescence, slowly freeing herself from emotional bias, gradually gaining the capacity to take a perspective on her feelings, her thoughts, her self, and the world.

Over the course of several centuries, this capacity for objectivity became more widespread, gradually becoming a predominant shaping force in society. At first, the new attitude of perspective-taking did not involve a denial of subjectivity, only an attempt to minimize its distorting influence. By the nineteenth century, science had gained a great deal of prestige due to the enormous success and pervasive influence of technology. As a result, the objective approach that had been so successful in the sciences was gradually applied to virtually all spheres of life. The view associated with this approach came to be known as "materialism" (or, more recently, "physicalism")—the idea that the basis of everything that exists is purely objective matter and energy, devoid of consciousness or intelligence.

Whereas the materialistic view had once been understood to be only one view among many, it gradually came to be seen as the best, and ultimately the only valid view. Philosopher Thomas Nagel coined the phrase "the view from nowhere" to describe the detached point of view that has come about as a result of the attempt to abstract all subjective factors from our understanding of the universe.

Physicist and astronomer Sir Arthur Eddington provides us with a vivid illustration of how this process of abstraction works by describing a typical problem one might encounter on a high school physics exam:

> The problem begins: "an elephant slides down a grassy hill-side…" The experienced candidate knows that he need not pay much attention to this; it is only put in to give an impression of realism. He reads on: "The mass of the elephant is two tons." Now we are getting down to business; the elephant fades out of the problem and a mass of two tons takes its place. What exactly is this two tons, the real subject-matter of the problem?… Two tons is the reading of the pointer when the elephant was placed on a weighing-machine. Let us pass on. [The candidate continues in this way to abstract further measurements from the world of experience.] And so we see that the poetry fades out of the problem, and by the time the serious application of exact science begins we are left with only pointer readings.[1]

Any feelings about the elephant, how it looks or feels sliding down the hill, any interest the creature may take in the scenery it encounters

along the way, have all effectively been eliminated from the calcula-
tion. The view from nowhere is an attempt to describe the world without subjective distortion. However, with the subject or viewer eliminated, the world can have no qualities. That is to say, it can be neither
friendly nor unfriendly, kind nor cruel, moral nor immoral—as these
are values requiring a point of view. Thus we are left with a world of
quantity—Eddington's pointer-readings.

The "view from nowhere"—viewing the world in terms of what
can be measured—is not in itself problematic. What makes it a problem is the added attitude that only that which can be measured is real.
As some economists put it, "If you can't count it, it doesn't count." In
the attempt to avoid bias and subjectivity, modern thought is in danger
of eliminating the subject altogether.

The effect of the view from nowhere in the field of psychological
science has been to make human experience—which cannot be easily
measured—an inexplicable mystery. The very existence of consciousness and free will has become a matter of widespread dispute. This
development is of more than purely intellectual concern. Because our
view shapes the way we think and feel and act, it has far-reaching consequences for the kind of society we create. One of the consequences
of ignoring the subjective element can be seen in the misuse of cost-
benefit analysis. Such misuse allows us to pursue a particular political
or economic goal without taking into consideration the number of
people who may get sick, injured, or die, as long as the material benefit
outweighs the cost. We may destroy whole species of wildlife and vast
stretches of forested land, but if the economic gain is seen to justify the
cost, we consider the destruction merely collateral damage.

The denial of the importance of subjective experience in the economic and environmental spheres reflects a deeper split within our
psyche. To the extent we are cut off from the part of ourselves that
connects us to other people, animals, and the greater physical universe, we are deprived of those aspects of our experience that have
always been the source of joy, beauty, meaning and purpose. We live
our lives unnourished by the feelings, insight, and creative imagination
that have their roots in subjective experience. Our world, our lives,
are deprived of their deeper meaning and value. It is not surprising

then that we have come to see the universe as having arisen through a meaningless process of random physical occurrences, indifferent to our hopes and dreams as well as our pain and suffering. Basing our actions on a view that does not take the subject into account, we create a world in which no subject would wish to live.

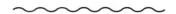

Having just arrived at her father's house, Sharon is looking for some way to understand the persistence of the powerful feelings of emptiness and futility that have dogged her since she came back from Vietnam. She has tried again and again to understand why, even after having achieved so much, and having surrounded herself with so many caring people, the intensity of her longing for "something more" only continued to grow.

The despair she feels would not be alleviated by an explanation involving genetic predisposition or malfunctioning neurotransmitters. She needs desperately to believe in something, and can't understand why, over the years, whatever she had invested with interest or enthusiasm soon lost its savor. Unable to comprehend what has been happening to her, Sharon only knows that she has to stop, take stock, and look at the forces that have been driving her into deepening despair.

Several weeks after arriving at her father's house, Sharon had an experience that set in motion a series of inner and outer changes that completely transformed her whole view of herself and the world. In order for us to make sense of what happened to her, and to understand the view at which she arrived, we need to become aware of a number of beliefs and assumptions that may impede us in our exploration of that view.

For example, we generally assume the physical "world" to be simply "out there," existing essentially as we perceive it. However, physicists tell us that what is really "out there" is nothing more than colorless, featureless waves of physical energy and/or particles of physical matter. The various shapes, sounds, and other sensations that we experience are not, according to them, inherent characteristics of the world,

but only the response of our brain to whatever it is that is "out there."
But does the physicists' portrayal of what is really "there" reflect actual
scientific knowledge, or is it in some way shaped by "the view from
nowhere"?

What *is* really "out there"—or "in here"?

CHAPTER 4

First Challenge To the View: Questioning the Assumptions of Materialism

> What if you dreamt that you went to heaven, and from there plucked a rose of exquisite beauty? And what then if you woke up and found that rose in your hand? Ah, yes, what then?[1]
>
> —Samuel Taylor Coleridge, *Anima Poetae*

Angela woke up one morning. She went to the bathroom, splashed some water on her face, then looked in the mirror. As she was looking at her face, she saw in her reflection a quality of luminosity, as if it were lit up from within. Scanning the room slowly, she noticed a subtle feeling of delight growing inside her as she took in the quality of aliveness in everything she saw. In that moment she realized she was dreaming, and awoke, finding herself once again in bed.

Angela sat up on the edge of the bed and pinched herself to check whether she was awake. She felt the pain of the pinch. She looked around the room; everything looked normal. She felt clear-headed and alert, appreciating the lingering feeling of calm happiness that had arisen in the dream. Satisfied now that she was awake, she went to the bathroom, looked in the mirror, and again saw the reflection of her face glowing with a soft luminosity. Still feeling calm but now somewhat confused, Angela wasn't sure what to think. As she searched for a way to understand what was happening, she once again awoke to find herself in bed.

Now, with a growing sense of uneasiness, she began to scrutinize her surroundings, looking for some clue to help her understand what was happening. She realized she could not think of any way to determine whether in that moment she was awake or dreaming. The feeling of uncertainty as to the nature of her state of consciousness persisted with some force for several minutes, and, though gradually the intensity of the uncertainty diminished, it returned periodically for some days and months afterward.

~~~~~~~~

Can you be sure, at this moment, whether you are awake or dreaming? Angela was once certain she could tell the difference. After this dream, she could no longer take that feeling of certainty for granted.[2]

Those who assume that all dreams are vague and "dreamy" and thus easy to distinguish from the waking state may find Angela's confusion hard to grasp. Research regarding lucid dreams (dreams in which one is aware one is dreaming) shows that it is possible to engage in the full spectrum of cognitive activities—reasoning, logic, etc.—with utmost clarity while in the dream state. Angela's experience is quite common among people learning the skill of lucid dreaming. It is referred to as a "false awakening," and frequently occurs several times in a row, as it did for her.

According to the view from nowhere, the physical world of matter and energy—existing independent of consciousness—is the primary reality. In our ordinary, everyday experience, this assumption of the view from nowhere is taken to be common sense. We assume that the sun, the planets, and the stars are simply "out there," independent of our or any consciousness. We assume this because this is the way the world feels to us. It is exactly this feeling that Angela lost in the moments when she was uncertain whether she was awake or dreaming. She could not say for certain whether the mirror, the water, or the bed were dream images existing solely in relationship to her consciousness or were material objects external to her (or any) awareness.

Rephrasing the question above: Can you be sure, even in this moment, whether the material objects around you exist apart from you or exist only in relationship to your consciousness? As psychologist William James has pointed out, since consciousness is the means by which we know anything, it is impossible to know for certain if there are material objects that exist entirely apart from it.[3] To the extent we allow for this uncertainty, it will be easier to consider the possibility that all objects—whether material or dream objects—have their existence solely in relation to consciousness.[a]

In this chapter we are inviting you to leave your ordinary sense of things open to question in order to more easily consider the view from infinity. Like the fish who has lived always surrounded by water, we are so immersed in our worldview—our ordinary sense of things—that it can be difficult, if not impossible, to be aware of it. In order to step even a little outside this view, we need first to look more closely at the way we construct the world of our experience.

CONSTRUCTING THE BODY, CONSTRUCTING THE WORLD

> Reflection will show that the physical body... is but the focus in which the forms or data of our sense-experience are, as it were, collected. The materialist's idea of the body as standing in its own right, as a collection of flesh, bones, nerves and so forth, is an artificial mental construction obtained by abstraction from conscious experience.[4]
>
> —Sri Krishna Prem, The Yoga of the Bhagavad Gita

Psychologists tell us that the solid, three-dimensional world we ordinarily take to be "reality" is actually a representation of the external world,

---

a. We are not saying that matter doesn't exist or that it's only an illusion. Nor are we saying that it is impossible for an unconscious, nonintelligent matter (or physical energy) to exist entirely apart from any kind of consciousness. However, we do suggest that to believe in such self-existent matter requires a leap of faith at least as great as alternative views that, in one way or another, consider consciousness to be primary.

which our minds begin constructing in the first few months of life. As infants, we must bring together in our mind an inconceivably large amount of information. We have to learn to judge distance and perspective, and to attribute solidity to objects we have never touched. By the time we are toddlers, this process of world-construction takes place effortlessly, subconsciously, and almost instantaneously—in a way so fast and so far from our surface awareness that we are unable to see that the solid world we take to be "out there" is not so solid as we believe.

In a sense, infancy can be seen as a rite of passage that induces us into a collective hypnotic trance that, by its very nature, is self-sustaining. From a very young age, every person with whom we come into contact—parents, teachers, friends, and relatives—and every element of our culture—television, movies, billboards, and shopping malls—becomes part of our initiation into the predominant belief structure of our social and cultural milieu. We are repeatedly told in one way or another what is real and what is not, what we should pay attention to and what we should ignore. By the time we are three, we have entered fully into what psychologist Charles Tart calls "the consensus reality"[5]—the worldview a society takes to be unquestionably real. In this culture the consensual worldview tells us that solid, inert, unconscious matter is what's real and what matters.

One sign of the pervasiveness of this worldview is the widespread interest among cognitive scientists in what has been called the "hard problem of consciousness." In 1995, philosopher David Chalmers published an article in *Scientific American* entitled "The Puzzle of Conscious Experience."[6] He proposed two basic dimensions to the problem of consciousness. On the one hand, he identified an "easy" problem—discerning the relationship between physical brain processes and various aspects of cognition and emotion. For example, when I react with anger to a driver cutting me off, what happens in my brain? How does the brain recognize and process the situation, and what is the means by which the neural reaction occurs? Then there is what Chalmers called the "hard problem"—understanding how the purely physical brain gives rise to conscious experience. Or, to put his question in the context of the view from nowhere, how does a universe of purely unconscious, nonliving matter and energy give rise to consciousness?

Looking at it from within the consensus worldview into which we have been initiated, Chalmers' question makes sense to us. The presence of matter is obvious, we might think—we can feel its solidity. Consciousness is not something we can touch or see, so how can we be sure it exists?

Stepping back momentarily from everyday "common sense," we might be just as likely to take the opposite perspective: Consciousness is the one thing, the only thing, we can be sure of because we have direct experience of it[a]; we only know that matter exists because it appears to us in our consciousness. From this perspective, we seem to be up against a different hard problem—the hard problem of matter: how, given the all-pervasive nature of our experience of consciousness, did we come up with the idea of a world made of matter that is separate from it? To believe that matter exists in this way seems to require a rather dramatic leap of faith.

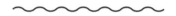

It may not yet seem credible to consider matter as the harder problem. So let's look a little more closely at what we usually take to be solid matter "out there," and see how it relates to the consciousness we usually take to be confined to the small space of our brain.[b]

Look at an apple. Where is it located? "Out there"? What makes it appear red? Is redness "out there," in the apple?

Neuroscientists tell us that the red we see when we look at an apple is not "out there" in the apple itself. What we experience as "red" is actually an interpretation of invisible light rays[c] that are reflected

---

a. "Consciousness" meaning not "I think," but the experience of being aware.

b. We are presenting the scientific data here without suggesting we agree or disagree with the conclusions that scientists reach. We are not challenging here the general scientific consensus that the "external" world—that is, the world external to animal or human perception—is in itself invisible, inaudible, or otherwise imperceptible. The aim here is to look at our assumptions about how things are, not offer speculations as to the nature of "reality" (if there is such a thing).

c. In other words, we don't actually see the light waves themselves. Rather, from the perspective of present-day neuroscience, we are aware only of our brain's response to them. The same is the case with sound waves and other waves of energy that our brain translates into our familiar sensory experience. This is why physicists tell us that the "real" world is invisible, inaudible, and so on.

off the piece of fruit, enter our brain through our eyes, and there are translated into the experienced color. And what about the apple? We can see it, smell it, touch it, taste it, so how can we doubt its existence? Neuroscientists tell us that our perception of space as well as our sense of the solidity of objects is similarly constructed in our brain.

Listen to a piece of music. Does the sound of the singer's voice exist outside you?

Not according to the physicist, who says that outside you there is nothing more than movements of air. These atmospheric disturbances,[a] projected toward your ears by the movement of stereo speakers, set into motion various parts of the ear. These vibrations are then transmitted down the auditory canal into different areas of the brain where, somehow, miraculously, the experience of sound emerges. The same is true for tastes and scents—in fact, for the entire "feel" of the world. The "real" world, as disclosed to us by modern science, thus seems to be an invisible, inaudible, intangible, odorless, and tasteless collection of waves of energy.[7] Oddly enough, it seems science may be pointing toward the same conclusion as some schools of Indian philosophy—that the world we experience is Maya, an illusion.[b]

Psychologist Charles Tart suggests that our relationship to the world is like that of a pilot in a flight simulator. Novice pilots learn to fly by sitting inside flight simulators that are designed to create an experience that is nearly indistinguishable from the actual experience of flying a plane.[8] Similarly, as Tart develops the metaphor, we "sit" inside our brain, responding to an invisible, untouchable world that we take to be entirely separate from and external to us, whose nature is unknown.[9] Our brain does the job of the flight simulator in constructing an experiential world of sights and sounds. We may be comfortable with the idea that it does this when we are sleeping, but it is perhaps discomfiting to contemplate that it does so equally when we are awake.

---

a. Twentieth-century French composer Edgard Varese, when asked his profession, replied, "I am a disturber of the atmosphere."

b. Some schools of Indian philosophy take the position that the world is an illusion in the sense that it doesn't exist. However, there are others that take the world to be real, while giving consciousness and matter equal reality status.

~~~~~~~~

This examination of the way we experience an isolated piece of fruit or piece of music *may not* challenge us to the point where we feel the need to more fully question our ordinary point of view. Looking at the whole context of experience might help us see more clearly the way in which deeply entrenched habits of mind shape the world we perceive.

Think back to the image of Sharon sitting on a bench near the pond with a tree overhanging the water. Imagine the solid wood bench, the play of light on the surface of the pond, and the sound of the leaves of the tree rustling softly in the breeze. A bird alights on one of the branches of the tree and begins to sing. A grasshopper plays by the edge of the water. Now picture Sharon getting up from the bench and walking away. The bird flies off. The grasshopper hops onto the bench, then exits the scene altogether.

How did everything look and feel to you when you first imagined it? Did you imagine the environment as existing in itself just as you perceived it? If so, according to what science tells us, you would have been wrong—without a consciousness present to receive and trans-late the waves of energy into visual images, there would have been no visual image. The only thing that would be left if you abstracted consciousness altogether—at least, according to the prevailing under-standing of the science of perception—would be orderly movements of physical energies that are invisible, inaudible, intangible, odorless, tasteless, unintelligent, and unconscious.[a]

Did your image of the scene change significantly after Sharon left... then again after the bird left... and again after the grasshopper left? If the scene looked and felt the same to you throughout, you have unwittingly constructed it based on your own human consciousness.

---

a After having taken some time to deconstruct your sense of "Sharon," the "bench," the "tree," and so on, you might try rereading the story about Sharon in chapter 1 and doing the same exercise of deconstruction. Keep in mind the ten-dency to take the things, places, and events described in the story as solid, mate-rial things existing entirely independent of consciousness. Later, when reading about Sharon, repeating this exercise may make it a little bit easier to understand her experience from the perspective of the view from infinity. You might also want to try this exercise with experiences in your own life.

Whenever we visualize something, we tend to forget that the appearance of the objects we imagine is dependent on our human viewpoint. The green of the grasshopper, the shimmering of the light, the solidity of the bench, and the fluidity of the water all exist relative to a particular set of sensory, emotional, and mental faculties. Each of these qualities would appear quite different to Sharon, the bird, and the grasshopper. Their minds and sense organs are so different that it is almost possible to speak of three different benches and three different ponds and, in a sense, three different worlds (or, to put it in a slightly less provocative manner, three different experiences of the world).

Take the tree overhanging the pond. Does the tree—as experienced by a person or animal—exist "out there"? We might think of the tree as an external or outer pattern of energy, and the seeing of it is an internal or subjective act of consciousness. Described in this way, it may seem that the tree that is experienced exists apart from the person or animal observing it, but as we've seen, the tree *as we experience it* has no existence independent of a conscious observer. The experienced tree *is* the relationship between a conscious act of knowing and a pattern of energy. A bird flying toward what we see as a "tree," a squirrel climbing it, and a termite burrowing through it will all see something very different. Then what is the "tree" apart from the perspective of the person, the bird, the squirrel and the termite?

> In itself [the tree] is nothing, it only becomes something through the shaping, selecting, presenting consciousness. And since the kinds of possibilities of consciousness are infinite, we can go a step further and say the [tree] is the sum of all ... possible ways of perceiving it. [10]

Where and when did you imagine this scene to be taking place? You may not have been fully conscious of it, but if you examine your mental image closely, you may notice a subliminal sense that the scene was located at some general point in time and space. How solid and reliable is our sense of time or space? Suppose you are sitting on the bench by the pond, watching a leaf fall from the tree. Consider your image of the leaf at any particular moment. The "leaf" that you see in that moment is actually more than 1/100 of a second old. It takes several billionths of a second for the light to travel from the leaf to your eyes, then more time for your brain to process the light and construct the image of the leaf. So the leaf you "see" is a fraction of a second out-of-date. Where is the leaf at the moment you "see" it? Since the earth is moving around the sun at approximately 67,000 miles per hour, the leaf has moved quite a distance from where it was when the light that reached your eye was first reflected off of it.

Perhaps it is hard to get a sense of the relativity of space and time perception on this small a scale. Consider a distant star. When you look at the night sky, the stars you "see" may actually be thousands of light-years away from the point where you "see" them. Or, they may have ceased to exist many years ago. Not only do we forget that the sensory qualities of everything we see exist only relative to our human consciousness, but the time and place within which we see them is also relative to the way our mind functions.

Perhaps looking at our world construction in a still larger context of space and time could be helpful. Take a moment to imagine what the universe might have looked like as it took form after the Big Bang...

You may have come up with something along the lines of what Alan Wallace writes here:

> As we attend to cosmology's description of the evolution of the universe from the Big Bang up to the emergence of life on our planet, a series of images of these events are brought to mind. We may imagine something like a cosmic firecracker at the beginning, red-hot gases expanding in space; the formation of radiant, bright stars; a molten, lifeless planet; and finally nucleotides that mysteriously transform into living, conscious creatures.

Now, consider Wallace's further comments:

> Upon reflection, it becomes obvious that none of these images existed in nature, for they are human constructs based

upon our conscious, visual experience. While texts on cosmology may display vivid artist's portrayals of the formation of stars and planets, such images may be profoundly misleading. They presumably depict these events as they would have appeared if humans had been on the scene to witness them. But cosmology denies that human consciousness was present, so they never looked like those illustrations. Indeed, in a cosmos devoid of consciousness, *they never looked like anything at all*. [emphasis added] No images are appropriate. Nevertheless, they do come to mind; and the tendency is to reify them, to assume that they existed in a mindless universe all on their own. [11]

THE FILMIEST OF SCREENS

If the world we experience is in some way constructed, what is it in us that gives shape to that world? Ordinarily, we have no awareness of the world being a construct of the mind. Clearly then, it's not what we're accustomed to thinking of as the mind that puts together the world as we see and feel it. Scientists now believe that the processing responsible for the construction of our representation of the world takes place in a domain outside the ordinary consciousness, in what they call the "cognitive unconscious."

More than a century ago, William James contemplated the existence of realms of consciousness beyond the ordinary:

> Our normal waking consciousness… is but one special type of consciousness, whilst all about it, parted from it by the filmiest of screens,[a] there lie potential forms of conscious-

a James's phrase has sometimes been written as "filmiest of screens," other times as "flimsiest of screens." We found examples of both, but, to our surprise, "filmiest" was the more common spelling.

ness entirely different. We may go through life without sus-
pecting their existence; but apply the requisite stimulus, and
at a touch they are there in all their completeness... How
to regard them is the question... At any rate, they forbid a
premature closing of our accounts with reality.[12]

The nature of this apparently unconscious realm has long been the
subject of dispute among psychologists.

In the early days of psychological science, many thought the
unconscious to be a state superior to "normal waking consciousness."
In 1869, philosopher Eduard von Hartmann, familiar with and influenced by Indian thought, described the unconscious as "far-seeing
and clairvoyant... superior to all consciousness, at once conscious and
supra-conscious."[13] This Romantic view was fairly common in the late
nineteenth century.

Psychotherapists of the time, many of whom were also influenced
by Indian ideas and practices, sought to invoke the powers of the
unconscious in their patients' healing process. In the last decade of
the century, however, Sigmund Freud proposed a very different idea of
the unconscious. Strongly influenced by Darwin's theory of evolution,
his theory reflected a more conservative, pessimistic view of human
nature. Freud characterized the unconscious as a kind of nether realm
made up of a seething mixture of sexual and aggressive drives, ever
ready to overwhelm the superficially civilized rational mind.

In the early twentieth century, when behaviorism was the dominant
force in psychology, there was no place for the conscious mind, much
less the idea of unconscious mental processing. By the mid-twentieth
century, the eminent behaviorist B. F. Skinner had depicted the human
being as entirely the product of mechanical forces, "beyond freedom and
dignity."[14] Gradually, however, many psychologists came to feel that a
psychology without consciousness was lacking something essential.

With the revival of interest in the study of consciousness, new research
methods were developed to explore the relationship of unconscious and
preconscious processes to conscious perception, memory, and learning.
Researchers were able to show, for example, what kinds of information
could be acquired when an individual was unconscious. Sophisticated

brain imaging procedures revealed a complex and dynamic picture of the neural activity that accompanies conscious experience.

A *New York Times* article on recent discoveries within cognitive science entitled "Your Unconscious Is Smarter Than You Are" reflects a new twist on the Romantic notion of the unconscious. No longer considered the repository of great or transcendent wisdom, it is seen by some as the processor of stunning amounts of information. According to psychologist John Kilhstrom, the *Times'* characterization of the cognitive unconscious is inaccurate. In spite of the fact that cognitive scientists have identified a number of psychological functions—perception, memory, and learning, among others—which go on outside of conscious awareness, Kilhstrom asserts that none of the higher-level thought processes can function without the participation of consciousness. Thus he counters, "Your unconscious is stupider than you are."[15]

What theorists of the unconscious generally agree on is the idea that some kind of mental activity occurs outside the spotlight of our full conscious attention.[16] Some mental activity takes place outside waking consciousness altogether. For example, when we watch a film, it appears to us that we are observing a seamless flow of moving images, but what is actually being presented to us is a series of rapidly changing still photographs (approximately twenty-four frames per second). Research shows that part of our brain is in fact capable of distinguishing one frame from another. However, no matter how hard we might try, we would not be able to consciously distinguish the separate images.[17]

Some of this mental activity takes place initially on the fringe of awareness and later enters into full consciousness. For example, until we are directed to notice it, we are usually not aware of all the sounds in our environment, or the feeling of our body sitting in a chair. However, such fringe or preconscious phenomena do affect us, as is evident to anybody who, lost in thought, has found themselves putting on a sweater before they consciously realized they were cold.

~~~~~~~~

We now invite you to participate in a few experiments that may help illumine the workings of your preconscious and unconscious mental processes.

Look at the following paragraph:

> Aoccdrnig to a rscheearchr at Cmabrigde Uinervtisy, it
> deosn't mttaer in waht oredr the ltteers in a wrod are, the
> olny iprmoetnt tihng is taht the frist and lsat ltteer be at the
> rghit pclae. The rset can be a tatol mses and you can sitll raed
> it wouthit porbelm. Tihs is bcuseae the haumn mnid deos
> not raed ervey lteter by istlef, but the wrod as a wlohe.[18]

You probably didn't need to rearrange the letters of these words in order to understand the meaning of the paragraph. Some kind of mental processing took place outside of conscious awareness that enabled you to understand the misspelled words.

One of the more interesting things psychologists have discovered about the relationship of conscious to unconscious activity is that it is a complex, dynamic one. Consciousness is not a simple, digital, on-off phenomenon. Rather, it seems to be a continuum. Consider the next paragraph. Read it as quickly as possible, then cover it up before reading further.

> A newspaper is better than a magazine. A seashore is a better place than the street. At first it is better to run than to walk. You may have to try several times... Once successful, complications are minimal. Birds seldom get too close. Rain, however, soaks in very fast. Too many people doing the same thing can also cause problems. One needs lots of room. If there are no complications it can be very peaceful. A rock will serve as an anchor. If things break loose from it, however, you will not get a second chance. [19]

Please don't uncover the paragraph yet. Do you remember the feeling you had as you read it? Were you at all confused or disoriented? Now try reading the paragraph, again doing it as quickly as possible, but this time with the idea that all the sentences are referring to a fairly common object used both by adults and children. Cover up the paragraph again as soon as you read it, and then go on to the instruction below.

Read the paragraph one more time, again going through it quickly, but this time holding in mind the idea that the subject of the paragraph is a kite.

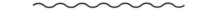

As you read through the above paragraph several times, you may have noticed a gradual dawning of understanding, and perhaps a moment when the full meaning suddenly emerged into awareness. As we saw in chapter 1, the progression in each moment from unconsciousness to consciousness is a complex process, with overlapping strands of unconscious activity gradually emerging into consciousness.

Pierre Janet, a nineteenth-century psychiatrist, described how some of these strands of pre-conscious experience can operate simultaneously in a person as noncommunicating streams of consciousness. Many decades later, Ernest Hilgard made use of Janet's observations to help explain phenomena he witnessed in hypnotized subjects. He coined the term "hidden observer" to describe a separate strand of awareness that remained active even when the conscious mind was apparently not functioning.[20]

Hilgard performed several experiments in which subjects in a hypnotic state were told they would not respond to various stimuli, such as the painful feeling of ice-cold water or the pungent smell of ammonia.[21] As suggested, they experienced neither the pain of the cold nor the pungency of the smell. However, he then demonstrated that these separate streams were not so separate after all. He later instructed these same subjects, while still under hypnosis, "When you are in this state you have a hidden part of you that knows… what is really going on." They were then told that, on the count of three, "this hidden part will no longer be hidden and you will be aware of things that you were not aware of or did not know before."[22] After receiving this instruction, the majority of subjects were able to describe the sensations of which they had not been previously aware.

To counter the criticism that subjects may actually have been consciously aware while allegedly under hypnosis, experiments were conducted in which physiological measures were used to substantiate subjects' verbal reports. In one such experiment, subjects were told that a box would occlude their line of vision such that they would not be able to see a screen on which a series of colored lights would be flashing. Although no box was actually there, the brain's response to the visual stimuli was nevertheless suppressed as a direct result of the hypnotic suggestion.[23]

BEYOND THE FILMY SCREEN

It is perhaps becoming clearer now why cognitive scientists tell us that the apparently solid world we experience is actually a representation constructed[a] by the mind. This representation is constructed gradually over the course of a brief moment—from an apparently unconscious stage, through James's "fringe" experience to full consciousness. The mind that does the constructing seems to be something quite different from our ordinary waking consciousness.

Are we then trapped in this mental construction? Are we like the novice pilot in Charles Tart's "flight simulator" metaphor, forever restricted to a representation of a world that we cannot know directly? Both William James and contemporary psychologists assert that the boundary between the ordinary and nonordinary consciousness is permeable. How might it be possible, then, to gain direct experience of the world beyond the "filmy screen" of our ordinary consciousness? Tart's systems theory of consciousness may help shed some light on how the boundary can be crossed.[24]

Tart explains that any particular state of consciousness is maintained by various stabilizing forces that include events, images, thoughts, beliefs, or feelings that function to keep the attention limited to a particular range of experience. When these stabilizing forces are disrupted in some way, the conscious state begins to undergo a transformation. A common example that everybody experiences is the transition from the waking state to sleep. Wakefulness is a state main-

---

a. A construction, not a creation of the mind; perhaps still more accurately, a co-creation of consciousness and energy.

tained by thinking and activity. It can be destabilized by lying down, closing one's eyes, turning out the lights, and relaxing the mind and body. Another example is the state of depression that may be stabilized by a particular interpretation of events, a physiological state, or by a matrix of feelings related to the overall mood of depression. It can be disrupted by shifting attention away from those feelings, changing one's interpretation of events, or changing the physiological state through medication, among other possibilities.

How might our ordinary waking consciousness be destabilized to allow for a conscious awareness of what lies behind James's "filmy screen"? There are individual factors such as beliefs, attachments, and desires that keep our attention locked in a narrow range of awareness. In addition, the entire society acts as a stabilizing force, every moment serving to reinforce the general cultural consensus. Such powerful forces require equally powerful disruptive forces to shift one's attention from its habitual absorption in the ordinary view. Tribal societies have for thousands of years employed rhythmic drumming and dancing as well as intoxicants as a means of redirecting their attention and thus destabilizing their ordinary state of consciousness.

However, external means such as drumming and intoxicants may be problematic. While they may be effective in shifting state, they bypass the conscious process that makes the connection between ordinary and nonordinary states of consciousness. If we are to gain direct knowledge of a state of consciousness beyond the filmy screen of our ordinary waking state, we need to remain alert during the process of destabilization.

In fact, it is possible to retain full conscious awareness during the transition from one state of consciousness to another. Every night when we go to sleep, we leave behind the waking state and make the transition into the dream and sleep states. A person who has trained himself to remain conscious during the process of falling asleep will experience the consensus reality slowly dissolving. The sensations that contribute to the feeling of having a solid body existing in a solid external world, the coherent thoughts, ideas, memories, images, and feelings that create a sense of being a solid self—all begin to come apart.

To remain conscious at the same time that one's world and very sense of self are coming apart can be anxiety-provoking, to say the least. The degree to which this will be upsetting depends on two things. For one, our fear will be intensified to the extent our identity has been caught up in the constructed self and world that are dissolving. Another factor relates to our belief about the nature of whatever is beyond our ordinary waking state. If it is primarily stupid, as Kihlstrom characterized it, we might very well fear ending up like a helpless infant or animal. But if, like the Romantic poets, we believe there is a vaster, more beautiful state of consciousness beyond, our natural fear of the unknown will be tempered by the anticipation of something greater.

Perhaps both Kihlstrom and the Romantics were correct. William James speculated that beyond that "filmy screen" lie many different forms of consciousness. Some may resemble the consciousness of our distant evolutionary ancestors. But there may also be states outside the ordinary waking consciousness that are in some way greater than it.

If we were able to become aware of the entire process by which the world is constructed, and in doing so were able to gain access to a more profound state of consciousness, our whole sense of ourselves and the world might radically change. According to yoga psychology, such a different consciousness exists and is accessible. However, before we can begin to explore what Sri Aurobindo has called the "rich and inexhaustible kingdom within," we need to examine some of the beliefs and assumptions that serve to anchor us in our present state of consciousness. Once seen, we will have the option of setting them aside long enough to gain a glimpse of another kind of consciousness, and to consider what value it may have to our individual and collective lives.

CHAPTER 5

Second Challenge To the View: Exploring Hidden Assumptions about Matter, Life, and Mind

> We all agreed that your theory is crazy. The question which divides us is whether it is crazy enough to have a chance of being correct.[1]
>
> —Niels Bohr, addressing a colleague regarding his theory on quantum physics

According to the view from infinity, the floor on which you stand, the pages of this book, and the cells that make up your body, are all meaningful, purposeful formations of an infinite intelligent consciousness. You may already hold this view as your personal philosophy, or you may think it utterly unscientific nonsense. In either case, it is likely that you have some unconscious assumptions about the world that will make it difficult to take the view from infinity seriously—in its totality. We explore those assumptions here in order to bring them to awareness and clear the way for a serious consideration of the view from infinity.

Many believe that a perspective that sees the universe as alive, intelligent, and pervaded by consciousness is in conflict with scientific data. We believe this is not the case, and that it is only thought to be so because of a mistaken association of the scientific method with the philosophic doctrine of materialism.

In these times, science is generally considered the court of final appeal for determining what is real—and what is even worth considering as real. And its view that reality is composed of essentially nonliving, nonconscious, nonintelligent fields of energy holds great sway.

However, this view was not arrived at by scientific means.

The scientific method cannot determine the ultimate nature of reality. Scientists observe physical events, and from these observations develop theories to account for what they observe. These theories are very useful in helping us become aware of the repeating, orderly patterns that make up the world of our experience. However, they do not tell us how those patterns came to be or what maintains them. As neuroscientist Donald Hoffman points out, scientific observations and theories are compatible with a number of different seemingly contradictory views of reality—including the idea that everything can ultimately be reduced to matter *(materialism)*, that everything can ultimately be reduced to mind *(idealism)*,[a] or that everything is made up of some combination of mind and matter *(dualism)*.[2]

This limitation on the part of science has been perhaps its greatest strength. The scientific spirit of free and open inquiry has helped foster a desire for liberation from authoritarian religions and governments, and has thus helped bring about more open societies. However, if science is, in fact, unable to determine the ultimate nature of reality, then it is very important that it maintain a clear and consistent neutrality in that regard.

But the human mind has an almost irrepressible tendency to hold on to one view as absolute truth and to fight to have that view predominate. A story is told of a group of people who were granted a vision of God. They were stunned by the beauty of this vision and were filled with great peace and joy. Some of them began to speak among themselves about what they had seen. As one was describing his experience, another person said, "Yes, I saw God, too. He was wearing a red hat." The other person said very gently, "Oh no, I think you're mistaken, his hat was blue." Slowly, sects began to spring up, the red hat and blue hat sects that existed at first in a state of somewhat benign tension, but which gradually escalated into holy wars over who had the true vision of God.[3]

---

a. It will be important to keep in mind later that the view from infinity, as presented here, is not compatible with a philosophy of idealism that considers matter to have a lesser status than mind.

We tend to think that this kind of conflict occurs only within the religious sphere. And it is true that neither holy wars nor crusades have been initiated by molecular biologists or astrophysicists. It's also true that for several centuries, scientists for the most part refrained from making pronouncements regarding the ultimate nature of the universe. However, in the last century or so, science has unwittingly fallen prey to the very habit of mind it was designed to avoid. In its desire to distance itself from doctrine in order to delve dispassionately into the nature of things, science has come dangerously close to advocating a doctrinaire materialism.

How did the materialist view come to be associated with science? According to Richard Dixey, it was the result of a kind of confidence trick played several centuries ago, back when scientists agreed to leave matters of God and spirit to the Church. Dixey describes the result as a cosmic version of the card game three-card monte. Often played on a city street, three-card monte begins with a dealer asking a passerby to pick one of three cards laid out on a cardboard box. He then turns all three cards facedown, moves them around at great speed, and for a small bet challenges the unsuspecting customer to point to the card he had picked. The dealer "allows" the customer to win the first round, but from then on the dealer takes all. How does he pull it off? By surreptitiously removing the card the customer chose and replacing it with another.[4]

Scientists who claim the universe to be the result of blind chance, devoid of consciousness, may in a way be unwitting victims of their own confidence trick. Having deposed God (and along with him, consciousness of any kind) as creator and maintainer of the "laws of nature," they were left with no way to account for the apparent regularities of our experience.

Consciousness cannot be found in the universe because the "consciousness-card" had been removed, along with God, as a prerequisite to scientific investigation. And by the early twentieth century, the "chance-card" was inserted in its place. However practical at the time, it was this sleight of hand rather than any empirical data that eventually led scientists to see the universe as "the outcome of accidental collocations of atoms,"[5] unintelligent and unconscious—yet somehow mysteriously well ordered.

This conclusion—which was not arrived at by scientific means—has come to be taken as scientific fact. Since we live in a culture strongly influenced by science, this materialistic view colors every aspect of our experience. Even if we consciously hold beliefs that are nonmaterialistic, our sense of ourselves and the world may still be powerfully affected by materialistic assumptions lodged deep in the cognitive unconscious. We will examine some of these assumptions in order that they may present less of a barrier to considering the view from infinity in an impartial manner.

TAKING AN AGNOSTIC STANCE TOWARD THE ORIGIN OF THE LAWS OF NATURE: EXPLORING OUR ASSUMPTIONS ABOUT MATTER

> The whole modern conception of the world is founded on the illusion that the so-called laws of nature are the explanation of natural phenomena.[6]
>
> —Wittgenstein, *Tractatus Logico-Philosophicus*

Is consciousness or intelligence of some kind responsible for bringing about the orderly patterns of the world we refer to as "laws of nature"? Or did they simply arise by chance? Passionate arguments have been made by scientists and philosophers in support of both views. Science and religion writer Roy Abraham Varghese writes, "There has to be intelligence in the laws of the universe or it would not exhibit the kind of rationality shown by the success of science... Not simply the existence of the world but its thoroughgoing rationality demand an explanation, and Infinite Intelligence as the ground and matrix of the world is the only satisfactory explanation."[7] According to physicist Henry Stapp, "The physical world described by the laws of physics is a structure of tendencies in the world of mind."[8]

In striking contrast to these views, philosopher Daniel Dennett suggests that the laws of physics "could themselves be the outcome of a blind, uncaring shuffle through Chaos."[9] Biologist Richard Dawkins, pointing to the pervasive suffering in the world, writes, "In a universe of blind physical forces and genetic replication, some people are going to get hurt, and other people are going to get lucky, and you won't find any rhyme or reason in it, nor any justice. The universe that we observe has precisely the properties we should expect if there is, at bottom, no design, no purpose, no evil, and no good, nothing but blind, pitiless indifference."[10]

But how do scientists who assert the latter view develop their conception of the way laws of nature came into being? According to physicist Stephen Hawking, a law of nature is nothing more than a theory, which "is just a model of the universe... It exists only in our minds and does not have any other reality."[11] A model in our mind can certainly help describe the behavior of patterns we see in nature, but how can it explain their existence? Biologist Rupert Sheldrake observes, "In the face of this problem, most scientists (usually implicitly, often unconsciously) fall back on the idea that mathematical laws of nature do indeed exist independently of human minds, that they are objective realities, whether we can describe them or not. Then the problem of what these immaterial laws actually are, and how they work, is usually avoided by flipping back to the idea that they are just models in our minds."[12]

In fact, science, as currently practiced, cannot provide an explanation for the origin or persistence of the regularities of nature we refer to as "laws." Physicists, when pressed, will acknowledge that they are not only unable to explain the laws of nature, but that they can't even tell us what matter or energy is. Richard Feynman, considered by many to be one of the most brilliant physicists of the twentieth century, has said: "It is important to realize that in physics today, we have no knowledge of what energy is."[13] Chemist A. G. Cairns-Smith further elaborates: "It is a fundamental mistake to identify a model with reality... Force, field...mass, energy... space, time... particle, wave, [are simply elements in the scientific model]... We know now for sure that we do not know at all what matter is."[14]

Given that scientists have no idea how the patterns in the universe they call "laws of nature" came about, the most appropriate stance would be one of open-minded agnosticism. Yet, we may still feel that it somehow conflicts with science to assert that consciousness is in some way involved in the workings of matter. To the extent this is the case, it should alert us to the fact that we hold some erroneous assumptions regarding what is and what isn't science.

Even if we were to develop an intellectual understanding of the essentially agnostic position of science,[a] it might still be emotionally difficult to let go of the view from nowhere, and thus maintain a truly neutral position with regard to the view from infinity. We tend to be uncomfortable with the sense of mystery this would entail. When we come across something that seems to violate our sense of how things work, we anxiously seek to explain it away, restoring as soon as possible our confidence in a knowable, predictable world. Yet, there was a time in our lives when we had a feeling for this mystery. As the poet G. K. Chesterton writes, "When we are very young children we do not need fairy tales: we only need tales. Mere life is interesting enough. A child of seven is excited by being told that Tommy opened a door and saw a dragon. But a child of three is excited by being told that Tommy opened a door."[15]

Since science as currently practiced can only be agnostic when it comes to the question of whether consciousness is involved in the laws of nature, it is not in conflict with the view from infinity. However, since we tend to hold subconscious assumptions about the world that are conditioned by the view from nowhere, it will be important to remain mindful of these assumptions while considering the universe from the perspective of the view from infinity. This doesn't necessarily require that we effortlessly scrutinize our every passing thought and feeling. We can instead become more like the little child who embraces the mystery of even the most ordinary details of experience, willing—at least temporarily—to suspend our need for clear and precise answers.

TAKING AN AGNOSTIC STANCE TOWARD THE CAUSE OF MUTATIONS: EXPLORING OUR ASSUMPTIONS ABOUT LIFE

In recent years there has been much public discussion regarding the causal factors underlying the evolutionary process. The "intelligent

---

a. Agnostic, that is, in regard to the ultimate nature of matter and consciousness.

design" movement claims to have proven that the mutations that occur in evolution could not have arisen by chance. Intelligent design theorists such as William Dembski rely in large part on statistical analysis to show that certain patterns of mutation cannot be random. Apart from these essentially philosophic arguments[a] (buttressed by mathematical computations), they offer no specific mechanisms by means of which intelligence might play an active role in evolution.[16]

Scientists, meanwhile, have conducted some interesting experiments that seem to suggest something is occurring beyond purely random mutation. Biologist John Campbell claims to have detected environmental sensors in bacteria "which can feed back to the activity and organization of the genes,"[17] directing a reprogramming of the whole genetic system. Biologist Barry Hall has carried out rather remarkable experiments with the intestinal bacteria *Escherichia coli (E. coli)*. As described by scientific theorist Howard Bloom, Hall placed the bacteria in a solution of salicin—a pain-reliever "squeezed from the bark of willow trees which, to the E. coli bacterium, is inedible as pitch. An individual bacterium can crank nourishment out of this unpalatable medication only if it undergoes a step-by-step sequence of two genetic breakthroughs, none of which entails making a giant step backward. The odds of pulling this off through random mutation are less than 1 in 10,000,000,000,000,000,000,000—or, to put it in English, more than 10 billion trillion against one."[18]

Physicist Eshel Ben-Jacob used insights from the mathematics of materials science to study what he felt were learning patterns in colonies of bacteria. Summarizing Ben-Jacob's conclusions, Bloom[b] writes, "A 'creative net' of bacteria, unlike a man-made machine, can invent a

---

a. In making a distinction between philosophy and science, we're neither assenting to nor dismissing Dembski's arguments. Had Dembski merely claimed that mutations leading to new species could not have arisen by chance, his argument would have remained within the realm of science. He entered the realm of philosophy when he offered "intelligent design" as the ultimate cause of evolutionary change.

b. Bloom's colorful use of anthropomorphic language should not be taken as an indication that he literally believes, for example, that bacteria "think" in the same way as race-car designers.

new instruction set with which to beat an unfamiliar challenge. Some colony members feel out the new environment, learning all they can. Others 'puzzle' over the genome like race-car designers tinkering with an engine whose power they are determined to increase. Yet others collect the incoming 'ideas' passed along by their sisters and work together to alter the use of existing genetic parts or to turn them into something new." [19] One bacteria colony can even learn from others, by means of which, according to Ben-Jacob, it "designs and constructs a new and more advanced genome" thus "performing a genomic leap." [20]

These experiments go beyond philosophic argument to provide empirical data from which some may infer the working of conscious intelligence of some kind. However, again, none of the methods used in these experiments provide direct evidence of consciousness at work.

Some scientists and philosophers of science go to the opposite extreme. Observing correctly that current research methods provide no direct empirical evidence of intelligence as an agent in evolutionary change, they conclude that science has therefore *proven* that natural selection in combination with mutations is a wholly nonintelligent, nonconscious process. For example, both philosopher Daniel Dennett and biologist Richard Dawkins argue quite vehemently against the idea of intelligent design, and for the idea that evolution is a process entirely without purpose. Claiming to base his argument on the evidence provided by physics and biology, Dennett concludes that evolution is a designerless process: "It is the wonderful wedding of chance and necessity, happening in a trillion places at once, at a trillion different levels. And what miracle caused it? None. It just happened to happen, in the fullness of time. You could even say, in a way, that the Tree of Life created itself. Not in a miraculous, instantaneous whoosh, but slowly, slowly, over billions of years."

Just as Dembski, Hall, and Ben-Jacob cannot provide direct empirical evidence of the working of consciousness in evolution, neither can Dawkins and Dennett provide direct evidence to the contrary. Realizing this, some contemporary biologists wedded to the idea of physicalism[a] resort more directly to philosophic arguments. In Darwin's

---

a. The philosophy that the ultimate basis of the universe is mindless and purposeless matter-energy.

time, arguing *for* the existence of God based on the complexity of the world was known as "natural theology." Contemporary biologists, by contrast, sometimes engage in what physicist Richard Thompson has called "negative theology,"[21] arguing that the allegedly problematic design of many creatures constitutes evidence *against* the existence of God. Paleontologist Stephen J. Gould presents such an argument, saying, "Odd arrangements and funny solutions are the proof of evolution—paths that a sensible God would never tread but that a natural process, constrained by history, follows perforce."[22] Gould and others who offer similar arguments rarely acknowledge that their concept of a sensible "God" may not bear much if any resemblance to that of sophisticated theologians. In any case, as with the others mentioned, Gould does not offer evidence of the absence of intelligence in the process of evolution—and of course, it is not possible to do so.

Both arguments—for or against the involvement of conscious intelligence in the process of evolution—rely on assumptions about chance that cannot be proven by current scientific methodology. Does consciousness create and maintain the laws or patterns of nature? Is it responsible in any way for the mutations that take place in evolution? Or did the laws of nature just happen to have happened "in the fullness of time" as the result of purely material causes, as Dennett suggests? And is Dawkins right that evolution is also a wholly mindless, purposeless physical process? Since current scientific methods cannot detect the presence or absence of consciousness, it seems that the appropriate stance for scientists to take—at this point in time—is one of consistent, rigorous agnosticism.[a]

Given that science itself is agnostic about the ultimate cause of mutations, there is no inherent conflict between the scientific understanding of evolution and the view from infinity. We have thus far explored some

---

a Again, agnostic with regard to the ultimate nature of matter, energy, and consciousness, and agnostic in regard to questions about the role of consciousness in creating and maintaining the laws of nature and its role in the evolutionary process. The scientist himself may personally hold materialist, dualist, idealist, or other philosophic or religious views. However, if it is correct that scientific findings do not in themselves prove or disprove any philosophic or religious position, the scientist as scientist must remain agnostic about the questions raised here.

common assumptions about what constitutes the scientific view regarding the laws of nature governing matter and the cause of evolution, and have found them to be ungrounded in scientific fact. We will now look at the field of parapsychology (psi) in order to challenge some common assumptions about something a little closer to home—the nature of the mind. The underlying assumption of the view from nowhere is that the mind is no more than a function of the brain. The findings of psi research provide empirical data that suggest—though do not prove—that the mind can function in some way independent of the brain.

Because the findings of psi research are so challenging, many critics have made strenuous efforts to find fault with them, questioning the research methodology and even accusing the researchers of outright fraud. To counter this, we will devote some space to showing that psi researchers have actually developed some of the most refined methods in the entire field of science, and, contrary to the assertions of many critics, have attained undeniable and repeatable results.[23]

The subject matter of psi challenges our subconscious assumptions in a more powerful way than the questions we've asked regarding the laws of nature or the source of evolutionary change. Psi research questions the norms of space and time we take for granted. It challenges us to drastically reconsider what our minds are capable of. And perhaps most daunting, it challenges the physical and psychological boundaries that we believe make us essentially separate from each other and the world. Thus, the findings of parapsychology challenge us to reconsider much of what we have assumed about the relationship between mind and matter. For these reasons, more than anything we've looked at so far, an exploration of psi research can help prepare the way for an open-minded consideration of the view from infinity.

KEEPING AN OPEN MIND? EXPLORING OUR ASSUMPTIONS ABOUT MIND

> Neither the testimony of all the Fellows of the Royal Society; nor even the evidence of my own senses, would lead me

to believe in the transmission of thought from one person to another independent of the recognized channels of sense.[24]

—H. L. F. von Helmholtz, psychophysiologist, late nineteenth century

Why do we not accept extra-sensory perception as a psychological fact? [Parapsychologist] Rhine has offered us enough evidence to have convinced us on almost any other issue… I cannot see what other basis my colleagues have for rejecting it… My own rejection of his views is in a literal sense prejudice.[25]

—Psychologist Donald O. Hebb, 1951

This is a subject that is so intellectually uncomfortable as to be almost painful… I end by concluding that I cannot explain away Professor Rhine's evidence and I cannot accept it.[26]

—Warren Weaver, mathematician, 1963

There are some things we know are not true, and precognition [foreknowledge of the future] is one of them; therefore, in this case, experimental data is irrelevant.[27]

—Director of a major nuclear physics institute, sometime in the 1980s

I wouldn't believe it even if it were true.[28]

—Contemporary scientist speaking to researcher Willis Harman upon being told of successful remote-viewing [formerly known as "clairvoyance"] experiments

In the previous two sections, we questioned the extent to which consciousness is involved, if at all, in the laws of nature and the process of evolution. More specifically, we looked at the question of whether consciousness is in some way responsible for creating and maintaining the laws of nature, and for bringing about the mutations involved in the process of evolution. Extending this question to the human being, we now ask, to what extent is consciousness responsible for generating brain activity?

For many years in the field of psychology there was a taboo on the very mention of the word "consciousness," a taboo that made it impossible to address this question. However, in the past decade, consciousness has become one of the hottest topics in science. Some, like neuroscientist J. Allan Hobson, assert definitively that consciousness is nothing more than a by-product of brain activity.[29] Others acknowledge that the relationship between consciousness and the brain is not yet understood, but remain confident that consciousness will eventually be found to be no more than a result of the complexities of brain functioning. Still others say the relationship between mind and brain is a mystery that is unlikely to ever be resolved. Given these disparate views, where might we look for answers?

William James once described psychology as the science of consciousness. One might expect therefore that it would shed some light on the nature of consciousness. However, psychologists have not yet been able to offer much insight on this subject. According to psychologist Ronald Melzack, "The field of psychology is in a state of crisis. We are no closer now to understanding the most fundamental problems of psychology than we were when psychology became a science a hundred years ago... some neuroscience and computer technology have been stirred in with the old psychological ingredients, but there have been no important conceptual advances... We are adrift... in a sea of facts and practically drowning in them. We desperately need new concepts, new approaches."[30]

Archmaterialist Francis Crick, in spite of having once declared, "You are nothing but a pack of neurons," grudgingly acknowledges that even neuroscience, at present, cannot explain how experience arises in the brain.[31] Psychologist and linguist Steven Pinker, when asked how scientists might go about studying consciousness, commented, "...beats the heck out of me. I have some prejudices, but no idea of how to begin to look for a defensible answer. And neither does anyone else."[32] Jerry Fodor acknowledges that philosophy may not be of much help either: "Nobody has the slightest idea how anything material [such as the brain] could be conscious. Nobody even knows what it would be like to have the slightest idea about how anything material could be conscious. So much for the philosophy of consciousness."[33]

Given how readily scientists acknowledge their limited understanding of consciousness, one might expect the skeptical among them would hesitate before asserting with absolute certainty that telepathy, remote viewing, and other parapsychological events are impossible. If there were no valid evidence for such phenomena, this readiness to dismiss them might be more understandable. But thousands of research studies have been conducted over the past century providing indisputable evidence that individuals have been able to acquire information without the use of their physical senses. Parapsychologists have so refined their experiments that some of the most hardened skeptics have been unable to find flaws in their methodology.

In his 1978 address to the American Psychological Association, psychologist Charles Tart reported that more than 600 experiments had been conducted providing "first-class scientific evidence for the existence of ...extrasensory perception (ESP) ... that cannot be explained in terms of brain processes..."[34] By the 1980s, leading scientific journals were publishing articles demonstrating evidence for telepathy, clairvoyance, and other parapsychological phenomena. These included reputable periodicals in such varied fields as physics *(Physical Review and Foundations of Physics)*; psychology *(American Psychologist* and *Psychological Bulletin)*; neuroscience *(Brain and Behavioral Sciences)*; and engineering *(Proceedings of the Institute of Electronic and Electrical Engineers)*.[35] British psychologist Julie Milton of the University of Edinburgh analyzed seventy-eight studies published between 1964 and 1993 "in which people attempted to acquire information [by means that cannot be explained in terms of our ordinary understanding of the working of] the physical senses. These experiments had been reported in fifty-five publications by thirty-five different investigators and involved 1,158 subjects... Milton found the overall effects to be highly positive, with odds against chance of 10 million to 1."[36]

Since the first psychic researchers began reporting their results in the late nineteenth century, skeptics have voiced a number of concerns as to their validity. Henry Sidgwick, founder and first president of the

Society for Psychical Research, showed remarkable foresight when he called upon the members of the society to reach for the very highest level of experimental integrity:

> We must drive the [skeptic] into the position of being forced either to admit the phenomena as inexplicable, at least by him, or to accuse the investigators either of lying or cheating or of a blindness or forgetfulness incompatible with any intellectual condition except absolute idiocy.[37]

Sidgwick's comment accurately predicted what would come to be the major criticisms of skeptics over the subsequent 123 years—fraud and incompetence. Charges of fraud dogged psychic researchers from the time they published their first results. One of the more stunning accusations was presented in an article by chemist George Price in a leading scientific journal. Unable to find any errors in the parapsychological experiments he examined, he concluded that the only possible explanation was that the researchers were lying. He did not feel it necessary to present a single piece of evidence for this conclusion.[38]

Following this, psi researchers so tightened the controls against fraud that skeptics were forced to find other bases of criticism. By the early 1990s the goal that Henry Sigdwick called for had been achieved. Psi researchers had so refined their methodology that it surpassed the standards of research in many other scientific fields. An increasing number of skeptics were unable to find any way to deny that some kind of inexplicable phenomena were taking place.

In 1995 the CIA released the results of twenty years of remote-viewing[a] experiments and subjected them to careful scientific scrutiny. One of the principal reviewers, statistician Jessica Utts of the University of California-Davis, wrote the following:

---

a. Remote viewing—formerly known as "clairvoyance"—refers to the ability to obtain information regarding distant events without the use of any known physical sense.

The statistical results of the studies examined are far beyond what is expected by chance. Arguments that these results could be due to methodological flaws in the experiments are soundly refuted. Effects of similar magnitude to those found in government-sponsored research...have been replicated at a number of laboratories across the world. Such consistency cannot be readily explained by claims of flaws or fraud...It is recommended that future experiments focus on understanding how [remote viewing] works, and on how to make it as useful as possible. There is little benefit to continuing experiments designed [simply] to offer proof [of the validity of remote viewing].[39]

The other principal reviewer was Ray Hyman—one of psi's most loyal and well-known critics. He fully agreed with Utts's primary conclusion that "the statistical results of the experiments 'are far beyond what is expected by chance.'" He also acknowledged that he could not "provide suitable candidates for what flaws, if any, might [have been] present."[40] In a journal article about these experiments, Hyman further commented, "The case for psychic functioning seems better than it ever has been. The contemporary findings... do seem to indicate that something beyond odd statistical hiccups is taking place. I... have to admit that I do not have a ready explanation for these observed effects."[41]

After several decades of ardently challenging the findings of psi research, Hyman acknowledged that the research was indeed impeccable. He did not, however, conclude that these findings proved that consciousness transcends time and space. Taking a stance of strict neutrality, he simply acknowledged that these phenomena cannot be explained—at the moment—from within the view from nowhere.

As we proceed to examine some examples of psi research, we invite the reader to adopt Hyman's agnostic stance—that is, to consider the findings themselves with an open mind, without committing to any specific philosophic view.

SOME PARAPSYCHOLOGICAL EXPERIMENTS

Psi phenomena generally make use of unusual capacities of consciousness in any one of its three aspects—knowing, willing, or feeling. The kind of phenomena people usually associate with psi research involve knowing something or effecting (i.e., willing) something that is out of reach of our physical senses. For example, telepathy involves knowing what someone else is thinking. Precognition involves knowing what will happen in the future. Psychokinesis involves willing a change in something physical without the use of physical means. Clairvoyance—now more commonly referred to as "remote viewing"—involves gaining information about something that is too far away to be seen by the naked eye.

Some of the least-known but most interesting examples of psi research involve feeling rather than knowing or willing ("feeling" in the following instances refers to being affected on a physiological level by acts of knowing and/or willing). In recent years the medical community has somewhat reluctantly come to acknowledge a strong connection between the mind (i.e., "knowing" and "willing") and the physiological response in the body (i.e., "feeling"). The following experiment takes this connection to a new level.

In 1993 the U.S. Army Intelligence and Security Command (INSCOM) did an experiment in which white blood cells were taken from the mouth of a volunteer and placed in a test tube in a different room from where the volunteer was seated. The donor was then shown a television program with a great deal of violent content. In the test tube containing his blood cells, researchers inserted a probe to monitor the level of cellular activity. They found that in the same moments the volunteer was watching scenes of fighting or killing, his blood cells, though situated in a room down the hall, showed signs of extreme excitation. They found the same results even when the donor and his cells were separated by up to fifty miles and up to two days after the cells were removed from his mouth.[42]

The INSCOM experiment examined the effect of a person's mind on part of his own body many yards or even miles away. In 1994 neurophysiologist Jacobo Grinberg-Zylberbaum published the results of more than fifty experiments that suggested the possibility of one person's mind having an effect on another person's body.[43] In these experiments Grinberg-Zylberbaum had subjects meditate together for twenty minutes. They were then placed in separate rooms known as "Faraday cages," which are both soundproof and electromagnetic radiation–proof. One of the subjects (Subject A) was presented at random intervals with a series of one hundred stimuli including flashes of sound and light. The other subject (Subject B) received no stimuli. He was instructed to stay relaxed, to try to feel the presence of the other, and to signal the experimenter when he was relaxed and believed he was able to feel the other's presence.

When the experiment was completed, the EEG brain wave records of the two subjects were examined and compared. The brain wave patterns of Subject A showed the expected responses to the stimuli of light and sound. What is remarkable is that the brain waves of Subject B showed responses corresponding in time to the responses of Subject A, even though Subject B had not been presented with any stimuli. One of the most interesting outcomes occurred in the brain wave patterns of a young couple who reported "feeling deep oneness… Their EEG patterns remained closely synchronized throughout the experiment."

If such connections are possible, why aren't we more aware of them? Some researchers suggest it has something to do with the nature of our ordinary waking consciousness.

IN A CLEAR MIND YOU CAN SEE FOREVER

During the initial phase of psi research, the biggest concern of parapsychologists was the inability to get consistent results. Even when there were consistent results, the effect size tended to be minimal at best. On occasion—as in the remote viewing experiments conducted by the CIA—certain individuals seemed to consistently obtain remarkable results, but such individuals have been rare. Beginning in the 1960s, researchers started paying more attention to how they might facilitate the development of psi abilities. In harmony with the spirit of the times, they focused on inducing altered states of consciousness in research subjects by means of sensory deprivation, relaxation, and other related techniques. While this did lead to some small improvements, results remained marginal.

In subsequent attempts to get better results, two approaches proved to be particularly successful. One approach was to measure different kinds of results. Previously, researchers were dependent on verbal reports, which relied on the conscious mind of the subject. Some researchers, like Grinberg-Zylberbaum, looked instead for results in the body—which reflected workings of the subconscious mind—thus bypassing the conscious mind altogether.

The other approach has been to train the conscious mind to be more receptive to psi phenomena. In other words, to get better results, they found they had to either bypass the conscious mind or train it.

Both approaches developed as a result of the growing recognition that the activity of the ordinary conscious mind presents an obstacle to the experience of psi phenomena. Researchers gradually came to see that the constant chatter of the mind blocks access to a type of consciousness that is naturally more receptive to extrasensory information. They discovered that the key to getting reliable results was to establish a calm, quiet, and stable state of mind. This quietude enables an individual to be receptive to the subtle feelings and images that carry extrasensory impressions.

In order to get a sense of how the conscious mind might present an obstacle to psi phenomena, try the following exercise, *"Stopping" the Mind* (you can do it with eyes open or have someone read the instructions to you):

> Sit quietly with your eyes focused on a neutral (not overly distracting) object. Start by focusing on the sensations of breathing, feeling the flow of air as you breathe in and out. This will help focus your attention. Do this for about 60 seconds.

> Now, let go of your focus on the breath. Try as hard as you can for about 10 seconds to stop thinking—that is, try to have no verbal thoughts...

Most likely, you will only be able to stop your thoughts for 1 or 2 seconds, if at all. Try again—now for about 30 seconds—to stay strenuously focused on the task of trying to stop thinking…

Pause for a moment… Take about 10 seconds to relax… Try once more to keep all your attention focused on the task of attempting to stop thinking. This time, while you're engaged in this effort, notice that various thoughts, feelings and images continue to arise in your awareness. Your main aim now is to remain mindful of the fact that these thoughts, feelings and images come into your mind without requiring any conscious effort on your part.

Once you have some sense of the fact that most of the content of your mind arises on its own—without conscious effort—go on to the next step: Do nothing. Thoughts, feelings, images, sensations will continue to arise and pass through your mind. Let them come and go, recognizing that "you"—the conscious "you"—are not calling them forth or controlling them in any way. To the extent the content of the mind is allowed to simply "be," there may arise a momentary sense that there is no "doer" or "thinker."

Most people who attempt this exercise for the first time (and usually, for the thousandth-and-first time as well) find it very difficult. People who have been successful in experiencing psi phenomena say that good results depend on being able to evoke a mental state of utmost clarity and transparency. To get a sense of this state of mind, you might imagine being in a remote forest, listening for the distant song of a rare bird. Trees are swaying in the wind, leaves are rustling, small animals are running through the forest. In order to hear the bird's song, you have to be so fully attentive—so still in both body and mind—that you feel almost as though "you" are not there at all.

Based on your experience a moment ago—attempting to sustain

this state for as little as ten seconds—it should be clear that it would require a great deal of training to maintain that state for a substantial period of time. To the extent psi results rely on a sustained state of mental quietude, it makes perfect sense that psi experiments using untrained or poorly trained subjects would fail to get good results.

If it were more obvious that achievement of significant psi results required extensive training of the mind, skeptics would have less basis for critiquing the difficulty of obtaining or replicating results in para-psychological research. The fact is, since the 1960s, psi researchers have known that training can improve psi abilities. Even modest training programs have produced significant improvements in experimental results. However, no program of sufficient depth or rigor to make a decisive difference has yet been developed.[a]

Why hasn't this been done? For one thing, there is extremely little financial or institutional support for parapsychology. Skeptics often claim that parapsychology has had poor results in spite of more than 125 years of research. According to parapsychologist Dean Radin, the combined funding available to the field of parapsychology during that period of time is equivalent to approximately two months of funding in mainstream experimental psychology.[44]

Targ, Radin, and others believe that, in addition to the noisy chatter of the mind, there is another barrier to successful psi experiments—the extent to which our minds have been thoroughly conditioned by a society steeped in the "view from nowhere." Believing that our consciousness is limited in time and space, we tend to unconsciously filter out anything that challenges this view. In fact, one might say most of us have received years of intensive training in deleting the subtle cues that might afford a wider accessibility to psi phenomena. According to Ervin Laszlo,

> ordinary waking consciousness is a strict censor: most
> people have been "brainwashed" to filter out all experience

---

a. Russell Targ has already developed a fledgling program to train people in remote viewing. See chapter 10 for a description of Alan Wallace's Samatha Project, which among other things may one day be successful in training expert subjects for psi research.

not clearly and evidently conveyed by eyes and ears. Parents tell their children not to imagine things, teachers insist that they should stop dreaming and be sensible, and peer groups, already brainwashed, laugh at the child who persists. As a result, modern youngsters grow up to be commonsense individuals for whom everything that does not accord with the dominant materialist idea of the world [the view from nowhere] is denied and repressed.[45]

As we become more detached from the conditioning of the view from nowhere, as well as from our identification with the movements of the surface mind, we can learn to shift our attention. As the "filmy screen" of our ordinary waking consciousness thins, we might more easily learn to notice the subtle thoughts, feelings, and images that take us to the still subtler thoughts, feelings, and images that are the stuff of psi phenomena.

THE MEETING OF MIND AND MATTER?

Most scientists agree that the results of parapsychological research are difficult to understand in the context of our current notions regarding the relationship between mind and matter. Some parapsychologists suggest that the idea of "nonlocality," derived from quantum physics, might help us better understand psi phenomena. "Nonlocality" refers to findings in quantum physics that seem to conflict with our conventional understanding of how things work. According to the laws of classical physics, nothing can travel faster than the speed of light. "Nonlocality" refers to the idea that "objects that are apparently separate are actually connected instantaneously through space-time."[46]

In the early 1960s, physicist John Stewart Bell worked out mathematical calculations showing that nonlocality was an unavoidable implication of quantum theory. According to Larry Dossey, Bell showed that:

> if two particles that have once been in contact are separated, a change in one results in a change in the other—immediately

and to the same degree. The degree of separation between the particles is immaterial; they could theoretically be placed at opposite ends of the universe. Apparently no energetic signal passes between them, telling one particle that a change has taken place in the other, because the changes are instantaneous; there is no time for signaling. The distant particles behave as though they were united as a single entity—paradoxically, separate but one.[47]

Physicists were hesitant to accept Bell's findings, but in 1982, Alain Aspect performed an experiment that definitively showed nonlocality to be an aspect of the workings of matter. His experiment was replicated in 1997 by Nicolas Gusin.[48]

The discovery of nonlocal connections is leading scientists to a radically new understanding of matter. Biologist Mae Wan-Ho claims to have found many examples of nonlocal effects in biological organisms as well. She uses the term "quantum coherence" to describe a process by which all components of the organism are in instant and continuous communication.[49] According to Ervin Laszlo, this instantaneous, systemwide correlation cannot be explained according to the laws of classical, nonquantum physics.

Parapsychologists and other scientists believe that ideas like nonlocality and quantum coherence suggest that matter is more mindlike than we have previously thought. For example, earlier we mentioned Freeman Dyson's characterization of atoms as behaving "like active agents rather than inert substances," making "unpredictable choices between alternative possibilities according to the laws of quantum mechanics."[50]

Some parapsychologists—observing that nonlocality challenges the classical understanding of time and space—suggest it might be used to explain psi findings that seem to imply that consciousness is capable of transcending time and space. By transforming our understanding of how matter works, quantum physics has presented us with a view of the universe more compatible with psi phenomena than that of classical physics. But physical theories—quantum or otherwise—can give us, at best, only an indirect understanding of the nature of consciousness. Dyson himself is careful to say that he is not claiming that his view "is supported or proved by scientific evidence... [but] only... that it is consistent with scientific evidence."[51] And, as physicist Arthur Zajonc points out, the objective approach of physics "remains silent on... the experience of a perceiving subject."[52]

If neither psychology nor the findings of physics provide us with any fundamental understanding of consciousness, where might we look—and how should we look—to gain a new view? We can start by looking directly at the subjective experience of the individuals engaged in parapsychology experiments.

For many years psi researchers have noticed that subjects who are passionately involved in an experiment tend to be the most successful. We saw in the Grinberg-Zylberbaum experiments that the young couple in love showed the highest level of brain wave synchronization. While this may not be so surprising with regard to communication between humans, experiments show this to be the case even in the relationship between a human being and a machine.

Robert G. Jahn, as director of the Princeton Engineering Anomalies Research laboratory (PEAR), observed hundreds of trials in which individuals successfully influenced the workings of highly sensitive electronic instruments. As described on the PEAR website:

> In these studies human operators attempt to bias the output of a variety of mechanical, electronic, optical, acoustical, and fluid devices to conform to pre-stated intentions, without recourse to any known physical influences. In unattended calibrations all of these sophisticated machines produce strictly random data, yet the experimental results display increases in information content that can only be attributed to the consciousness of their human operators.[53]

Jahn, explaining these results, writes, "The most common subjective report of our most successful human/machine experimental operators is some sense of 'resonance' with the devices—some sacrifice of personal identity in the interaction—a 'merging,' or bonding with the apparatus."[54] Larry Dossey adds, "The highest scores are seen when emotionally bonded couples, who share unusually deep love and empathy, interact together with the electronic devices. They achieve scores up to eight times higher than those of individuals who try to influence the devices alone."[55]

In a rather radical departure from the typically impersonal stance of the view from nowhere, Dossey suggests there may be an extremely close relationship between the nonlocal connections of subatomic particles and the feelings of empathy described above. "Nonlocal connectedness... is manifested between subatomic particles, mechanical systems, humans and machines, humans and animals, and humans themselves. When this nonlocal bond operates between people, we call it love. When it unites distant subatomic particles, what should we call this manifestation? Should we choose a safe, aseptic term such as nonlocally correlated behavior, or bite the bullet and call it a rudimentary form of love?" Dossey is not claiming that human beings and subatomic particles have the same experience of love. Rather, he suggests that what manifests as a purely impersonal connection at the level of matter may be, in essence, the same phenomenon as that which occurs between loving human beings.

Perhaps this is what William James was hinting at when he wrote:

> We with our lives are like islands in the sea, or like trees in the forest. The maple and pine may whisper to each other with their leaves...but the trees also commingle their roots in the darkness underground, and the islands hang together through the oceans' bottom. Just so there is a continuum of cosmic consciousness, against which our individuality builds but accidental fences, and into which our several minds plunge as into a mother sea... [56]

WHEN A VIEW IS NOT A VIEW

Even if we are sympathetic to what Dossey is suggesting, it is important to recognize that scientific methodology as currently employed cannot answer the question that he raises. Scientific methods that measure the observable, quantifiable correlates of experience can say nothing about the ultimate nature of a phenomenon; they can only describe it and develop concepts that help us understand and predict certain aspects of its behavior. As Feynman and Cairns-Smith have pointed out, current methods of science describe the workings of matter and energy but do not provide us with a way of understanding what they are.

Some scientists have suggested that the solution may lie in a "view from within," one that involves the development of more refined methods for the study of subjective experience. However, from the perspective of the yogic tradition, if these methods are employed by the ordinary untrained mind, they will not take us much further on the road to understanding consciousness. The yogis say that it is not possible by means of the ordinary surface consciousness to comprehend the ultimate nature of objective or subjective reality.[a]

If we acknowledge that science—as currently practiced—is by nature neutral with regard to the superiority of one view of reality over another, how would we determine which view to choose as the best guide to understanding the universe and ourselves? Before we can address this question, we need to clarify what we mean by a "view." Rather than intellectual ideas or mental beliefs, the "view from nowhere" and the "view from infinity" might each be thought of as referring to a particular way of looking.

As described somewhat whimsically by Alan Wallace, the view from nowhere attempts to determine what the universe would look like if nobody were looking. His answer is, "Nothing." It would not

---

a. By developing a way of knowing other than the ordinary conscious mind, it may be possible to develop a scientific method that could discern directly the workings of consciousness in the material universe and in the process of evolution. This possibility will be discussed at length along with its usefulness for scientific research in Appendix A.

even contain what Arthur Eddington referred to as "pointer readings," because in a universe without a conscious observer there would be no one present to read the pointer. It does not seem likely that a way of looking that denies the existence of the looker can tell us much about the nature of consciousness. In fact, the view from nowhere might more aptly be thought of as a way of not looking.

Rather than asking which view to choose, perhaps the better question would be: Is there a way of knowing that is not bound by any particular intellectual view? The "view from infinity" is more about how we look than about what we see. Though in another way, it is about both, because what we see depends on how we look. What might we see if we were to look through the eyes of infinity?

BOOK III

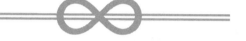

The Journey

If mankind could but see though in a glimpse of fleeting experience what infinite enjoyments, what perfect forces, what luminous reaches of spontaneous knowledge, what wide calms of our being lie waiting for us in the tracts which our animal evolution has not yet conquered, they would leave all and never rest till they had gained these treasures. But the way is narrow, the doors are hard to force, and fear, distrust and skepticism are there, sentinels of Nature, to forbid the turning away of our feet from her ordinary pastures.[1]

—Sri Aurobindo, *Essays on Philosophy and Yoga*

THIRD CHALLENGE

Consciousness is… the fundamental thing in existence—it is the energy, the motion, the movement of consciousness that creates the universe and all that is in it.[1]

—Sri Aurobindo

We invite you to take this point in the book as a point of departure from the terra firma of your familiar worldview. From here on, we proceed on the assumption that consciousness *is* fundamental—in fact "*the* fundamental thing" in the universe. For the duration of "The Journey," we invite you—*as an experiment*—to accept this assumption as a working premise, to join us in looking at everything we see, know, feel, think, hear, as being in some way a movement of consciousness.

If you are intrigued by the challenge of "trying on" this dramatically different view, it will be helpful to notice old habits of mind when they arise, to notice the tendency to dismiss something based simply on an old assumption (such as the idea that consciousness is confined to a few cubic centimeters of gray matter). If you notice this happening, see if you can come back to the feeling of taking part in an experiment, of opening to the possibility of a completely different way of seeing.

PART I

THE VIEW FROM INFINITY

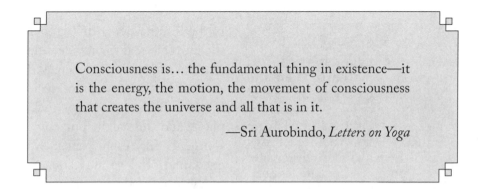

Consciousness is… the fundamental thing in existence—it is the energy, the motion, the movement of consciousness that creates the universe and all that is in it.

—Sri Aurobindo, *Letters on Yoga*

CHAPTER 6

The View from Infinity

INTIMATIONS OF INFINITY

While India—the home of yoga psychology—has always placed great value on intellectual understanding, the yogic tradition takes direct spiritual experience to be the foundation for any valid intellectual view. In the chapters that follow, we will describe the vision of yoga psychology in terms of the spiritual experience at the core of the Indian tradition—the experience of an infinite Consciousness,[a] an infinite Being in whom the entire universe has its existence.[2] But it is important to remember that the description of the vision is not itself the view from infinity. It is meant only to be a pointer to an experience or way of knowing that cannot be captured in words.

The story we are about to tell of the evolution of consciousness should not be taken solely as an intellectual account of evolution. It is primarily intended to help direct attention to the various workings

a. We capitalize words such as "consciousness," "being," and "soul" when we are using them specifically to refer to an Infinite Reality beyond our ordinary consciousness.

While the Indian spiritual tradition has perhaps been the one to speak most openly of the all-pervasive, all-embracing nature of the Infinite Divine Being, all spiritual teachings have—at least at their mystic core—pointers to this experience. In the New Testament, St. Paul describes God as "He in whom we live and move and have our being."[3] In the Koran, Allah is referred to as being closer to us than life itself, closer than "the jugular vein." In the Hebrew Bible, God, speaking to Moses, gives His name as "I Am That I Am."[4] Native American and other indigenous peoples recognize Spirit to be present and active throughout the universe.

of the Infinite Being throughout the universe, and to provide intimations of Its Presence here and now, in our every thought, feeling, and sensation, every rock, plant, and animal in our environment, and each person we encounter. The various streams of the yoga tradition are one in their agreement that the ordinary human mind is not capable of perceiving the Infinite. However, yogis of all traditions have always made use of words to evoke something beyond the mind, to open a window onto the richness, beauty, and vastness of that Reality which is the very substance of all we experience.

Jewish scholar Abraham Heschel describes a state of mind that can make the experience of this greater Reality more accessible. He suggests cultivating an attitude of awe that is "itself an act of insight into a meaning greater than ourselves... [enabling] us to perceive in the world intimations of the Divine... to sense the ultimate in the common and the simple; to feel in the rush of the passing the stillness of the eternal."[5]

But how can we cultivate an attitude of awe? For some, a "thinning of the veil" that opens us to the sense of awe can occur in communion with the power and beauty of nature: listening to the gentle, unearthly silence of a large metropolis blanketed in snow... watching the play of light dancing on the windswept surface of Lake Geneva... walking down Fifth Avenue in the hush of twilight, lost in thought, suddenly catching sight of the deep orange sunlight setting fire to skyscraper windows. The awesome quality of these experiences tends, to some extent, to calm the disjointed play of our ordinary thought, bringing about an openness and tranquility that allows for something deeper to emerge from within.

Literature, painting, dance, theater, cinema, and religious ritual have all, since prehistoric times, been at heart a means of softening the boundaries of our ordinary awareness, thus helping us experience something that transcends our limited selves. In the solemn intonation of a priest's chanting of a sacred text, our hearts softened, our minds stilled, we feel a mysterious Presence spreading throughout the cathedral... we are transported with Sri Aurobindo's Savitri, as she voyages "through worlds of splendor and of calm"[6] ...in a darkened theater, we face death with Sir Thomas More, at peace in the noble equanimity of a high ideal.

The various practices of the yoga tradition are designed to make it possible for us to enter into this deeper experience at will, without need for external triggers. Ultimately these practices can help dissolve the filmy screen altogether so that the "stillness of the eternal," the soft and luminous presence of the Infinite, is always and everywhere present in our experience. All yogic practice calls upon us to shift our attention—to step back from the familiar round of thoughts, feelings, and sensations that tend to absorb us, and to gently redirect our attention inward. We invite you to join us in doing just that.

SHIFTING ATTENTION

THE SPACE OF AWARENESS

Bring your attention to the sensations of your body. Let your eyes remain open, taking in the words of the text with a gentle, nongrasping awareness. Move your attention to different parts of the body, noticing the different sensations that arise...

As you attend to various sensations, notice that there is no clear boundary in your awareness between the sensations that make up the body and the space around the body...

As you release the sense of a clear boundary, begin to notice the larger space in which these sensations move...

Allow the sense of this larger space to continue to expand until you lose the sense of it having a beginning or ending, just open space...

As your sense of this space expands, see if you can notice a quality of stillness and calm associated with the unchanging nature of the space, the feeling of simply being that remains unchanged while the sensations continue to move and change in various ways...

Notice any sounds that are occurring, notice that they all occur within this larger space... notice whether near or far, the sounds all exist within the same open space ...

Notice images arising in the mind... these too are moving and changing in various ways, all within this larger space ...

Thoughts arise in space, move through it, dissolve back into it, the space remains, unchanged by whatever moves through it...

Feelings come and go—whether feelings of happiness, sadness, anger, joy, liking, or disliking—constantly changing, leaving the space untouched, unchanged...

Staying aware of sensations, images, thoughts, and feelings arising and passing away, notice the tendency of the mind to hold on to them, to harden them into solid objects... Releasing this tendency, see if you can become aware of a sense of ease and calm that may emerge as the sense of spaciousness expands... As the feeling of wide open space continues to expand, a feeling of quiet joy may enter into awareness...

Notice how everything moves, changes constantly within this space—sensations, thoughts, feelings—all patterns of moving energy, contained within the space, but leaving the space undisturbed...

THE FIELD AND THE KNOWER OF THE FIELD

Within various spiritual traditions, there are many words to describe these two aspects of experience—the changing, shifting field of sensations, thoughts, and images, and the still space of Consciousness in which they exist. The sacred yogic text, the *Bhagavad Gita* (literally "the song of God") refers to these, respectively, as the "Field" and "Knower of the Field."[7]

The Knower (or "Conscious-Being") refers to that Infinite Being that holds the entire universe within Its Awareness. It is also That which, at this very moment, is seeing through our eyes, but which—in the words of the *Kena Upanishad*—"our eyes cannot see... which hears through our ears, but our ears cannot hear."[8] It is seeing and hearing equally through all eyes and ears—those of an ant as well as those of a cat or human being. It remains aware whether we are awake or asleep. We can get a sense of it by looking for that in us which is unchanging from infancy through all the changes of life, that core feeling of "I am" in the depths of our psyches.

This Infinite Conscious-Being is frequently referred to as "God," but that word has so many images and associations attached to it, it rarely serves as a portal to experience. Describing the advantage of a simple word like "Being," Ekhart Tolle writes:

> The word "Being" explains nothing, but nor does "God." Being, however, has the advantage that it is an open concept. It does not reduce the infinite invisible to a finite entity. It is impossible to form a mental image of it. Nobody can claim exclusive possession of Being. It is your very essence, and it is immediately accessible to you as the feeling of your own presence, the realization "I am" that is prior to "I am this" or "I am that." So it is only a small step from the word "Being" to the experience of Being.[9]

The Field (or "Conscious-Energy") includes all that we sense— sights, sounds, physical sensations, tastes, and smells; all that we feel— pleasure and pain, liking and disliking, anger, joy, love, sadness; and all that we think—our beliefs, memories, plans, worries, ideas, and the images passing through our minds; everything that exists within space and time. All are forms of Conscious-Energy, movements of Conscious-Energy arising out of the Being of the Knower—over billions of years of evolution, throughout our lifetimes, and in this moment and every moment of experience.

All that exists is the interaction of the Knower and the Field. Every atom, every tree, bird, rock, and mountain range are movements of Conscious-Energy within the Consciousness of the Being at the center of all things. But these two—the Knower and the Field, Conscious-Being and Conscious-Energy—are not actually two. They are inseparable aspects of one unbroken Infinite Reality—one aspect being the still, changeless, witnessing Consciousness, the other an ever-moving, ever-changing Consciousness—outside of which nothing exists.

Related Terms

Knower:[a] The Infinite, the Divine, Conscious-Being (and on an individual level, the individual Soul), *He*

Field: Nature, Conscious-Energy, *She*

Knower + Field: The Infinite, the Divine, the One, He and She

The *Gita* does not mean to imply by the word "Knower" that the Infinite Knower is solely, or even mainly, an intellectual. The "Knowing" of the Knower includes feeling, willing, and sensing—all the ways in which it comes to know Itself as the Field.

In the Indian tradition, the Infinite can be approached in infinite ways—through wisdom, love, or service, as an intimate friend, and even as a lover. The relationship of the universe to the Infinite beyond is often imaged as that of a child held in the womb of the Consciousness of the Mother, who gives birth to the universe and holds it in Her embrace throughout the ages.

AN INTUITIVE EXERCISE

In the chapters that follow, we're going to be looking at the same events we described in chapter 1—the evolution of consciousness in the uni-

---

a. It will be helpful, as you read through the book, to bear in mind the extreme limitation and misleading nature of words. We will frequently be using terms such as "the Infinite Knower," "the Individual Knower hidden in matter," "the evolving Soul," etc. When we do, it may seem as if we're talking about an entity of some kind. But the word "Knower" is only a symbol for that which is indefinable, immeasurable, and infinite.

verse, the unfolding of consciousness over the course of a lifetime, and its emergence in each moment—as expressions of the interaction between the Field and the Knower of the Field. We describe the different grades of consciousness in spiders and amoebae, humans and salamanders, as well as the shifts in consciousness from infancy through adolescence, and from Australopithecus to *Homo sapiens* in this light.

We'd like to invite you to engage with this story as an intuitive exercise, attempting to keep a sense of the stillness behind as you read. To help connect with this experience of calm stillness, we offer at various points an evocation of the Silence that is there behind all movements of consciousness.

This way of looking provides an alternative to the view from nowhere that gives us no basis upon which to unravel the mysteries of consciousness —where it comes from, how it exists, how it manages to unfold in such an apparently orderly manner, how all this amazing intelligence, beauty, and diversity emerged out of apparently nonconscious, nonliving matter. Virtually every aspect of our experience changes when it is seen as the expression of the Knower, existing within that Infinite Consciousness, unfolding for the pure joy of creative Self-expression. Everything changes when we look through the eyes of infinity.

> Once seen in the substance and light of... eternity, the world... becomes other than it seems to the mind and senses; for then we see the universe no longer as a whirl of mind and life and matter... but as no other than [the] eternal [Divine Reality]. The universal Being in whose embrace we live... [is] a spirit who immeasurably fills and surrounds all this movement with himself—for indeed the movement too is himself—and who throws on all that is finite the splendor of his garment of infinity, a bodiless and million-bodied spirit whose hands of strength and feet of swiftness are on every side of us, whose heads and eyes and faces are those innumerable visages which we see wherever we turn, whose ear is everywhere listening to the silence of eternity and the music of the worlds.[10]
>
> —Sri Aurobindo, *Essays on the Gita*

So we proceed...*for the time being*...upon the assumption that we are living in a universe that is made of, infused with, and held within an infinite Consciousness...

PART II

THE EVOLUTION OF THE FIELD

OVERVIEW

Introduction

If our minds were sharp enough, we would see that our consciousness in the first moment of awakening from sleep emerges not all at once, but in a series of rapid stages. First there is a simple registration of sensation—sound, light, the touch of the body against the mattress. Along with this a primitive feeling tone arises accompanied by a reaction of attraction or aversion. Within the space of less than a second, more complex feelings, thoughts, and intentions come into play. Finally, our ordinary "self" is fully reconstructed and we "awaken."

If we were to expand each of these periods of milliseconds to billions of years, we would see a remarkable parallel to the unfolding of consciousness in the universe over the course of evolution. From a state of apparent sleep, the universe "wakes up" to the consciousness of matter, then in plants and animals gradually becomes conscious of primitive feelings and reactions. In mammals and primates, the capacities of knowing, willing, and feeling become progressively more complex until, in the human being, thoughts, intentions, and feelings come together to form a "self." [a]

---

a. Strictly speaking, it is not the universe, but the Knower "within" the universe who is awakening.

Behind the entire play of universal conscious-energies, there is the ever-wakeful Knower who remains present, fully conscious, beyond all time and space—the Timeless Being, unchanging throughout the ceaseless change of evolution. However, He allows an infinitesimal spark of Himself, a tiny spark of His Consciousness to enter into the Field of evolution. The consciousness of this spark is at first almost wholly absorbed in the whirling of subatomic particles, oblivious to its Divine Source. This spark is the Soul at the heart of matter, which slowly—over the course of billions of years—awakens from its slumber: dreaming in plants and animals, coming to partial wakefulness in human beings, and one day fully awakening to its oneness with the Infinite Knower.

How can we understand the relationship between the Knower—ever-awake, beyond time and space—and what seems to be a different Knower, hidden and almost wholly asleep in Matter? Is there anything in our own experience that might help? [a]

CONTACTING THE KNOWER WITHIN: CULTIVATING INNER SILENCE

It is possible to feel a distant reflection of that Infinite Knower by shifting attention away from the ever-changing sensations, feelings, and

---

a. It is the custom in the tradition of yoga psychology to use the same term to refer to one aspect of being or consciousness manifesting at different levels. For example, the same word "atman" is used to refer to the individual Knower, the cosmic Knower, and the transcendent Knower beyond time and space. This multiple usage reflects the yogic understanding that the Infinite is present, in Its fullness, at each and every point of the universe.

thoughts in which your consciousness is usually absorbed. Letting the play of the surface consciousness become softer and more porous, the Light of that vast, open Space becomes more apparent. Keeping your attention, as much as possible, on that larger space of Consciousness behind, you can discern the Silent Presence of the hidden Knower deep within your heart:

There is a background for everything. Every movement moves upon something.

And that something is a Silence which upholds everything, including your own mental activity. All the thoughts and mental movements come and go, against a base that is ever stable. That is Silence...

Suspend for a moment your thought-activity and you'll become conscious of this presence.

...Think of this Silence again and again and try to become aware of it. By a steady digging in of this idea in your consciousness, this fact will become a reality to you—not merely for the mind but for the rest of the being.

Into this Silence you must learn to relax yourself.

Instead of trying to get at it, simply relax, call, and let yourself lie in the folds of the Silence.

That will slowly come over you and claim you.[1]

—Kapali Sastry, paraphrasing Sri Aurobindo

Throughout the unfolding of the various grades of consciousness over billions of years of evolution, the Infinite Knower is always present behind, the Knower in whose Being the whole universe of moving, flowing Conscious-Energy resides. And the apparently limited Knower, the soul-spark absorbed at first in the whirling of matter, slowly awakens as the play of evolution proceeds. This is the story of that awakening.

> Consciousness is... the fundamental thing in existence—it is the energy, the motion, the movement of consciousness that creates the universe and all that is in it... When consciousness in its movement... forgets itself in the action it becomes an apparently "unconscious" energy; when it forgets itself in the form it becomes the electron, the atom, the material object. In reality it is still consciousness that works in the energy and determines the form and the evolution of form.[1]
>
> —Sri Aurobindo, *Letters on Yoga*

CHAPTER 7

Matter: The Birth of the Universe: Awakening of the Physical Consciousness

THE DREAM OF THE KNOWER: A FABLE

Before the universe was born, the Knower had a dream, a dream of an extraordinary adventure in which He would play all the parts. He saw within His own vast Being the possibility of infinite worlds in which He could endlessly explore different ways of expressing Himself. He saw His Consciousness taking the form of stars, planets, and living creatures. And He saw Himself becoming absorbed in the play of these stars and planets and living creatures, temporarily forgetting his true nature. He foresaw the evolutionary journey as a joyous opportunity to rediscover himself, slowly, gradually, in billions of ways over billions of years.

However, the timeless, silent, Infinite Consciousness of the Knower is also there, changeless, behind the vast ever-changing Field of Conscious-Energy. Even after the dream gives birth to the physical universe, the Silent Consciousness remains, just as it was, eternally calm, beyond time and space. Even after the universe is born, the Infinite Being beyond the universe continues to dream, each moment dreaming the physical universe into existence. And He remains still, calm, and silent even now, as the dream of the universe continues to take shape. Calm and still, he enjoys both the dream and its manifestation as the universe, lending his Infinite capacities for knowing, willing, and feeling to the evolutionary adventure.

THE AWAKENING OF THE PHYSICAL CONSCIOUSNESS IN THE UNIVERSE

Cosmologists tell us that the universe began "as an unimaginably hot and extremely compact region of pure energy."[2] The patterns we know as "laws" seem to have emerged when the universe was less than a trillionth of a second old, and about the size of a grapefruit. In another fraction of a second the universe expanded to approximately 10^{50} times its prior size. [a] Over the hundreds of thousands of years that followed, as the universe gradually cooled to the "moderate" temperature of about 3,000 degrees, the first atoms—hydrogen and helium—began to form. By the time the universe was a billion years old, galaxies had begun to take shape.

You may wish to pause for a moment to notice whether, in reading this scientific description of the early universe, you conceived of it in the conventional way—in other words, as purely physical events taking place in a purely "material" time and space. Try rereading the description, this time tuning your awareness to the Silence that is present here and now behind your surface awareness, keeping in mind that the words refer to movements of conscious-energy taking place within the Consciousness of an Infinite Being.

a. That's 10,000,000,000,000,000,000,000,000,000,000,000,000,000 times larger than it was a fraction of a second before.

According to the view from infinity, the energy of the Field of the Knower is always a Conscious-Energy. Thus the "extremely compact region of pure energy" that was the embryonic universe had a consciousness associated with it. And wherever there is consciousness, it will always express itself with some degree of knowing, willing, and feeling.

What kind of consciousness could possibly have been present at this early stage in the existence of the universe? Sri Aurobindo refers to it as the "physical consciousness," that aspect of the consciousness of the Knower that is associated with "matter."[a] Yogis who have a highly developed intuitive capacity have had a direct experience of the consciousness of matter. Within the atom, they are able to detect a simple, primitive kind of knowing, a capacity to register—in a way unimaginable to our complex minds—the presence of other atoms. Similarly, these yogis perceive a primitive form of feeling in the polarity of attraction and repulsion that manifests within and between atomic particles. And they can discern the working of a primitive form of will in the response or reaction of one atom to the impact of another.

But it is not this primitive physical consciousness that is responsible for the large rhythmic patterns known as "laws of nature," or the incredibly complex interactions that led to the formation of galaxies. It is the infinitely greater Consciousness of the Infinite Being behind, which at every moment is making use of the limited surface physical consciousness to orchestrate the unfolding evolution—to establish order and coherence, and to develop the more complex material forms needed to express increasingly complex forms of consciousness.

THROUGH A GLASS DARKLY

Here we see through a glass darkly; there we see fully.[3]

—Paraphrase of St. Paul

---

a. That is, conscious-energy in the form that we perceive as "matter."

Sometimes just before awakening from sleep, we have a dream of uncommon clarity and astonishing beauty, as if all were illumined by an unearthly light. Usually we find upon awakening that all that remains is a pale reflection of that experience. It is as though our ordinary, dull surface consciousness cannot hold on to the richness of the heightened dream consciousness.

In much the same way, the physical consciousness that first emerges along with the birth of the physical universe is only a dim reflection of the dreaming consciousness of the Knower behind. In that dream "prior" to the Big Bang, the physical consciousness associated with the "dream-planets" and "dream-stars" is infinitely stable, and calm, reflecting the stability and calm of that which is unborn, beyond time and space. We sometimes get a glimpse of this "deeper" aspect of the physical consciousness when we contemplate the imposing presence of a giant redwood tree, the immensity of a Himalayan peak, or the vast calm of the Pacific Ocean. We can also get a sense of this essential stability by focusing on the pure feeling of "I Am" deep within—the feeling of essential Being-ness that remains unchanged through the ever-changing experience of our lives.

The "I" who ordinarily wakes up out of sleep is only the dimmest reflection of the Infinite "I Am" in the depths of our consciousness. Similarly, when the Soul—the seemingly limited portion of the consciousness of the Knower—first awakens in matter, it possesses only the dimmest reflection of the consciousness of the Infinite Being ever awake beyond the universe. The Soul is almost wholly asleep, unable to manifest the clear, calm stability of the vaster physical consciousness of the dream out of which the objects of our universe are continuously arising.

THE NATURE AND INFLUENCE OF THE PHYSICAL CONSCIOUSNESS

One might describe the physical consciousness that emerges along with the birth of the universe as sleepy, not unlike ours when we first awaken from a deep sleep. This consciousness at the beginning of the universe was so very dim, vague, and amorphous that it seemed to be absent altogether. The "world," as known by this barely awakened consciousness, was equally dim, vague, and amorphous, devoid of anything we would recognize as form. For that consciousness, there were no gaseous clouds swirling through the blackness of space. There was no "blackness." There was only the faintest awareness of anything at all.

Emerging as it did, out of near total self-forgetfulness, the physical consciousness remained almost wholly "unconscious." It is for this reason that matter appears to be inert, mechanical, and repetitive in its expression. If you bring to mind one of those mornings when you had great difficulty rousing yourself out of a deep sleep, you may get some sense of the nature of the physical consciousness. Reflecting back on those moments, perhaps you will recall something like this: Your body felt heavy and immobilized, your energy dense and sluggish. As you struggled to emerge into a semblance of clarity and alertness, you had to fight a tremendous undertow pulling you back into the oblivion of sleep. It may have taken a heroic effort to resist that force, to simply get yourself out of bed. And when you finally did manage to extract yourself from the gravitational pull of sleep, you were probably still barely awake, hardly able to move through your habitual morning wake-up routine.[a]

The various physical objects in our environment as well as the stuff of our own bodies are made, in part, of the same conscious-energy as that which composed the newborn universe. This present-day physical consciousness continues to bear the imprint of its sleepy origins at the dawn of the evolutionary journey. But this is not a bad thing. The mechanical, repetitive nature of the physical consciousness in matter is what makes possible the stability of physical forms in the environment, the continuity of species from generation to generation, and the consistency of behavioral patterns in individuals. It is thanks in part to the inert nature of matter that we are able to navigate a world that is

---

a. This is not meant to suggest that the physical consciousness is inherently inert, dull, and so forth. The description here is of its present condition. According to Sri Aurobindo, the physical consciousness has the potential to be radically awakened and transformed.

relatively constant, stable, and predictable, to recognize ourselves and each other from day to day, and ultimately to perceive change against the backdrop of that stability.

In human beings, the physical consciousness helps maintain the proper functioning of the atoms and cells of our body, thus providing a stable basis for the mental and emotional nature. However, having the physical consciousness as the basis for our thoughts and feelings carries with it an evolutionary challenge. Its mechanical, repetitive nature can affect our thinking, making it stereotypical, conformist, or prejudicial in nature. It is in part the dull, repetitive, and mechanical nature of the physical consciousness that makes it so difficult to overcome habits and destructive addictions such as smoking, compulsive eating, and drug or alcohol abuse. When particularly strong, the mechanical quality of the physical consciousness might take the form of obsessive-compulsive behaviors in which people repeat certain actions, or repeat the same thought again and again for no apparent cause.

We've all been aware of the dulling influence of the physical consciousness on days when our mind is cloudy or sluggish, making it difficult to follow a conversation, to keep track of the task we're engaged in, or remember where we've put things from one moment to the next. In its extreme form, this kind of dullness might manifest as Alzheimer's disease or other forms of dementia. When the dullness of the physical consciousness affects the emotions, we may experience it as an indifference to the suffering of others, or a lack of responsiveness to the beauty in things. In a more extreme form, the heaviness of the physical consciousness can lead to the emotional darkness and despair of depression.[a]

Under the strong influence of the physical consciousness, our will may be adversely affected, making it difficult to concentrate, make decisions, or hold on to our goals and our sense of purpose. We are more likely to give in to passing impulses, finding ourselves engaging in actions that we know are not good for us or that we believe to be wrong.

On a cultural scale, it is to some degree the dull insensibility of the

---

a. These comments regarding the relationship between the physical consciousness and various psychological disorders are meant to be taken as intuitive hypotheses.

physical consciousness that overwhelms us when we are caught up in the whirlwind of rapid societal change. As a result, we may avert our eyes to things like the slow accumulation of toxic waste or the distant suffering of starving children. We become inured to incremental changes for the worse—like the frog in water that is being slowly heated to a boil, comfortable with the status quo until the change becomes threatening enough to jolt it into action, but only after it is too late.

THE WORKING OF THE PHYSICAL CONSCIOUSNESS IN OUR DAY-TO-DAY EXPERIENCE

Sharon is sitting on the wooden bench by the pond in the backyard. Having arrived at her father's house just a few days before, she is feeling a sense of numbness and resignation. Her eye is drawn to a falling leaf slowly making its way to the ground. As it falls, a series of disjointed memories pass through her mind—she sees the truck pulling into the medical compound, hears the sound of gunfire, and remembers the feeling of being jolted into action, falling to the ground, her body trembling, fearful of a surprise attack from a group of Viet Cong soldiers rumored to be in the area.

The image slowly shifts as her mind goes back to that night during the riots. She can almost feel the bodies of her younger siblings as they lay pressed to the floor under her arms the night the riots took place.

"Willie, Clarissa, keep your heads down!"

She remembers holding her breath, praying that the bullets from the street would not ricochet through her window. Piercing sounds filled the air—sounds of police sirens and fire engines, breaking glass and people shouting. Her arms stiffen against the side of the bench as she recalls the pervasive sense of danger. Feeling the roughness of the wood against her hands, her attention returns to her surroundings. She becomes aware of the large oak tree to her left, and as her gaze moves upward along the trunk, she has an almost visceral sense of its strength and solidity.

Her mind, momentarily calm, is drawn back to more recent images of her life in the city and the sense of emptiness that filled her days. Feeling again the painful heaviness of despondency, her body slumps into the bench, numb and drained of energy.

As we contemplate this scene from the yogic perspective, we see that it is taking "place" completely within the consciousness of the Divine Knower. We see also that there is nothing there other than His conscious-energies moving within, surrounded and supported by His vast, calm, Being. We see the physical conscious-energy taking shape as what we perceive to be a tree, a bench, a pond. This conscious-energy is at work in Sharon's body, below the level of her surface awareness, supporting her every movement, helping (in concert with other layers of conscious-energy) to maintain its physiological processes. We see also the relative dullness of her surface physical consciousness, still bearing the imprint of its sleepy, nearly unconscious origins at the birth of the universe.

In the moments before Sharon began to focus on the falling leaf, her state of mind was being influenced by the dull, inert quality of the physical consciousness which was shaping the various thoughts and feelings that emerged. Under its influence, her mind was drawn to dwell on the negative memories that had plagued her, and the sense of danger and underlying insecurity that had haunted her for so much of her life. She was feeling little energy or motivation, helplessly resigned to her current state, and without hope for the future.

For a moment, her mind fell quiet as she gazed at the trunk of the tree and experienced the simple solidity of its presence. This feeling of solidity reflects in part the working of a purer physical consciousness to which we sometimes gain fleeting access when our surface mind is stilled in moments of great intensity. Just a few seconds later, Sharon succumbs to the inertia and dullness of the ordinary physical consciousness as her thoughts turn once again to feelings of despair about the emptiness of her life.

THE EVOLUTION OF PHYSICAL CONSCIOUSNESS IN THE INDIVIDUAL

There is, as we have seen, a rough parallel between the emergence of consciousness over billions of years of cosmic evolution and its unfolding within the first few milliseconds of a human being awakening from sleep. There is also a rough parallel between these two patterns of unfolding and the development of consciousness over the course of an individual human lifetime. The consciousness of the human infant is largely absorbed in the physical sensations associated with the movements of her body, though she does not know they are "her" sensations or "her" body. To the extent she has a "self," it is largely a "physical self," as is the "self" that emerges in the first instants of awakening from sleep, as was the "self" of the early universe before the advent of life.

According to yoga psychology, there are a number of centers of conscious-energy associated with various regions of the physical body. These centers are referred to in Sanskrit as *chakras* (literally, "wheels"— so-called because to the subtle vision of the yogi, they appear as whirling wheel-like vortices of energy). They act as conduits and transducers for the vaster energies of the Cosmic Dream, enabling them to emerge as the more limited energies of the surface awareness. The physical consciousness in human beings is associated with the center or chakra located at the base of the spine. This center regulates the flow of physical energy to the surface, allowing only an infinitesimal portion of it to emerge. In moments when the physical consciousness is predominant in our awareness—as when Sharon's mind is being pulled to revisit the habitual images of her past—it is this chakra that is most active.

TABLE 1: THE PHYSICAL CONSCIOUSNESS

Grade of Consciousness	Expression Over Course of Cosmic Evolution	Expression In Individual Human Being		Center of Consciousness (Chakras)
		Full, Clear Expression	Limited and/or Distorted Expression	
Physical: The stabilizing con-sciousness associated with matter	The consciousness first associated with subatomic particles, atoms, molecules, rocks, streams, etc; later associated with the physical bodies of plants, animals and humans	Calm, stable	Dull, inert, mechanical	**1st:** Base of spine

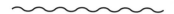

For evolution to proceed, something was needed to move the consciousness of the universe forward. Similarly, something is needed to further awaken the consciousness of the infant, and something is needed to prod the groggy sleeper to wakefulness. What is that something?

> Consciousness is... the fundamental thing in existence—it is the energy, the motion, the movement of consciousness that creates the universe and all that is in it... When consciousness in its movement... forgets itself in the action it becomes an apparently "unconscious" energy; when it forgets itself in the form it becomes the electron, the atom, the material object. In reality it is still consciousness that works in the energy and determines the form and the evolution of form. When it wants to liberate itself... out of Matter, but still in the form, it emerges as life.[1]
>
> —Sri Aurobindo, *Letters on Yoga*

CHAPTER 8

Life: The Evolution of Life: Awakening of the Vital Consciousness

SETTING THE STAGE FOR THE BIRTH OF LIFE

"**B**ehind" and supporting every movement of the universe, even in this very moment, is the Infinite, still, silent Consciousness of the Knower. It is there in the depths of our being, this vast calm that is the foundation of every movement of thought, feeling, and sensation. It is "dreaming" the world into existence at every moment. "Before" the universe was born, it dreamed of an immense, complex world of material forms, a Field of Conscious-Energy existing entirely within its own Consciousness.

The Infinite Knower saw, in this dream, that something was needed to animate these forms. We tend to think of rocks, clouds, and other physical things as made of purely material energy. But from the yogic perspective, a life energy—or vital consciousness[a]—existed throughout the universe from the beginning. Without it, the planets would not circle their suns, nor would molecules combine to form the building blocks for more complex physical forms.

By taking a different perspective, it may be easier to get a sense of the pervasive activity of the vital consciousness—equally active in what we take to be inanimate matter as it is in living creatures. Lewis Thomas, imagining himself viewing the earth from a distant point in space, writes that

> the astonishing thing about the earth, catching the breath, is that it is alive… If you could look long enough, you would see the swirling of the great drifts of white cloud, covering and uncovering the half-hidden masses of land.[2]

Thomas further suggests that if we were to speed up the flow of geologic time, we would see

> the continents themselves in motion, drifting apart on their crustal plates, held afloat by the fire beneath. [The earth itself would have] the organized, self-contained look of a live creature, full of information, marvelously skilled in handling the sun.[3]

Novelist H. G. Wells, in his book *The Time Machine,* draws a vivid picture of the dramatic change in perspective experienced by his time

---

a. "Prana" in Sanskrit. This is not the same as the "vital force" proposed by some nineteenth-century biologists. The vital force was a theoretical construct designed to account for phenomena that contemporary biologists now attribute to purely physical causes. The yogis, on the other hand, are describing a direct perception of the energy that animates physical forms.

traveler observing changes in the world around him as he hurtles into the future:

> As I put on pace, night followed day like the flapping of a black wing… I saw the sun hopping swiftly across the sky, leaping it every minute, and every minute marking a day… I saw the moon spinning swiftly through her quarters from new to full… the jerking sun became a streak of fire… I saw trees growing and changing like puffs of vapor, now brown, now green; they grew, spread, shivered, and passed away. I saw huge buildings rise up faint and fair, and pass like dreams. The whole surface of the earth seemed changed— melting and flowing under my eyes.[4]

But we do not need a time machine to become aware of the pervasive working of the vital consciousness. By refining our own consciousness, we can become directly aware of its presence in rocks as much as in a rose or a rabbit. However, the refinement necessary to achieve this level of perception would require painstaking discipline and an unusual ability to quiet the noise of the ordinary waking consciousness. An easier way to get a sense of how the vital consciousness works—and the role it plays in the process of evolution—is to look once again at what happens as we awaken from sleep.

The Sleeper Awakening

At the moment of awakening, there is at first no more than an extremely dim awareness of the physical environment. At this point there is little distinction between various objects, or between "self" and "other." Almost imperceptibly a vague feeling emerges, an indistinct sense of things being "pleasant" or "unpleasant." In a flash this is followed by a slightly more conscious impulse to reach out to that which is "pleasant" and avoid or change what is "unpleasant." These primitive vital reactions then become elaborated into more complex emotional responses. According to yoga psychology, these three dimensions of responsiveness to the environment—(1) the initial awareness of "pleasant" or "unpleasant"; (2) the more conscious impulse to control or change it; and (3) more complex emotional responses to it—represent three distinct levels of the vital consciousness.

Expanding this sequence from milliseconds to billions of years, we see the emergence of the same levels of vital consciousness in the universe. Following the Big Bang, at first all that was awake was the physical consciousness. During this early period in the life of the universe, the Soul—that "part" of Infinite Being that entered into and forgot Itself in matter—had only a dim awareness of Its environment. Billions of years later, with the emergence of the first level of the vital consciousness in plants and animals, the Soul was able to respond to things as pleasant or unpleasant.

Over time, the Infinite Knower beyond the universe continued to "dream" up new and more complex material forms. As these forms developed, the vital consciousness was able to emerge more fully, becoming intensely dynamic and far more complex in its capacity to respond.

THE NATURE OF THE VITAL CONSCIOUSNESS

The story of the emerging vital consciousness in plants and animals is our story as well. The vital consciousness that began to awaken in the earliest living organisms is the same conscious-energy that fuels our body, desires, feelings, and thoughts.[5] The vital consciousness that moves human civilizations—that motivates countries to reach out and develop complex trading systems, to express themselves through art, to discover the world through science, to conquer and possess through war—is the same energy that billions of years ago animated the newborn universe.

What are the essential characteristics of the vital consciousness as it manifests in the course of evolution? According to Sri Aurobindo, the "vital"[a] manifests in living creatures as a will to possess, master, and enjoy. On the one hand, it seeks to develop the capacities of the individual. On the other hand, it attempts to reach out, to absorb, assimilate and master what is external to the individual. In living creatures,

---

a. The use of the term "vital" to mean the vital consciousness is analogous to the use of the word "mind" to mean the mental consciousness.

from the amoeba to the human being, the vital seeks pleasure and delight in all experience. As evolution proceeds, it seeks this pleasure and delight in experiences that are increasingly varied and intense.

When the vital consciousness first emerged in the course of evolution, it was in a state of near slumber, like the matter in which it arose. It woke up to find itself seemingly cramped in the inert stuff of matter, apparently cut off from everything around it, and without access to its full energy and power. The vital consciousness in the living creature, dependent upon the body, is subject to the sense of limitation and incapacity that is characteristic of the relatively dull and inert physical consciousness. Throughout the course of evolution, the vital has had to struggle against the inertia and apparent unconsciousness of matter.

In addition to its struggle with the limits of the physical consciousness, the vital has been limited by its identification with a finite physical body. Whether identified with a one-celled amoeba or a complex multicellular human body, the vital feels itself to be limited, separate from and at odds with other creatures as well as its environment. Unable to fully master either itself or the world around it, the organism feels threatened by everything. As a result, its attempts toward self-expansion tend to take the form of struggle and conflict. It needs to attack in order to protect itself, and to seize upon that which it feels it is lacking. Thus, what is in essence a joyful movement toward possession or mastery becomes distorted as a movement of domination and self-aggrandizement at the expense of others.

THE EVOLUTION OF THE VITAL CONSCIOUSNESS

According to yoga psychology, the three levels of the vital consciousness mentioned above correspond to the second, third and fourth chakras associated respectively with the lower abdomen, the solar plexus, and

a. The terms "lower" and "higher" are not value judgments. They indicate the order in which these levels evolved. They also refer to the fact that the different levels of the vital consciousness are associated with lower or higher parts of the physical body. No one would think that the center of the chest is in any way superior to the abdomen—both are equally necessary. So it is with the levels of the vital.

TABLE 2: THE VITAL CONSCIOUSNESS

Grade of Consciousness	Expression over Course of Cosmic Evolution	Expression in Individual Human Being		Center of Consciousness (Chakras)
		Full, Clear Expression	Limited and/or Distorted Expression	
Vital (*prana* or life): The consciousness that animates matter, supports and links the mental and physical consciousness	Higher Vital: more complex emotions emerging in mammals	Divine Love, Compassion, Delight	Deeper feelings — human love, hate, joy	**4th:** heart
	Central Vital: will to mastery emerging in reptiles, mammals, birds, primates	Mastery and power in service of the Infinite	Ambition, powerful desires	**3rd:** solar plexus
	Lower Vital: impulses and instincts emerging in earliest animals	Enjoyment of the Divine in everything without personal craving or desire	Desire, greed, impulses, fear	**2nd:** below navel
Physical: The stabilizing consciousness associated with matter	The very primitive consciousness first associated with subatomic particles, atoms, molecules, rocks, streams, etc; later associated with the physical bodies of plants, animals, and humans	Calm, stable	Dull, inert, mechanical	**1st:** base of spine

the heart (center of the chest). Sri Aurobindo refers to these simply as the lower, central, and higher vital.[a]

Having charted these levels in such a neat and orderly manner, we want to caution the reader to be wary of the mind's tendency to assume that the Infinite Reality is parceled out in similarly neat packages.

The working of the lower vital is evident in primitive creatures like the sea anemone, which has the capacity to respond to only a very limited range of external stimuli. Its vital reaction to the stimulus is hardly more than a simple positive or negative feeling, characteristic of the lower vital. The working of the central vital can be seen in the activity of reptiles, birds, and mammals when choosing a mate, protecting their young, and defending their territory. The functioning of the higher vital can be seen clearly in the complex relationships that it makes possible—between animals, and even between an owl and a human being.

Bernd Heinrich, professor of zoology at the University of Vermont, found a young horned owl buried in the snowfall of a late spring storm and nursed him back to health. For the following three summers, the owl, whom he named "Bubo," lived in the woods surrounding the professor's log cabin, choosing to spend time with him on a regular basis.

As Professor Heinrich described their interaction:

> Bubo wakes me at 4:34 a.m. by drumming on the window beside my ear. He joins me for breakfast, sharing some of my pancake . . . He hops onto the back of my chair, making his friendly grunts while I caress his head, and he nibbles on my fingers endlessly... He plays rough, and so do I, but eventually he tires of it and lies down on my arms. Looking at the clock I see that we have played for one and a half hours... It is the many varied soft and hushed sounds that Bubo makes that I find most fascinating. I hear them only when I am next to him; they are his private sounds, reserved for intimacies... It is these intimate details that bond friendship and promote empathy and understanding, and you learn such things from wild animals by living with them.[6]

As is apparent in the story of Bubo, in more complex animals such as mammals, birds, and primates, all three levels of the vital consciousness are active. For example, in the simple acts of play described below, we can intuit the sheer pleasure associated with vigorous movements *(lower vital)*, the joy of mastering a game *(central vital)*, as well as feelings of affiliation and affection for one's playmates *(higher vital)*.

According to Richard Carrington, elephants who have been trained to play cricket and soccer "play the game with the enthusiasm of boys... on the village green."[7] Journalist Laura Tangley[8] describes young dolphins who "routinely chase each other through the water like frolicsome puppies and have been observed riding the wakes of boats like surfers." Primatologist Jane Goodall, who studied chimpanzees in Tanzania for four decades, tells of chimps who "chase, somersault, and pirouette around one another with the abandon of children."[9] In Colorado, biologist Mark Bekoff once watched an elk race back and forth across a patch of snow, leaping and twisting its body in midair on each pass—even though there was plenty of bare grass nearby on which he could have run. According to recent research, play serves to help young animals develop the skills they will need when full-grown. However, in Bekoff's opinion, there is no question that it's also fun, that "animals at play are symbols of the unfettered joy of life."[10]

Behind the emergence of these three levels of the vital consciousness is the desire of the Knower to express more of his infinite power and delight of Being. The focus through which this greater power is expressed is the awakening Soul, that "portion" of the Knower that is participating in the evolution. As evolution proceeds, the Soul becomes progressively more individualized. The evolving vital consciousness contributes to this process of individualization by helping to give shape to the emerging personality.

British musicologist Len Howard, in the course of more than ten years of studying birdsong, described the birds with whom she became intimately familiar as "distinct individuals who she could easily recognize and with whom she could form close friendships."[11] She found that even birds of the same species "can be distinguished because, like humans, they each have distinct movements, postures, emotions,

In this cosmic adventure of hide-and-seek we call "evolution," what is the purpose of the development of personality and the ultimate awakening of the individual soul? The yogis say this is a question that cannot be answered in terms the mind can understand. However, since our minds are persistent in asking questions we are not capable of understanding, yogic and other spiritual traditions have offered various stories and myths that can provide at least a clue.

In the Koran, Allah is supposed to have said, "I was a hidden treasure, and sought to be known."[12] The story behind this poetic statement is that of the Knower entering into and hiding Himself in the Field of matter[a] slowly awakening over billions of years. As he awakens, the Infinite Being "beyond" time and space gains a new window through which He (as the subject) can look out upon Himself as the universe (the object). He is then able to see this vast Field of Conscious-Energy (which is Himself in a particular form) in an entirely new way, from an entirely different perspective. As this window becomes more fully individualized, He is able to know His Infinite Being in infinite ways—as the bird choosing a mate, as the elephant playing cricket, as the writers writing this book and the reader who is reading it.

behaviors, and personalities." According to psychologist Theodore Barber, individual birds act "with great flexibility... in choosing their mates, in building their nests, in protecting and teaching their young, in defending a territory, and in other activities that were assumed to be stereotyped or instinctual." They have been shown to be capable of forming "true friendships with birds of their own and other species and also with humans and other animals."

---

a. Actually, there is no "entering into"—since matter, as much as anything else in the universe, is nothing else but the Knower in a particular form.

THE WORKING OF THE VITAL CONSCIOUSNESS IN OUR DAY-TO-DAY EXPERIENCE

Sharon is sitting by the pond enjoying the cool air, the colors of the tree, and its leaves. It's now been a little more than a week since she came to her father's house. Watching the light play on the surface of the pond, thoughts and images flow through her mind. She feels enjoyment tinged with sadness. As she continues dwelling on memories, her sadness grows deeper. Feelings of anxiety arise, mixed with feelings of anger, remorse, and despair. She remembers Vietnam and her growing sense of meaning-lessness amidst the bloodshed and violence of war…Bobby Thompson's voice suddenly comes into her mind. In her imagination, she can see his thin, boyish face, his smile as clear as if it had been yesterday that she was nursing his wounds…

"May I have some water?"

As Sharon hands Bobby a cup, her fingers brush against his. She notices the coldness of his hand.

She watches his face as he speaks of his brothers and sisters back home growing up in a neighborhood plagued by poverty and crime. As he goes on talking of his hopes and dreams and the possibility of returning home to help bring about change in his community, she begins to feel a kinship with him that is reassuring. She speaks to him of her dream of returning to her own community to serve as a doctor, and they talk and laugh about the possibility of working together one day.

Bobby's hand moves down to his side where the bullet had entered. He grimaces in pain, then smiles again at Sharon. She senses a strength in him, a resiliency and powerful will to live. But she has seen so many men die, she wonders if he will be strong enough—or lucky enough—to survive. For several weeks after Bobby returned to combat, Sharon watched anxiously each evening as the truck rolled into the compound carrying the bodies of dead soldiers, hoping that he would not be one of them.

She never saw Bobby again in Vietnam. Some years later she heard that he had returned to the city where he grew up. Not long after setting up a community center for inner city children, he had been killed—an innocent bystander in a gang-related shooting.

In the period of time that Sharon sits reminiscing, the vital consciousness plays through her in many varied and rapidly shifting ways. If we stop at any moment to look at our own consciousness, we can observe a similar array of varying, often conflicting vital emotions and feelings. Recognizing the three different levels of the vital can help us sort out these various strands of experience. In order to understand how these levels operate in Sharon as well as in ourselves, it will be helpful to relate them to their origins in the evolutionary process.

The first level of the vital to emerge in the course of evolution *(the lower vital)* was a further development of the positive-negative polarity present in matter. The same polarity manifests as attraction and repulsion in the earliest living organisms, pleasure and pain in more complex animals, and in human beings as liking and disliking. This aspect of the vital tends to be absorbed in habitual, semiconscious reactions to things. Desire for praise, anger at blame, annoyance and irritation at perceived inconveniences—a constant round of reactivity characterizes this level of the vital consciousness as it generally manifests in human beings.

As Sharon is consciously enjoying the simple sensations of colorful leaves and cool air, she is at the same time subconsciously responding with various forms of like or dislike to many other aspects of her environment. For example, while watching the play of light on the water, she is most likely unaware that she is constantly reacting to the changing patterns of light and shade. She is also probably unaware of a fleeting feeling of annoyance at the sound of someone in the distance laughing a bit too loudly, and perhaps dimly aware of a feeling of irritation that arises in response to occasional twinges of mild pain on the left side of her lower back.

The feeling of strength and resiliency that Sharon sensed in Bobby, the powerful ambition they shared to make a difference in their communities, are characteristic of the next, more complex level

a. In the amoeba, the energy of the central vital, though active, is not yet evolved on the surface.

of the vital consciousness *(the central vital).* At all levels of evolution, it is this layer of the vital that is most involved in the attempt to master oneself and one's environment. The amoeba reaching for its food, the bird improvising new songs to impress its mate, Sharon's desire to bring about a transformation in her community—all are manifestations of this vital urge toward mastery.[a] The central vital is also what brings drama to life. It is the source of great and noble heroism as well as cruel and ruthless conquest. It drives equally, without discrimination, the scientist who spends years researching the cure to a deadly disease, and the one who avidly pursues the next line of biological weapons.

The tenderness that Sharon feels toward the wounded soldier, her feelings of affiliation and kinship as well as her concern for his well-being, are all expressions of the third level of the vital consciousness *(the higher vital).* What manifests as affinities between elements, and attraction and aversion in primitive organisms, emerges as care for one's offspring in mammals, and develops into still more complex feelings of love and hatred in human beings. Kindness and cruelty, joy and despair, compassion and hardheartedness are equally the expression of the higher vital, just as nobility and ruthlessness coexist as expressions of the central vital.

The three levels of the vital consciousness are constantly interacting. For example, what we take to be "love" is usually made up of a combination of all three. Our affection for a lover *(higher vital)* may be intertwined with sexual desire *(lower vital)* and a passionate desire to possess the other person *(central vital).* Compassion for the pain of others—which can be a relatively pure movement of the energy of the higher vital—is usually mixed with pity, which has elements of fear and aversion to suffering *(lower vital).* It can also be mixed with ambition to change the circumstances that lead to suffering *(central vital).* What makes this even more difficult to sort out is the influence of the pure love and feeling of connectedness that are native to the Soul, and which are always fully present behind, though only partially expressed in the surface consciousness. It requires a long and careful study of the action of the vital consciousness to discern this subtle intermingling of levels.

THE EVOLUTION OF THE VITAL CONSCIOUSNESS IN THE UNIVERSE AND THE INDIVIDUAL

Early in the evolutionary journey, the vital consciousness served to help awaken matter and support the creation of organisms that could express more of the Divine Consciousness. Its qualities of passion and dynamism as well as its indiscriminate seeking for intensity and variety of experience were essential for furthering the evolutionary journey.

The growth of the vital in the child is in some ways similar to the evolution of the vital consciousness in the universe. Just as the attention of the Soul is first almost wholly absorbed in the play of matter, the infant's attention is initially caught up in its discovery of the physical world. And, just as the awakening Soul gradually develops the capacity to become aware—if only dimly—of physical sensations, so the growing infant learns to step back and develop an awareness of her body and the physical environment.

As the Soul continues to evolve in plants and animals, the various levels of the vital consciousness awaken. Similarly, in the developing child, these levels awaken over time. The toddler's desires and impulses *(lower vital)* slowly become more distinct. As the child grows older, she develops more control over herself and her environment *(central vital)*. In adolescence, as interpersonal relationships grow in importance, more complex emotions *(higher vital)* begin to emerge.

The vital consciousness in both the universe and the individual enjoys drama, intensity, and experience of all kinds for their own sake, without regard to their value or consequence. However, at a certain point something else was needed. In the course of evolution, the mind working behind the scenes emerged into conscious awareness, developing the capacity to make value judgments, to assess the meaning and purpose of different actions. The long and meandering process by which the mind emerged was one that took billions of years.

> Consciousness is… the fundamental thing in existence—it is the energy, the motion, the movement of consciousness that creates the universe and all that is in it… When consciousness in its movement… forgets itself in the action it becomes an apparently "unconscious" energy; when it forgets itself in the form it becomes the electron, the atom, the material object. In reality it is still consciousness that works in the energy and determines the form and the evolution of form. When it wants to liberate itself…out of Matter, but still in the form, it emerges as life, as animal.[1]
>
> —Sri Aurobindo, *Letters on Yoga*

CHAPTER 9

Animal Mind: The Evolution of the Physical Mind and Vital Mind

GIVING SHAPE TO THE UNIVERSE

Associated with the various manifestations of physical energy—from the whirling of the atom to the formation of a galaxy—is the physical consciousness of the Knower that pervades the entire universe. Still deeper than this physical consciousness is His dynamic vital consciousness animating matter, sustaining the various orderly and coherent patterns of the physical universe. What is it that gives shape to these forms, that is responsible for the regularities in their behavior?

According to yoga psychology, there is a still subtler mental consciousness that organizes the workings of the vital and physical consciousness. The so-called "constants" and "laws of nature"—reflected in the orderly movement of atoms and the circling of planets around their suns—are, from the yogic perspective, manifestations of the hidden mental consciousness of the Knower. It is the shaping of the vital and physical consciousness by His mental consciousness (and ultimately, a Consciousness beyond mind) that gives rise to the world as we experience it.

"Behind" all the activity of the Field of Conscious-Energy, the Infinite Being of the Knower remains, still, vast, and silent, beyond space and time. Without sacrificing in any way His eternal calm, the ever-wakeful Knower "dreams" a universe of infinitely varied forms. In this world He dreams into existence, the stable physical consciousness that supports the material forms is a reflection of His Being; the vital consciousness animating the forms is a reflection of his infinite Power; and the mental consciousness that gives shape and meaning to the forms is a reflection of his infinite capacity for Knowledge and Understanding.

The still Consciousness of the Silent Knower (He) and the active, moving Consciousness that is dreaming the universe into existence (She) are not two. He and She, the Silent Knower and the Field of Conscious-Energy, are inseparable aspects of one, indivisible Divine Reality.

AWAKENING FROM SLEEP

In the process of awakening, after a first dim awareness of the body arises accompanied by a vague feeling state, the mind comes more actively into play. If we could zoom in on the few hundred milliseconds that follow, we would see a wide range of unfolding mental functions. This same unfolding of consciousness occurs in each moment. However, most of us have not refined our awareness to the point where we're able to discern all that happens in a few thousandths of a second. Perhaps by looking at a fairly mundane experience and examining it in slow motion, we might get a better sense of how this process unfolds.

Suppose you're walking down a street at dusk, thoughts passing through your mind in a somewhat random manner. Out of the corner of your eye, you catch a glimpse of something moving. You begin to make out a shape, but you're not sure what it is. As the amorphous shape becomes clearer, you see what you recognize to be a puppy—not any particular puppy, just "puppy." From the first glimpse of something moving to the realization "It's a puppy" all happened within the space of a second or two.

Less than a second later, you recognize it as the puppy that belongs to the little girl who lives down the street. As you begin to think about the little girl and how happy she was several months ago when her parents gave her the puppy for her birthday, you pause. You notice the dark, rich blue of the sky, the clear air, and watch with a smile as the puppy dashes down the street toward her house. You observe that your mind has become quieter and your body feels more relaxed.

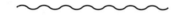

What's happening here in terms of the unfolding mind? There is first a simple undefined sensation *(a glimpse of something moving)*, followed by a clearer nonverbal perception *(you make out a shape)*. As the shape becomes clearer, there is a recognition *(ah, it's a puppy)*, and then some further conceptual elaboration *(the realization that the puppy belongs to the little girl down the street, she was so happy when she got it, etc.)*. There is then a moment of self-awareness, a kind of stepping back from the situation, creating some open space in the mind *(pausing to notice both the external environment and your internal state of mind and body)*.[a]

The emergence that occurred in the space of a few seconds—from the initial sensation through conceptual elaboration to self-awareness—is similar to what took place as the mental consciousness emerged over the course of evolutionary history. It began more than

---

a. Describing this process purely in terms of mental components may sound quite dry. In actual experience, it is not possible to separate out the feeling aspect from the workings of the mind. Though we are now focusing in on mental functions, all aspects of consciousness are active in every moment. For example, in the scenario above, though only the functions of the mind were described, the vital consciousness was active as well—from an initial reaction to a potential threat, to more complex feelings of happiness associated with the memory of the little girl's love for her puppy.

a billion years ago in one-celled organisms with the dim registration of an external stimulus and developed into the complex capacities of social intelligence and self-awareness of which primates and humans are capable. From the perspective of yoga psychology, this eons-long increase in complexity of the mental consciousness is a reflection of a deeper process—the awakening and individualization of the Soul. As the Soul awakens, it shifts its attention, progressively stepping back from its absorption in the workings of the Field. It is this freeing of attention that manifests as an increasingly complex mental consciousness, leading eventually to self-awareness.

THE NATURE OF THE MIND

The Upanishads[2] speak of four general functions of mind[a] that are inherent in the Mind of the Knower. It is these functions that manifest progressively over the course of evolution. We also see them working sequentially in the incident described above:

> (1) sensing (the initial glimpse of something moving); (2) perceiving (which includes both the initial perception of a shape and the subsequent nonverbal recognition of it as a puppy); (3) and (4) understanding and volition (the rest of the sequence, including the memory of the girl and the intentional pause that led to further self-awareness).

Sri Aurobindo identifies various parts of the mind that are associated with each of the four functions. He uses the term "physical mind"[3] to refer to the part of the mind that organizes sensory experience. It is what enabled you, in the example above, to sense the movement in the bushes, organize that sensation into the perception of a shape, and subsequently recognize that shape as a puppy. Because of its close association with the physical consciousness, the physical mind tends

---

a. Sanskrit: *sanjnana, prajnana, ajnana,* and *vijñana.*

Though every act of knowing involves all four functions, only the functions of sensing and perceiving are available to the surface consciousness in the earlier stages of evolution. Even in human beings, the four mental functions do not act in a harmonious, well-integrated fashion, as they do in the "mind" of the Knower, in which sensing, perceiving, understanding and willing are one simultaneous all-comprehending movement of consciousness.

to be characterized by dullness, inertia, and repetitiveness.[a]

The vital mind organizes vital and emotional experience. It is what enabled you to mentally recognize the young girl's reaction to receiving the puppy as one of joy. Being closely associated with the vital consciousness, this part of the mind is strongly influenced by the vital's predilection for drama, and its indiscriminate search for intensity and variety of experience.

The thinking mind[b] is that part of the mind that is relatively free from the influence of both the physical and vital consciousness.[4] It employs a more complex understanding and conscious will in order to comprehend the nature of an experience. In the example above, it was this part of the mind that understood the story of the puppy—how it got to be there and how it fit into the larger context of your life. It was also by means of the thinking mind that you chose to pause and reflect on your experience.

The chart below lists the four functions of mind in the order in which they appeared over the course of animal evolution. It describes the workings of the different aspects of mind—the physical mind, vital mind, and thinking mind—as they relate to the four mental functions. The last column describes the "experienced world" to which these various ways of knowing give rise. The details presented in the chart will be elaborated in the course of the chapter.

---

a. The dulling effect of the physical consciousness and the impassioned quality of the vital consciousness will become clear later in the chapter. As described here, the qualities of the physical consciousness, vital consciousness, and mental consciousness correspond roughly to what in Sanskrit are called the *gunas,* or qualities of nature: *tamas, rajas,* and *sattwa.*

b. Sanskrit: *buddhi.*

TABLE 3: THE EVOLUTION OF		
Mental Functions	**Working of Physical Mind**	**Working of Vital Mind**
(3) and (4) Understanding and Volition (conscious mental will)	Continues to have functions of sensing and perceiving, all changed due to the influence of the thinking mind	Organizes energy of the higher vital—i.e., the more complex emotions that develop as the thinking mind evolves. Function of organizing energy of central and lower vital remains; functions on all 3 levels changed due to the influence of thinking mind
(2) Perceiving	Object awareness: recognition of more complex stimuli by comparison with internal images; association learning	Organizes energy of the central vital—i.e., desires, strong vital impulses toward fight or flight, as well as the impulse for cooperation and collaboration
(1b) More Complex Sensing	Crude recognition, simple (conditioned) learning, crude mental maps	Organizes energy of the lower vital—i.e., the simple feeling awareness of a stimulus as pleasant or unpleasant (life-enhancing or threatening)
(1a) Simple Sensing	Barest registration of stimuli; awareness of vibration, heat, light	

THE MIND

Working of Thinking Mind	Animals in Whom These Functions are First Active	Experienced World Associated with This Way of Knowing
Enduring relationships, clearly defined social roles, complex communication, and flexible cultural traditions	Most intelligent primates and all humans	A "world" in the sense we think of it comes into being. This is the beginning of a "story" that defines the emerging "self" and "world"
Selective attention; associative "thinking" using nonverbal concepts; complex planning and problem-solving; increased flexibility of behavior	The most intelligent mammals and all primates	World becomes progressively more solid, defined, and enduring
Ability to construct complex mental maps, i.e., to recall and organize many details of one's experience and environment in the form of internal images	More complex birds and mammals	More complex relationships between perceived objects in the environment; the capacity to hold in mind past relationships gives greater solidity, definition, and endurance to the perceived world
Thinking mind emerges: Complex learning and problem-solving; greater ability to adapt; capacity to anticipate and plan; beginnings of cultural transmission	Birds and mammals	
	Amphibians and reptiles	Extremely limited groups of sensations combined into objects
	Insects	Relationships between poorly defined classes of sensations
	One-celled organisms	Formless vibrations

We have listed volition as the last mental function to emerge. Nevertheless, wherever some kind of knowing is manifest—even in the simplest one-celled creatures—it is accompanied by some degree of willing. However, at the earliest stages of evolution, whatever rudimentary mental will has evolved to the surface is most likely overshadowed by the more predominant impulses and desires of the vital will. Again, it is hard to adequately convey the dynamic, multidimensional nature of the evolution of consciousness in a static, two-dimensional chart.

THE EMERGENCE OF MIND OVER TIME

We will look here at a few milestones in the emergence of the mental consciousness of the Knower as it manifests in various animals over the course of evolution. Initially, the mind in animals is more or less wholly dominated by the physical and vital consciousness. The thinking mind, when it emerges in birds, mammals, and primates, is not so tethered to the movements of the physical and vital consciousness, so there is a corresponding increase in the capacity for flexible and creative behavior. This greater flexibility and freedom made possible by the emergence of the thinking mind enables the Soul to step back still further from its absorption in the workings of the Field, and ultimately to reawaken to its True Nature.

The Emergence of Simple Sensing

All four functions of the mental consciousness described above are active throughout the course of animal evolution. However, in the most primitive animals only the physical mind has evolved, and only the sensing function is active on the surface; the other functions are working, so to speak, "behind the scenes." For example, in one-celled organisms there is an extremely simple mental consciousness at work on the surface, an infinitesimal fraction of the Knower's infinite Intelligence. Creatures such as amoebae and bacteria have a rudimentary capacity to register external stimuli *(simple sensing)* and will move toward or away from an object depending on whether it is harmful or beneficial. They cannot integrate what they sense into a perception *(the second mental function)* as more complex animals can do. Neither can they learn or adapt *(the functions of understanding and volition)* beyond what they are genetically programmed to do.

However, some scientists are coming to see there is more going on in the behavior of bacteria than can be accounted for by their nearly somnambulant surface consciousness. In rather colorful language, Howard Bloom here summarizes the findings of Israeli physicist Eshel Ben-Jacob. Describing groups of bacteria, Bloom writes that they can

> invent a new instruction set with which to beat an unfamiliar challenge. Some [members of a colony of bacteria] feel out the new environment, learning all they can. Others "puzzle" over the genome like race-car designers tinkering with an engine whose power they are determined to increase. Yet others collect the incoming "ideas" passed along by their sisters and work together to alter the use of existing genetic parts or to turn them into something new.[5]

What does it mean to say these primitive creatures "puzzle" over the genome or "collect" incoming ideas? From a scientific perspective, how is this possible when animal psychologists tell us that bacteria—creatures that possess no brain of any kind—experience the world as little more than a blur of vibrations of heat and light?

From the yogic perspective, what Ben-Jacob is seeing is a reflection of the infinite Intelligence of the Eternal Knower who feels and senses the entire earth simultaneously within His own Being; who perceives the relationship of each part to every other part in infinite ways; who also understands what is needed at each particular moment in evolution within the larger context of the entire evolutionary spiral; and who possesses the will to effortlessly coordinate the workings of each point, including those represented by billions of bacteria. This infinite Intelligence, whether or not we're aware of it, is working through each bacterium, every star and galaxy, as well as through our own consciousness at this very moment.

Words like *hidden* and *behind* the surface may make it sound as though the Unborn Knower is somehow separate from the Field. On the one hand, we've identified an Infinite Intelligence hidden behind the surface, beyond time and space. We've also identified a Field of Conscious-Energy—galaxies, bacteria, puppies—in and through which He/She is somehow acting and interacting with Him/Herself. But the Knower and the Field are not two; they are One inseparable Divine Reality.

Why then do yogic texts so frequently use these spatial terms— within, behind, higher, lower, and so on? When people first begin to have glimpses of a greater Consciousness, they are usually still partially identified with their physical body. Because of this, the greater Consciousness and Intelligence is perceived to have a spatial relationship to that body: They feel deep within their hearts a yearning for some kind of awakening; they sense around them some kind of Force or Energy; they feel in the skies "above" some kind of Presence. These words—in, above, around, and the like—are not meant to be taken literally. Rather, they are meant to be portals through which we might gain a glimpse of the workings of something greater, vaster, Infinite. The Infinite Knower is all pervading—He/She is just as much outside as within; in front as behind; below as above.

The Emergence of More Complex Sensing and Perceiving

With insects there is an enhanced capacity to manipulate the environment. This comes as a result of the greater development in their surface consciousness of the first mental function of sensation. The spider, for example, is capable of making a crude mental map of its environment and using it as an aid for hunting prey. Neuropsychologist Merlin Donald recounts that

> [The jumping spider] will often "ambush" a potential quarry. Having spotted its prey perched on a flower stem, it will move away from it, rather than toward it, drop to the

ground, and climb up the other side of the plant, out of sight
of its victim. It will then approach it stealthily, always from
behind, and, once close, suddenly attack.[6]

It is not the surface consciousness of the spider that "strategizes"
how to ambush its prey. The surface consciousness of the spider is
probably only aware of a blurry "something" that resembles potential
food, and an urge to eat it.

In spite of this advance in behavioral complexity, the spider is limited
to actions that are controlled by genetic mechanisms. Beyond its genetically programmed activity, the spider's awareness of the environment
and its capacity to adapt are extremely limited. According to Donald:

> It seems blissfully unaware of the most significant objects
> in the larger environment. It goes on weaving webs and
> ambushing anything that resembles a prey, no matter where
> it is. It shows no signs of adapting its behavior to the larg-
> er scenarios that might be imposed by a wider world. The
> spider's world is tiny, restricted to a small number of play-
> ers and situations. It misses any feature that might demand
> significant... capacities to perceive or remember.[7]

In amphibians and reptiles there is still more of the previously hidden mind active on the surface, enabling these creatures to "synthesize
their sensations into a complex perception." However, frogs are able to
perceive only a limited range of objects—they "are designed to detect
bugs, but not cows, oak trees or Chevy Malibus."[8] The frog can also
respond to more complex events

> within a limited framework. This is evident in their very
> complex mating rituals, in which they must recognize not
> only their own kind but also the correct forms of the ritual
> itself.... They can deal with serious complexity in finding
> food, building nests, defending territory, hiding from preda-
> tors, finding escape routes, and so on.[9]

Even with this additional capacity for the perception of objects and events, the amphibian and reptile, like the insect, remain relatively inflexible, as there is yet only a very limited ray of the larger intelligence operating through their limited surface consciousness. These organisms "are designed to carry out certain specialized operations with great efficiency. But they cannot move beyond this and adapt to novel situations."[10]

The Emergence of Understanding and Complex Volition

The inflexibility of creatures such as frogs, spiders, bees, and bacteria is a reflection of the limitations of the physical and vital mind. Relying almost exclusively on the functions of sensing and perceiving to construct their experienced world, their mind has no capacity to step out of that construction. Consequently, their behavior patterns remain limited and largely repetitive in nature.

With birds and mammals, the functions of understanding and volition (the thinking mind) begin to emerge. These functions allow them to step out of their constructed world and relate to it in more flexible and creative ways. The new capacity of imagination ("new" only from the perspective of the surface consciousness) now becomes available. Combined with the ability to make complex mental maps of their environment, these animals are capable of solving problems that would confound a more primitive mind. Along with the emergence of the more complex thinking mind, the vital mind and physical mind also become more complex.

As a result of these new capacities, mammals and birds are more adaptable in a wider array of circumstances. For example, Merlin Donald notes that "raccoons are fiendishly clever at surviving in an urban environment and obviously carry around elaborate cognitive maps of entire neighborhoods. The locations of sources of food, and places of danger and safety are noted and stored for future use."[11] Some mammals are able to apply their sophisticated problem-solving abilities to anticipate the behavior of others. For example, one group of young elephants living in captivity on an African plantation stuffed mud into the bells they wore around their necks. This prevented the bells from ringing, allowing the elephants to sneak into nearby banana groves and steal bananas without being detected by the plantation owner.[12]

The capacity for selective attention—that is, the ability to intentionally focus on a particular facet of the environment—also emerges in birds and mammals. The extraordinary patience of a cat waiting with unwavering attention at a mouse hole is the envy of many a meditator aspiring to be present in the moment, undistracted by thought. Merlin Donald here describes the remarkable capacity for vigilance that can be seen in various predators: "There might be no immediate evidence of prey around them when they start, but they initiate their vigil autonomously of their environment because they harbor expectations. Hunting wolves can track a specific prey for long distances... often in the face of many potential distractors."[13] The consciousness of a cat or wolf actively focusing its attention is quite different from that of the spider waiting passively until his instinct is triggered by the appearance of a potential prey.

Along with greater capacities for knowing and willing came a greater capacity for feeling. Mammals have an increased ability to hold complex mental images of themselves and the environment than their reptile or insect predecessors.[a] With a more clearly defined self-image, the animal can have more clearly defined feelings in response to the events in its environment.

The thinking mind also brings to mammals a greater capacity for memory, allowing them to anticipate future events, and hold in mind, for hours or even days, images of events that occurred in the past. This makes possible a more complex and more enduring sense of themselves and a more complex world of objects, events and creatures to which they can respond with a wider variety of feelings and emotions. This sets the stage for a more coherent "story" of self and world to emerge.[b]

Elephants, for example, have been known to mourn fellow elephants who have died. Joyce Poole, an expert in elephant behavior, "has seen elephants keeping vigil over their dead compatriots."[14] She describes

a. Predecessor in terms of less complex consciousness, not in terms of evolutionary succession.

b. A story that the mind constructs about the world in which it lives.

the expression "on their faces, their eyes, their mouths, the way they carry their ears, their heads, and their bodies" as suggestive of what we would call grief. She also notes that "elephants have been observed to stop when walking past a place where a companion died—a silent pause that can last several minutes."[15] Such an emotion would not be possible without an enduring image of the deceased elephant and a memory of times past, which the thinking mind makes possible.

"That Damn Bird": The Transition from Animal To Human Mind

Scientists and yogis alike agree that there is a fundamental difference between animal and human consciousness. However, in practice, it has been extremely difficult to draw a distinct line between the two. It had long been thought that language was unique to humans, but this distinction has recently become blurred. Celebrated primates such as Kanzi the bonobo and Koko the gorilla have been taught basic sign language and have proven themselves to be capable of some human-like communication. Still, such capacities were generally thought to be limited to primates. In the past twenty years, the research of Dr. Irene Pepperberg has forced students of animal behavior to further reconsider their earlier assumptions.

More than a quarter century ago, Dr. Pepperberg became interested in studying the capacity for meaningful communication in birds, intending to use primate studies as a model for her own research. However, at the time nobody believed birds were capable of the same level of communication as primates, and her first grant application to the National Institutes of Health came back with comments "essentially asking me what I was smoking."[16] Undaunted, she developed a training program for parrots that after more than twenty years, has defied many previous expectations of what is possible in terms of animal communication and understanding. Because of Pepperberg's success, Mike Tomasello, one of her colleagues who lectures on primate intelligence, has been forced to add at some point in his talks that "the described behavior is found only in primates, except for that damn bird."[17]

That "damn bird" to which he refers is the African Grey parrot, Alex.

As a result of Dr. Pepperberg's training, Alex can demonstrate some remarkable cognitive abilities. As described by psychologist Theodore Barber, Alex

> proficiently uses more than 100 English words correctly to refer to all objects in his laboratory environment that play a role in his life including his fifteen special foods, his gym, the shower, the experimenter's shoulder, and more than one hundred other things. He at times refuses the experimenter's request ("No!") and may tell the experimenter what to do ("Go away." "Go pick up the cup." "Come here.") He also requests particular information ("What's this?" "What's here?" "You tell me." "What color?") After Alex had learned to use the numbers one through six and had learned a triangle is "three-cornered" and a square is "four-cornered," he spontaneously and creatively called a football a "two-corner" and a pentagon a "five-corner."[18]

Alex continues to surprise not only skeptical scientists, but Dr. Pepperberg herself. She described one occasion in which she was

> trying to get him to sound out refrigerator letters, the same way one would train children on phonics. We were doing demos... for our corporate sponsors; we had a very small amount of time scheduled and the visitors wanted to see Alex work. So we put a number of differently colored letters on the tray that we use, put the tray in front of Alex, and asked, "Alex, what sound is blue?" He answers, "Ssss." It was an "s," so we say "Good birdie" and he replies, "Want a nut."

> Well, I don't want him sitting there using our limited amount of time to eat a nut, so I tell him to wait, and I ask, "What sound is green?" Alex answers, "Ssshh." He's right,

it's "sh," and we go through the routine again: "Good parrot.""Want a nut.""Alex, wait. What sound is orange?""Ch."
"Good bird.""Want a nut."We're going on and on and Alex
is clearly getting more and more frustrated. He finally gets
very slitty-eyed and he looks at me and states, "Want a nut.
Nnn, uh, tuh."[19]

In fact, Alex displays some cognitive abilities that human children
usually do not demonstrate before the age of four or five. He is able,
for example, to clearly differentiate color, shape, and number. He can
look at a group of different objects of different color, shape, and material and tell you which one is round, which one is red, and which one
is made of wood.

As amazing as this may seem, it pales in significance when compared with the extraordinary complexity of the totality of cognitive
abilities we take for granted in a three-year-old human child.

Consider, for example, the following exchange:

Mother: What would you like for Christmas?

Three year-old child: A new bike.

In order to make that very simple statement, the three-year-old
child has to have an implicit (nonconscious) understanding that the
word "Christmas" represents a whole range of experience. Neither
Alex nor any other animal yet studied by scientists has demonstrated
the ability to use symbolic language in this way. When the three-year-
old hears his mother utter the word "Christmas," he is—at least subconsciously—aware that it represents a ritual involving the exchange
of gifts, the gathering of family members, the singing of certain songs,
and the recitation of particular prayers in church along with perhaps a
number of other associations.

How is it that a toddler has the capacity to take a simple sound
such as "Christmas" to represent such a complex range of experience?
From the yogic perspective, it is because he has developed sufficient
self-awareness to separate his "self"—at least to some extent—from
the ritual, the family gathering, and the experience at church. In other
words, he is able to step back from them and see them as events related

to each other and himself.

What about self-awareness in animals? The existence of some kind of self-sense is not altogether absent even in some less complex animals. Ethologist Frans de Waal suggests there is a continuum of self-awareness extending from fish to human beings.[20] According to science writer Robin Cooper, "centered experience" of some kind exists in early mammals, who have "a center upon which sensations seem to impinge, and from which actions seem to emanate... [there is a] central point [by means of which] all impressions and experiences can be knitted into a unity."[21] But for most animals, it is not possible to step back from and become objectively aware of this center—that is, to be self-aware. The first appearance of this stepping back capacity seems to be in primates (and possibly dolphins, a few other mammals, and maybe even "that damn bird" as well).

For the past several decades, scientists have used mirrors to help determine whether or not an animal has developed the capacity for self-awareness. Daniel Povinelli, director of the Laboratory of Comparative Behavioral Biology at the New Iberia Research Center in Louisiana, has been studying self-awareness in chimpanzees. Journalist Karen Wright describes here one encounter between Povinelli's chimpanzees and their mirrored reflections:

> Povinelli lugs a three-by-three-foot mirror into the chimp compound and gives his apes a chance to eyeball themselves for the first time in about a year... All the chimps are excited by the new arrivals, but some seem to understand better than others just who it is that has arrived. Apollo hoots and feints in an attempt to engage his reflection in play. Brandy fixes her gaze on the mirror while repeating a series of unusual gestures, apparently mesmerized by the simian mimic who can anticipate her every move... It is Megan, the Einstein of the cohort, who performs an eerily familiar repertoire of activities before the looking glass. She opens her mouth wide and picks food from her teeth, tugs at a lower lid to inspect a spot on her eye, tries out a series of exaggerated facial expressions.[22]

As Povinelli explained to Wright, chimpanzees do not at first recognize themselves in the mirror. Rather, they "act very much as if they were confronting another chimp." After initially attempting to interact with the mirror image, they "soon abandon such tactics and, like Brandy, begin to perform simple, repetitive movements, such as swaying from side to side, while watching their mirrored doubles intently." Povinelli suggests that

> at this stage… the animals may be apprehending the connection between their actions and those of the stranger in the glass; they may understand that they are causing or controlling the other's behavior. When they finally grasp the equivalence between their mirror images and themselves, they turn their attention on their own bodies, as Megan did.[23]

In describing the chimps' emerging self-awareness, Povinelli is careful to distinguish the glimmer of self-awareness present in apes from the more highly developed self-awareness of a human being. As Povinelli characterizes it, the self-awareness of an orangutan is nothing like, "'God, I'm an orangutan, and gosh, I was born 17 years ago, and here I am, still up in the trees, climbing. I wonder what my fate is?'"[24]

What exactly is the difference? The chimp and the orangutan, like the human infant or very young toddler, are able to objectify their body, but they cannot attend to their emotions, thoughts, or perceptions as objects.[a] It is not until approximately age four or five that the human child can step back from his impulses and emotions and become aware of them. And it is not until the child becomes an adolescent or an adult that he will (potentially) be able to have an awareness of his "self" as a complex organization of physical, vital, and mental characteristics.

What is happening here from the perspective of yoga psychology? How can we can explain the mysterious emergence of a sense of self out of what is apparently a collection of sensations, perceptions, feeling

---

a. It is not until approximately fifteen months that an infant can recognize herself in a mirror.

responses, and willful acts—that is, a particular configuration of the Field of physical, vital, and mental consciousness, itself having no clear, stable center. What makes it cohere, what gives it a sense of "identity"? It is the presence of the Infinite Being behind—in a particular focus (the individual Knower or Soul), taking a particular perspective on the totality of Himself—that creates the feeling of a center or "self" in the surface consciousness.

THE WORKINGS OF THE PHYSICAL MIND AND VITAL MIND IN HUMANS

How do the physical mind and vital mind typically function in human beings? The physical mind, which gives shape to our perceptions, is as a whole permeated by the relatively obscure and unawakened physical consciousness. Sri Aurobindo characterizes the physical mind as

> mechanical, inertly moved by habits... always repeating the same unintelligent and unenlightened movements... attached to the routine and established rule of what already exists, unwilling to change; or, if it is willing, then it is unable. Or, if it is able, then it turns the action into a new mechanical routine and so takes out of it all soul and life. It is... full of ignorance and inertia...[25]

An individual whose consciousness is focused largely in the physical mind would tend to act in a repetitive, predictable manner. He might be inclined, for example, to choose the same foods every day, the same restaurants, the same television programs each week, the same route to work. He would tend to think in rigid categories, making him particularly prone to prejudices of various kinds, to seeing things as black or white with little interest in shades of gray. He would probably also be reticent to seek out new information that might require changing his habitual point of view.

The vital mind, strongly influenced by the vital consciousness, mediates between pure vital impulse, desire, and emotion, and the thinking mind. In Sri Aurobindo's words,

> [The vital mind] expresses the desires, feelings, emotions, passions, ambitions... of the vital [consciousness] and throws them into mental forms (the pure imaginations or dreams of greatness, happiness, etc. in which men indulge are one peculiar form of the vital-mind activity).

> [The vital mind] has the passion for novelty and is seeking always to extend the limits of experience for the satisfaction of desire, for enjoyment, for an enlarged self-affirmation... It desires, enjoys, possesses actualities, but it hunts also after unrealized possibilities, is ardent to materialize them, to possess and enjoy them also... If there were not this factor, the physical mind of man left to itself would live like the animal, accepting his first actual physical life and its limits as his whole possibility... But this vital mind... comes in with its demands and disturbs this inert or routine satisfaction which lives penned within the bounds of actuality...creates a dissatisfaction, an unrest, a seeking for something more than what life seems able to give it: it brings...a constant demand for more and always more, a quest for new worlds to conquer, an incessant drive towards an exceeding of the bounds of circumstance and a self-exceeding.[26]

In its passionate seeking for intensity, the vital mind has a penchant for melodrama. In conjunction with the physical mind, it can hold on to an experience of anger, grief, or suffering, going over it again and again, flaming the attendant emotions, perhaps fantasizing about revenge, heroic restitution, or righteous recompense. Soap operas and reality TV are the product of the vital mind, and feed its insatiable need for drama. Neurologist Oliver Sacks offers a vivid portrayal of the colorful and unruly nature of the vital mind when it is unleashed by Tourette's syndrome: "the stream of thought… may lose itself, break into a torrent of superficial distractions and tangents, dissolve into a brilliant incoherence, a phantasmagoric, almost dreamlike delirium."[27]

The physical mind is lost in the slumber of sameness; the vital mind is lost in the drama of change. From the perspective of yoga psychology, both are meant, in the course of evolution, to yield to the guidance of the thinking mind[a] while continuing to perform their unique and necessary functions.

THE DREAMING CONSCIOUSNESS BEHIND THE WORKINGS OF THE PHYSICAL AND VITAL MIND

The Infinite Knower is, at this moment, "dreaming" the universe into existence. The dreaming is made up of vast subtle fields of mental, vital, and physical consciousness. In our ordinary surface mind, we are unaware of these subtle fields of consciousness out of which the physical world is formed. Because our minds are so busy and so full of chatter, our attention is absorbed in the end result—the physical world—and we are blind to the all-pervasive but subtle process of dreaming.

We suggested earlier that when human beings cultivate the ability to quiet their minds, they become more receptive to parapsychological phenomena. The reason for this is that the quiet mind allows access to the dreaming—the subtle fields of mental, vital, and physical consciousness. When we have access to this inner consciousness, it is entirely natural and normal to gain knowledge through direct contact with an event that is remote in time or space—knowledge we usually consider to be "paranormal." We also gain the possibility of being in direct contact with the thoughts, feelings, and sensations of others. Animals, whose consciousness is not filled with verbal chatter, are far more open to this inner realm than most human beings. In fact, animals live very much in contact with this larger, inner realm. A great

---

a. According to the Indian sacred text, the *Mundaka Upanishad*, the proper role of the thinking mind *(buddhi)* is to serve as "leader of the life and the body."

deal of their behavior as well as the evolution of animal species is associated with the workings of these subtle fields of conscious-energy.

Aimée Morgana, a New York City artist, has recorded some truly
remarkable examples of telepathic communication between herself
and her African Grey parrot, N'kisi. Between 2000 and 2003, Aimée
recorded 630 instances of telepathy on the part of N'kisi. For example,
one evening she and her husband were watching a Jackie Chan movie.
N'kisi was in his cage at the other end of the room, where he could see
neither the TV screen nor its reflection. According to Aimée,

> there was an image of [Chan] lying on his back on a girder
> way up on a tall skyscraper. It was scary due to the height,
> and N'kisi said, "Don't fall down." Then the movie cut to a
> commercial with a musical soundtrack, and as an image of a
> car appeared N'kisi said, "There's my car."[28]

Was this telepathy (N'kisi contacting those images in the minds
of Aimée and her husband), or was it clairvoyance (N'kisi picking up
on the TV images by some nonphysical means)? Or, was it perhaps
some combination of both? In what are clearer examples of telepathy,
N'kisi frequently responds to Aimée's dreams. As Aimée describes it,
"I was dreaming that I was working with the audio tape deck. N'kisi,
sleeping by my head [he usually sleeps by her bed], said out loud, 'You
gotta push the button,' as I was doing exactly that in my dream. His
speech woke me up."[29] Aimée describes another occasion, when "I was
on the couch napping, and I dreamed I was in the bathroom holding a
brown dropper medicine bottle. Kisi woke me up by saying, 'See, that's
a bottle.'[30][a]

According to Rupert Sheldrake, flocks of birds make use of such
telepathic abilities through what he refers to as morphogenetic fields.
For example, "birds like dunlins and starlings do not fly in lines and
do not follow leaders. They react to maneuver waves spreading from

---

a. You can hear N'kisi's voice at this website: www.sheldrake.org/nkisi/nkisi1_
text.html.

any direction, including from the back of the flock. This would not be possible if they had to see the other birds behind them. But if they sense changes in the field of the flock directly, then we can begin to understand their behavior."[31]

Sheldrake hypothesizes that these nonphysical "morphogenetic" fields hold a collective memory for the species, which also helps coordinate "the behavior of animal groups, such as termite colonies, flocks of birds, schools of fish and packs of wolves." What we have been referring to as the larger consciousness behind—the consciousness that confers an astonishing degree of instinctive intelligence on creatures as simple as the bacterium—would, in Sheldrake's language, be the result of a morphic resonance from past members of the same species.[a]

But these species-specific fields of conscious-energy are not the whole story. Associated with every formation of the Field is a portion of the Knower. As we saw, there is a diffuse, undifferentiated Presence associated with the conscious-energy of the atom. With animals, the Soul becomes more defined, taking shape as the group-soul of a species. This group-soul is the source of and support for the fields of conscious-energy by which a group of animals can communicate telepathically. In human beings, in part because of the full emergence of the thinking mind, the Soul becomes still further differentiated and we can speak of an individual Soul as well as a more defined group-soul of a family, nation, or people.

---

a. The yogis do not assert that this "instinctive intelligence" found in one-celled organisms is "conscious" in any way resembling more complex animals, much less human beings. We feel awe in contemplation of the beautiful manifestations of intelligence in these primitive creatures to the extent that we have an intimation of the working of the Divine Intelligence.

> Consciousness is... the fundamental thing in existence—it is the energy, the motion, the movement of consciousness that creates the universe and all that is in it... When consciousness in its movement... forgets itself in the action it becomes an apparently "unconscious" energy; when it forgets itself in the form it becomes the electron, the atom, the material object. In reality it is still consciousness that works in the energy and determines the form and the evolution of form. When it wants to liberate itself... out of Matter, but still in the form, it emerges as life, as animal, as man.[1]
>
> —Sri Aurobindo, *Letters on Yoga*

CHAPTER 10

Human Evolution I: The Nature of the Thinking Mind

THE NATURE OF THE THINKING MIND AND THE EMERGENCE OF SELF-AWARENESS IN THE HUMAN BEING

The emergence of the thinking mind in evolution brings with it many remarkable capacities including, among others, complex learning and problem-solving, selective attention, and the capacity for planning and decision-making. But the most remarkable by far is the capacity for self-awareness. Because self-consciousness arises so effortlessly for most of us as infants, it is something we tend to take for granted. Perhaps in looking at someone who, at a young age, lost that sense of self, we may begin to appreciate just how momentous it is.

Helen Keller was born in 1880 in Tuscumbia, Alabama. Bright

and lively as an infant, at the age of nineteen months she contracted an illness that left her both deaf and blind. As a result, within a few months she lost not only all use of language, but all sense of herself as a distinct individual. As she described it some years later:

> Before my teacher came to me, I did not know that I am. I lived in a world that was a no-world. I cannot hope to describe adequately that unconscious, yet conscious time of nothingness. I can remember all this, not because I knew that it was so, but because I have tactual memory. It enables me to remember that I never contracted my forehead in the act of thinking. My inner life, then, was a blank without past, present, or future, without hope or anticipation.[2]

Nearly six years after Helen's illness, Annie Sullivan, a graduate of the Perkins School for the Blind in Boston, came to live with the Keller family. Under her tutelage Helen slowly and arduously—with conscious effort each step of the way—not only regained her use of language, but reawakened to the sense of herself.

The story of the thinking mind—and its relationship to what we think of as our "self"—is very much about this process of waking up.

WAKING UP FROM SLEEP

After awakening from sleep, in hardly more than a few blinks of an eye, the whole sense emerges that: "I am here, with this body, with these feelings and thoughts, in this world." What took 10 to 15 billion years of evolution to make possible now happens within the space of a few seconds. And it is not just the sense of self that is miraculously recreated in this brief time, but the world[a] as well. What is the role of the thinking mind in bringing all this about?

Suppose as you open your eyes just after waking up, you notice in

---

a. That is, the experienced world.

your peripheral vision something shiny and red. As you continue to awaken, you realize it is an apple. This realization triggers your memory of having placed the apple there the night before as part of your intention to start eating a healthier breakfast.

Did the "red" you noticed exist "out there"? Earlier we saw that it is, in fact, the result of an interaction between your consciousness and some kind of external energy pattern.[a] What about the apple itself, not to mention the whole surrounding environment as well as you, the person who perceived it? What does the thinking mind bring to this entire construction?

Almost instantaneously, before the thinking mind comes into play, the sensing and perceiving functions of the mind (in conjunction with the physical and vital consciousness) construct what we take to be an externally existing object—one that is red and roundish. Because these first two functions have evolved over billions of years, they are well established in our consciousness and thus act with extreme rapidity (usually measured in milliseconds).[b] It is the speed with which they unfold that gives us the impression of a preexisting, solid physical object. If our consciousness were more refined, we would be able to see the subtle mental and vital consciousness forming the material object out of the subtle physical energy of the Knower's Dream.

To recognize this object as an "apple"—that is, to possess the ability to verbally identify it as such—requires the working of the thinking mind. Simply recognizing the "apple"—that is, applying the verbal concept to it—is already a momentous leap beyond the working of the physical and vital mind. But the thinking mind is responsible for far more, even in that initial moment of recognizing the apple as you awaken from sleep.

Along with the verbal, conceptual recognition of the "apple," an

---

a. External, that is, to your individual consciousness, not your "True Self." This will be clarified later in the book.

b. The "physical mind" and "vital mind" together contribute to this rapid process of sensing and perceiving.

enormous amount of subconscious[a] "thinking" takes place. Every experience you've ever had with an apple in some way contributes to the present-moment "apple" experience—all the rich complexity of social-emotional interactions you've had with people while eating, buying, picking, or dunking for apples; every fact you've ever learned about apples; every creative thought you've had or heard about what to do with an apple; the aesthetic awareness of the beauty, color, and shape of apples you've seen or tasted, ethical considerations about how to use apples to feed the poor, and more—all of that goes into the seemingly simple construction of the percept "apple" in that moment.

The richness of the simple experience of an apple comes so naturally, and so automatically, that it is hard to get a sense of the enormous amount of activity of the thinking mind that goes into it. Just to see an apple is an extremely complex subconscious mental process of which most of us have little awareness.

Some artists, through long years of practice, or natural proclivity, have sensitized themselves to this subconscious process and have thus learned to see things as if for the first time. Impressionist painter Paul Cézanne, describing this way of seeing, writes, "The same subject seen from a different angle gives a subject for study of the highest interest and so varied that I think I could be occupied for months without changing my place, simply bending more to the right or left."[3]

To get a sense of just how difficult it is to become aware of the process by which the mind constructs the world, you might try the following experiments. Try, for example, to look at the word LAND on the next page as if you were someone who had never seen the alphabet and had no notion of what a written word was. See if you can see it as series of meaningless marks and shapes, without having them cohere into something you recognize.

---

a. Nowadays this is referred to as the "cognitive unconscious" (some add the terms "affective" and "motivational" unconscious—taking into account feeling and willing as well as knowing). However, since according to yoga psychology, there is nothing in the universe that is "un" conscious, the term subconscious (including even much of the activity of the thinking mind) is more accurate.

First try looking at the word as a whole:

LAND

Now look at the letters separately:

L   A   N   D

Look at the parts of the letters:

|— /—\ |\| |)

Now look at the "word" again:

LAND

If you found that difficult, this may be somewhat easier:

> Hold your hand out at arm's length in front of you. Move the hand slowly toward your face, then away from you again. Try this several times. It's the same hand at a distance as it is up close to you, right? It doesn't change size. Or does it?

> Now try moving the hand again, this time, observing, if you can, how the hand seems to grow larger as you move it closer, and smaller as you move it away. If you're able to perceive the hand changing size, you've succeeded in at least partially overriding the perceptual habit learned in infancy, which psychologists refer to as "size constancy."

It might be easier to do this looking at a distant object like a parked car. When you have the opportunity, look at a car off in the distance. Hold your thumb up. Notice the entire length of the car is less than the size of your thumb.

Of course, you know better. You've spent your whole life adjusting size and distance. But what if you had never seen anything at a great distance. What would your estimation of the size of the car be then?

While exploring the Congo rain forest, anthropologist Colin Turnbull met Kenge, a member of the Ba Mbuti pygmy tribe. Kenge had lived his whole life in the rain forest, surrounded on all sides and above by thick foliage. He never had the experience of seeing objects at a great distance. One day,

> Turnbull took him to an area of open grasslands. A flock of buffalo grazed several miles away, far below where they were standing. Familiar with the size of buffalo in the forest, Kenge could make no sense of these tiny dots in front of him. He asked Turnbull, "What insects are those?" "When I told Kenge that the insects were buffalo," Turnbull wrote, "he roared with laughter and told me not to tell such stupid lies." When Turnbull tried to explain how far away they actually were, Kenge began scraping mud off his arms and legs, no longer interested in such fantasies. Later, as the men approached the herd in a car, Kenge became frightened. He could see the animals growing bigger and feared that a magic trick was being played on him.[4]

A moment ago, you experimented with undoing the subconscious process by which the mind automatically constructs the external world and maintains size constancy. However, this process is so ingrained, it is very difficult to fully undo. Perhaps the story of Kenge gave you some appreciation for the extent to which these subconscious processes shape our perception of the world.

By looking at those who either never developed or at an early age lost some of the mental capacities we take for granted, we may be able to get a clearer sense of the wide range of functions of the thinking mind. Beyond our construction of the world, the various aspects of the thinking mind are responsible—in ways we don't normally realize—for our most basic sense of who we are.

AWAKENING THE THINKING MIND: PUTTING TOGETHER THE WORLD AND THE SELF

Constructing the Visual World

Virgil had been functionally blind since the age of six. All that remained of his sight was the capacity to "see light and dark, the direction from which light came, and the shadow of a hand moving in front of his eyes."[5] At the age of fifty, he had an operation to remove the cataracts that which had obscured his vision for over forty years. The ophthalmologist who treated him had done many similar operations on people who had lost their vision fairly late in life. In virtually every case, these people were able to see without difficulty immediately following the operation. But Virgil was different. As he described it later to neurologist Oliver Sacks, at first

> he had no idea what he was seeing. There was light, there was movement, there was color, all mixed up, all meaningless, a blur. Then out of the blur came a voice that said, "Well"? Then, and only then, he said, did he finally realize that this chaos of light and shadow was a face—and, indeed, the face of his surgeon.[6]

For Virgil, every moment after his operation involved a painful struggle to literally "make" sense of the patches of light and color registered by his eyes. As Sacks explains it:

> When we open our eyes each morning, it is upon a world we have spent a lifetime learning to see. We are not given the world: We make our world through incessant experience, categorization, memory, reconnection. But when Virgil opened his eyes, after being blind for forty-five years—having had little more than an infant's visual experiences and this long forgotten—there were no visual memories to support a perception; there was no [visual] world of experience and meaning awaiting him. He saw, but what he saw had no coherence.

His retina and optic nerve were active, transmitting impulses, but his brain could make no sense of them.[7]

In order to bind together what were disparate sensations into familiar objects, Virgil had to spend hours consciously attending to the minute details of even the most common objects of his household, looking at them from various angles, trying with his mind to "figure out" what they were.

He found walking "scary" and baffling. With steps, "all he could see was a confusion, a flat surface of parallel and crisscrossing lines; he could not see them (although he knew them) as solid objects going up or coming down in three-dimensional space."[8] His dog, as he moved, looked so different from different perspectives, he at times wondered if it was even the same dog:

Sometimes he would get confused by his own shadow (the whole concept of shadows, of objects blocking light, was puzzling to him) and would come to a stop, or trip, or try to step over it.[9]

After years of blindness, Virgil was forced to use the more complex functions of the thinking mind in ways few of us ever do. In each moment he was required to use conscious reasoning and attention in order to quite literally make "sense" of his sensations.

Now we turn to someone who was diagnosed as a young child with autism and who learned through an equally strenuous and conscious effort to compensate for a cognitive deficit of a very different and, in some ways, more devastating kind.

Making Sense of People

Temple Grandin published her autobiography *Emergence: Labeled Autistic* in 1986.[a] It was a feat of self-reflection and self-analysis

---

a. These descriptions of Temple Grandin's experience are, like Virgil's above, taken from Oliver Sacks' book *An Anthropologist on Mars*.

thought at the time to be impossible for an autistic person.

The typical picture of autism includes at least three distinct types of behavior: (1) mechanical movements such as waving the hand repeatedly in front of the face, or continuously moving an object back and forth; (2) unusual use of language, such as the repetition of apparently meaningless phrases, often in a flat monotone; and (3) difficulty with social interaction, especially that aspect which involves nonverbal communication. While autistic individuals are often mentally retarded, this is not always the case. Some are able to develop normal social skills, and some may even be intellectually or artistically gifted.

In Temple's case, she was fortunate to have a supportive family and teachers who helped her, from the age of three, develop the linguistic and social skills necessary to become a very successful biologist and engineer. However, even as an adult, she continues to lack a visceral, emotional understanding of the ordinary social conventions and sociocultural matrix that most of us take for granted.

According to most recent theories of autism, one of the defining deficits of an autistic individual is their inability to "mind-read"—that is, to make inferences about what other people are thinking and feeling. Normally, we do this continuously with every person we meet, though the process is generally, at least partially, outside our awareness.

Imagine yourself in a job interview or on a first date. Almost everything you say, every aspect of your behavior, is based on your assumptions about the other person's state of mind. Suppose you were in such a situation but had absolutely no clue as to the appropriate way to respond—whether, for example, a particular comment warranted laughter or concern. Imagine you had no way of reading the person's expression or behavior to get an indication of what they thought of you—whether, for example, they thought you were clever or an idiot. You would have no idea whether they felt warmly toward you or disliked you. Even if they told you how they felt, you could only process this information in a purely rational, nonemotional way.

This implicit understanding of social and cultural context is precisely what Temple lacked. Because of this, she spent years consciously analyzing peoples' behavior and expressions in order to logically piece together what most of us understand automatically.

While Temple had enormous difficulty relating to people, she had no problem at all feeling the emotions of the animals with whom she worked. With them she feels "at home," secure and at ease in a way she cannot with other human beings. "When I'm with cattle, it's not at all cognitive. I know what the cow's feeling."[10] With people, she feels like "an anthropologist on Mars."[11]

One might think that Temple would have an easier time with infants and little children, who are less mentally complex than adults. However, both as a child and an adult, she has had much difficulty talking or playing with them. She even has trouble playing peekaboo with an infant, unable to get the timing right. By the time children are three or four years old, they have a tacit, emotional understanding of other people that is beyond anything she thinks she could ever learn. As a child herself, Temple felt that there was something mysterious taking place between normal children, some kind of easy understanding they shared that so totally eluded her, she imagined they were telepathic.

By means of extraordinary and persistent intellectual effort, Temple Grandin has learned to recognize the behaviors associated with the various states of mind underlying social interaction—an accomplishment made more remarkable by the fact that she is incapable of experiencing these states of mind herself.

We often take the thinking mind to be a very narrow instrument, made up primarily of the functions of logic and critical reason. As we see here, it encompasses far more—from construction of the world of visual objects to comprehension of the multifaceted world of social and emotional meaning. But it performs an even more essential function. As we will see in the case of Helen Keller, the thinking mind plays a fundamental part both in the construction of the world we experience and the essential sense of who we are.

Creating A Self and A World

Before Helen became ill, she was a bright, precocious infant. She had already learned to walk and had developed some vocabulary. After she lost her capacity to see and hear, she not only lost her capacity to use language, she lost her sense of herself. Looking back on that time, Helen referred to herself as "phantom." She wrote, "I was like an unconscious clod of earth. There was nothing in me except the instinct to eat and drink and sleep. My days were a blank... without interest or joy."

In 1887, when Helen was seven years old, her parents contacted Alexander Graham Bell, an activist within the field of deaf education. He arranged for them to visit the Perkins Institute for the Blind in Boston. Annie Sullivan, a recent graduate of Perkins, was selected to become Helen's tutor—and she was to remain by Helen's side for the next forty-nine years.

By the time Annie appeared on the scene, Helen had become extremely undisciplined. She had a limited repertoire of some sixty gestures with which she could communicate her needs and desires. Much of the time she was frustrated by her inability to communicate and would throw tantrums in order to get what she wanted. When Annie arrived, she realized that before Helen could become capable of learning, structure and discipline would need to be established. This was in part for the obvious purpose of managing Helen's unruly behavior. But more important, a stable pattern of interaction would provide the background against which Helen's sense of self and world could begin to take shape.

The chief method that Annie used to communicate with Helen is known as "finger-spelling." With her fingers, she would create patterns in Helen's hand that represented the letters of various words. Though she quickly learned the finger-spelling patterns and seemed to enjoy using them, Helen had no idea that they related to words or objects. Years later, in her autobiography, Helen described the moment when she reawakened to the meaning of language:

> We walked down the path to the well-house, attracted by the fragrance of the honeysuckle with which it was covered. Someone was drawing water and my teacher placed my hand under the spout. As the cool stream gushed over one hand she spelled into the other the word "water," first slowly, then rapidly. I stood still, my whole attention fixed

upon the motion of her fingers. Suddenly I felt a misty consciousness as of something forgotten—a thrill of returning thought; and somehow the mystery of language was revealed to me. I knew then that "w-a-t-e-r" meant the wonderful cool something that was flowing over my hand. That living word awakened my soul, gave it light, joy, set it free! I left the well-house eager to learn. Everything had a name, and each name gave birth to a new thought. As we returned to the house each object that I touched seemed to quiver with life. That was because I saw everything with the strange new light that had come to me.[12]

What happened in that moment when Helen finally made the connection between the letters W-A-T-E-R and her experience of flowing water? How did this simple experience awaken her "soul," give it "light, joy, set it free"?

The development of language is often understood to be a process of learning to attach particular sounds to particular objects. This view presumes that there is a preexisting world of objects "out there" waiting to be named. It is as though the Neanderthal living some 60,000 to 120,000 years ago inhabited a world very much like ours, to which he affixed increasingly complex verbal labels.

However, the "world" of objects and events—as modern human beings experience it—does not exist apart from our particular kind of consciousness.[a] In Helen's case, "water"—the cool, flowing substance that can be repeatedly drawn from a well, poured from a pitcher, or bathed in—had no existence prior to the moment her thinking mind reawakened and she connected the word to her experience. And simultaneous with the emergence of the object "water," the "world"—as we generally know it—came into being.

In that same moment, something even more momentous took

---

a. As we've seen, the "world" is so dependent on the way it is known that one could almost say there is one "world" for the jumping spider, another for the raccoon, and yet another for N'kisi. And as we'll see, the "world" of the Cro-Magnon was profoundly different from that of a twenty-first-century human being.

place. The "word"—the reawakening of the thinking mind—brought back to Helen her sense of self. She was no longer "Phantom." She was now someone in relationship to the "world"; she was a "self" with a past, present, and future.

From the perspective of the view from nowhere, there is nothing terribly momentous about Helen's experience. Psychologists say that the "self" is originally constructed from the preverbal experiences of the infant. As a baby begins to have some sense of herself as distinct from others and her environment, layers of verbal memories and associations accumulate, resulting in the rather complex adult self. In other words, from this point of view, there is no inherent reality to the "self" apart from this construction. So the return of Helen's sense of self may have been no more than the return of that construction, triggered by the association of a word to the sensation of flowing water.

But if we take seriously Helen's own description, we can see that something more was going on. Helen spoke of how her soul "awakened," how the word "gave it light, joy" and "set it free." If there is no "self" apart from the accumulation of experience, what was she talking about?

According to yoga psychology, the reawakening of the thinking mind in Helen did far more than bring back the capacity for language, construct a world, or restore a previously constructed "self." The thinking mind, at this critical juncture, provided a focus for the rays of the ever-free, ever-joyous, ever-luminous Divine Soul—the individualized Knower behind—to irradiate her surface consciousness. From the yogic view, it is a reflection of the Knower behind, the individual Soul, which provides the light of self-awareness to the "self" organized in the surface consciousness. And that individual Soul is itself a reflection of the Supreme Self of the universe, the vast, Infinite Reality in whom we "live and move and have our being."

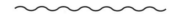

We've looked at the various functions of the thinking mind—how it can be used to augment the sensing and perceiving functions of the mind; how it plays an essential role in our emotional and social lives;

and the part it plays in constructing the world and our sense of "self." The moment of Helen Keller's awakening to self-awareness pointed to a deeper function of the thinking mind—that is, to be an instrument for the awakening of the Soul.

As we will see in the course of human evolution, the thinking mind, paradoxically, can create enormous obstacles to the awakening of a deeper consciousness. It can focus attention on the surface of things to such a degree that a wealth of inner experience is completely lost to our awareness. Its obsession with dividing up the world, reducing it to ever smaller and more meaningless pieces, can lead to an occlusion of the Soul so great that the world itself is seen to be a purposeless "collocation of atoms," a "sound and fury signifying nothing."

However, when the thinking mind attends to the "self" and the "world" with a certain kind of receptivity and clarity, it can become an instrument through which the Soul can gradually awaken.

CHAPTER 11

Human Evolution II:
The Evolution of the Thinking Mind

THE STORY OF HUMAN HISTORY FROM THE
PERSPECTIVE OF THE EVOLUTION OF CONSCIOUSNESS

In the course of cosmic evolution, the mental consciousness of the Infinite has been expressed in increasingly complex forms through the minds of various creatures, from the earliest one-celled organisms to human beings. This consciousness first manifested as the physical mind and vital mind in primitive organisms, then as the thinking mind in birds, mammals, primates, and human beings. On a smaller scale, with the appearance of *Homo sapiens*, there has been a collective unfolding of the thinking mind. It was initially dominated by the physical consciousness, then by the vital consciousness. In the last several thousand years, the thinking mind has begun to come into its own.[1]

The interaction of these various movements of consciousness is something too subtle and complex to be neatly classified. However, just as we were able to discern a general pattern of increasing complexity over the course of biological evolution, we can get a general idea of the evolution of the thinking mind throughout human history.

The following chart describes the progressive influence of the physical, vital, and mental consciousness on the thinking mind as it emerged over the course of human evolution. It relates these collective grades of consciousness to their expression in the individual human being and the time of their emergence in biological evolution.

Over the hundreds of thousands of years since the appearance of *Homo sapiens*, as the thinking mind grew progressively free of the influence of the physical and vital consciousness, it developed the capacity to assist them in functioning more harmoniously, more in line with their rightful roles. However, its newly won independence was

TABLE 4: INFLUENCES ON THE THINKING MIND IN HUMAN HISTORY

Grade of Consciousness Defined	Corresponding Center of Consciousness (Chakra)	Expression in Individual Human Being	Evolution of the Thinking Mind in Human History	Form in Which Each Grade of Consciousness First Emerged
Mental: Organizes the energy of life and matter; opens to and gives form to knowledge from below and beyond the mind	7th: crown of head, opening to conscious-energy above	Higher levels of thought	Emergence of the thinking mind in its own right: brings the capacity to think and reason relatively free of the distortions of the physical and vital consciousness; emerges in humans over last 5,000—10,000 years	Humans
	6th: forehead	Reasoning		Early stages emerge in higher mammals, birds, primates
	5th: throat	Speech, communication		Beginning to emerge in some mammals, birds, primates

Grade of Consciousness Defined	Corresponding Center of Consciousness (Chakra)	Expression in Individual Human Being	Evolution of Thinking Mind	Form in Which It First Emerged
Vital (*prana* or life): Animates and sustains the forms of matter; links together matter and mind	4th: heart	Higher Vital: deeper feelings—love, hate, joy	Thinking mind progressively shaped by the three levels of the vital consciousness: emerges in humans slowly over approximately the last 100,000 years	More complex emotions emerging in later mammals and birds
	3rd: solar plexus	Central Vital: ambition, powerful desires		The will to mastery emerges in reptiles, amphibians, early mammals
	2nd: below navel	Lower Vital: desire, greed, impulses, fear		Impulses and instincts in earliest animals
Physical: The stabilizing consciousness associated with matter	1st: base of spine	Consciousness associated with the body	Thinking mind shaped by the physical consciousness; emerges in humans several million years ago	The consciousness associated with subatomic particles, atoms, molecules, planets, stars, etc.

Given the complexity of human consciousness, it is important when looking at this chart to take into account the considerable limitations of such neatly delineated categories.

somewhat fragile. In order to avoid falling back under their sway, the thinking mind sought to dominate the physical and vital consciousness—as well as the natural world that embodies them—becoming something of a tyrant.

The desire to control nature kept the attention of human beings focused on things of the outer world. Over time, this increasingly external focus blocked access to the inner world, the dreaming consciousness of the Knower. In addition, the mind grew to rely increasingly on its rational, analytic capacities to the exclusion of its more creative and synthetic possibilities. The psychological and practical problems to which this narrow mental functioning has given rise are an indication that something more than the thinking mind will be needed to resolve and reintegrate our fractured lives and world.

THE INFLUENCE OF THE PHYSICAL CONSCIOUSNESS ON THE DEVELOPMENT OF THE THINKING MIND

To get some sense of what life might have been like for our earliest ancestors—hominids living approximately 1 to 5 million years ago known as Australopithecus—try the following experiment. Imagine that you have virtually no language with which to form thoughts or communicate to those around you. You use facial expressions and gestures to help express what you mean. You have no concept of country, world, solar system, or universe. Your sense of a "world" consists of all that exists within whatever small territory you can cover by foot within a couple days' time.

You have almost no sense of yourself as a distinct entity. All that happens to you is just an experience in the moment; it's not happening to a "someone" that you are. You are not burdened with a life story, with a self that needs to be improved, or a life that needs changing. Your memory is short-lived, so if something frightening happens, it is soon gone, leaving little conscious residue of fear. You are unaware of the passage of time; you do not anticipate, and thus have no fear of your own death. Your emotions and emotional ties are direct and very simple—you have no experience of anything as complex as romantic love that requires two "someones" and a story connecting them. Yet, you have an inner connection with others that is intimate, visceral, and without an overlay of language or thought.[a][2]

What movements of consciousness are reflected in these simple activities and experiences? The thinking mind is already active, given that there is some kind of extremely simple self-awareness present. But it is largely dominated by the influence of the physical consciousness. Emotions are simple, directly related to events in the environment; abstract conceptions of time are almost nonexistent. There is no distinct sense of self, and the mind is largely preoccupied with basic survival needs—food, water, warmth, sex (for procreation rather than pleasure), and safety.[3]

Beginning about 2.5 to 1.8 million years ago, with the emergence of the species *Homo erectus*, the vital consciousness began to have a greater impact on the evolution of the thinking mind. Over the next several million years the different layers of the vital consciousness— lower, central, and higher—each played a role in helping awaken and complexify the activity of the thinking mind.

INFLUENCE OF THE VITAL CONSCIOUSNESS ON THE DEVELOPMENT OF THE THINKING MIND

As the energies of the lower vital consciousness (second chakra) came to have more influence on the thinking mind, life became richer. In addition to tending to their basic survival needs, our *Homo erectus* ancestors began to pursue pleasure and enjoyment for their own sake.

The distinction between self and others was still minimal. However, when Neanderthal man appeared on the evolutionary scene, humanity collectively experienced something akin to what Helen Keller experienced the day she understood water—the emergence of a more defined sense of self, and with it a world more defined in terms of that self: "my clan," "my food," "my shelter."

An increasing influence of the central vital consciousness (third

---

a. Thanks to Duane Elgin, *Awakening Earth*, for this summary of the experience of early humanity.

chakra) led to further development of the thinking mind. Sometime between 70,000 and 40,000 years ago the Neanderthal species died out. During that period a new species of *Homo sapiens* appeared, the Cro-Magnon, who had a larger brain and a more complex thinking capacity. In conjunction with this greater thinking capacity, a still richer life became possible. The drive of the central vital for mastery and possession contributed to the development of a greater capacity for modifying the environment. Among other things, human beings of this period undertook migrations to various parts of the world creating expanded trade networks, and developed remarkably sophisticated forms of art, including painting, pottery, and music.

The increasing influence of the higher vital consciousness (fourth chakra) on the thinking mind led to still greater cognitive complexity and with it, a greater emotional intelligence. Human beings now became capable of developing complex social relationships and culture—the kind that Temple Grandin found so mystifying. The capacity for relationship and the richness of culture continued to grow over time, making possible, approximately 10,000 years ago in what is now the Middle East, the emergence of the first complex civilizations.

Over the next several thousand years the thinking mind continued to become more complex. As the thinking mind became freer of the influence of the physical and vital consciousness, the world (as it was perceived by human beings) became more intelligible. For example, humans during the first several thousand years before the common era began to discern the patterns that we now refer to as "laws of nature." The ongoing unfolding of the thinking mind led to a number of developments that provide the basis for our modern way of life, such as the formation of social classes, the division of labor, and the first instances of centralized political authority.

THE THINKING MIND COMES INTO ITS OWN

With the freeing of the thinking mind, there emerged a more clearly defined sense of self, one shaped by the more complex ideas, philosophies, and social and political views of the more complex thinking

mind. In ancient Greece the capacities of the newly emerging individual led to rapid developments in science, philosophy, the arts, and
the establishment of democratic institutions. Similarly, in India of the
first millennium B.C.E., these new capacities led to developments in
medicine and astronomy, mathematics, logic, and grammar, and to the
emergence of democratic forms of governance in many small cities.

Along with these developments there came about a growing sense
of separation between the individual and his environment that, for
many, was unsettling. Cultural historian Jean Gebser describes the
process as "an extraordinary event which is literally earth-shaking...
an event that fundamentally alters the world."[4] The growing sense
of a separate self severed the protective circle of nature, which had
afforded the human being an intimate relationship with the cosmos.
As the world lost its womblike protectiveness, fear was the natural
result—fear of the natural world as well as a growing alienation from
one's fellow human beings. This was reflected in new philosophies and
religious doctrines that rejected the gods of the natural world, looking to an abstract skyward god in their place. The human body, full of
instincts and unruly passions, as to some extent was the natural world
as well, were seen as threats to the fledgling reasoning mind.

Pessimistic philosophies and religious doctrines emerged in both
Greece and India around this time, exerting an immense influence
on both Asian and European cultures for more than fifteen hundred
years. There were ascetics on both continents who saw this world as a
"vale of sorrows." For them, the "pure aesthetic pleasure derived from
contemplation [of the beauties of nature was] as wicked as scientific
curiosity."[5] All thought was to be directed toward God, and all enjoyments of the senses were to be scorned.

During the Middle Ages in Europe, the pessimistic ascetic response
grew in ascendancy to the point where it came to stifle intellectual learning and expression as well as exploration of the physical world. However,
the evolving mental consciousness continued to press forward toward
manifestation. By the end of the first millennium A.D., a small but growing number of European merchants and artisans had become dissatisfied with the world-negating emphasis of the predominant religious
culture. At the same time, many European scholars, as a result of con-

tact during the Crusades with the highly sophisticated culture of Islam, were inspired to reexamine their views toward intellectual inquiry.[a] Similar developments reflecting more complex aspects of the thinking mind were taking place throughout the world, from India and China to Ghana and parts of what are now the Americas.

The slowly increasing liberation of the thinking mind from the dominance of the physical and vital consciousness led in Renaissance Europe to a powerful longing for greater freedom. As the individual self continued to become more well defined, there emerged a growing desire for freedom from religious dogma as well as the oppressive social and political authority that predominated during the Middle Ages. The thinking mind has continued to become more complex since the beginning of the modern era. Having relied on the thinking mind as our primary instrument, we have created a world of such complexity and disharmony that at this point, only a power of consciousness greater than the mind will enable us to survive.

THE INFLUENCE OF THE INNER CONSCIOUSNESS ON THE DEVELOPMENT OF THE THINKING MIND

The experience of our early ancestors, before the flowering of civilization, may seem dull and impoverished compared to our own. Yet, cultural historian Jean Gebser tells us that early human beings lived in a state of consciousness in some ways far richer than that of modern humanity.[6] According to social scientist and futurist Duane Elgin, they lived in an astonishing world, one wild with wonder and beauty:

> [Their] world was experienced as... a magical place filled with unknown and uncontrollable forces, unexpected miracles and strange happenings. Nature was known as a living field, an animated and vital presence without clear edges or

---

a. In addition to the many original contributions of Islamic culture, the study of Greek philosophy and art—which Islamic scholars had engaged in during the medieval era—was transmitted to Europe during the Crusades, contributing immensely to cultural changes that led ultimately to the Renaissance.

boundaries between the natural and the supernatural. Where contemporary humans see a world filled with separate and lifeless things, the awakening hunter-gatherer saw a world of living and interconnected beings.[7]

From the perspective of yoga psychology, the richness of the experiential world of ancient humans derived from their openness to what Sri Aurobindo calls the "subliminal" or "inner" consciousness—what we've been referring to as the "dreaming" consciousness of the Infinite Knower. The forces and energies of this realm are the immense conscious-forces that pervade the universe: a far greater physical consciousness than we ordinarily experience, a far vaster and more complex world of vital energies, and a still vaster world of mental energies. They are of such magnitude that even the most powerful forces we know of in the physical universe—from the eruption of Mount Vesuvius to the explosion of a supernova, to the fury of a hurricane—are only small reflections of the much greater forces of the inner realm.

In humanity's distant past, before the thinking mind had come to dominate the physical and vital consciousness, it did not block access to the inner worlds to the extent it does today. Because the world experienced by our ancestors was not so clearly defined by thought, they did not perceive it to be so neatly delineated and carved up into separate, distinct objects. Similarly, because their self-sense was more fluid than ours, they felt deeply interconnected with the world around them. From the yogic perspective, this greater transparency between the inner and outer realms of consciousness is what gave such richness, depth, and magic to their experience.

Because we in modern times are no longer in touch with the living forces and beings that characterize the inner realm, we tend to look at the "magical" rituals and symbolism of premodern cultures as primitive superstitions. But from the yogic view, the rituals and symbols of the early human being evoked something he felt to be intimately

> present behind himself and his life and his activities—the Divine, the Gods, the vast and deep un-nameable, a hidden, living and mysterious nature of things. All his reli-

gious and social institutions, all the moments and phases of his life [are] to him symbols in which he seeks to express what he knows or guesses of the mystic influences that are behind his life and shape and govern or at least intervene in its movements.[8]

From the perspective of the view from nowhere, the "Gods" are no more than naïve personifications of what we now take to be impersonal, purely physical forces of nature. Sri Krishna Prem, one of the great yoga psychologists of recent times, turns this perspective inside out with the following statement made from within the view from infinity:

It is simply not true that Osiris is a vegetation, or Apollo a solar myth. Rather, if we must talk like this, we should say that vegetation is an Osiris myth and the sun a myth of Apollo, since Apollo and Osiris and all such names refer to facts of a higher order than those with which physical scientists deal.[9]

From the perspective of yoga psychology, the inner "dreaming" consciousness, the world of larger-than-life conscious-forces, is the immediate source out of which all physical objects in the universe take form, now and in every moment.[a] It is one of the major sources of our thoughts, feelings, and sensations as well.

Assuming the validity of the yogic perspective—that is, taking seriously the existence of the greater forces and beings of the "dream" or subliminal realm—how did we so completely lose touch with the inner consciousness?

We've looked at the fact that it is the tendency of the thinking mind to create distinctions. This tendency has served many important evolutionary purposes. It has helped bring order to the physical and vital consciousness. It has helped the vital consciousness pursue mastery of the material world with greater efficiency and effective-

---

a. And, as we will see in the next chapter, there is a still greater consciousness than the Dreaming Consciousness.

ness. It has also been instrumental in allowing for the development of a more clearly individualized sense of self, with the ultimate purpose of creating a unique focus of consciousness through which the Infinite Divine Being can experience Himself in an infinity of ways.

However, as we've seen, as the thinking mind became more complex (along with the civilization to which it gave shape), it became alienated from other aspects of consciousness. In addition to cutting itself off from the body and emotions, the rational mind, wary of the power of the "Gods"[a] to overwhelm it, cut itself off completely from the inner realm. This resulted in an almost exclusive focus on the outer world—a focus that constitutes William James's "filmy screen."

In ancient times, cultures had developed rich and complex support systems to help individuals navigate their encounters with the inner realms. However, in order to maintain the "screen," there arose a powerful taboo, particularly in Europe, against having any knowledge of or contact with the forces and beings of this realm. In the latter part of the Middle Ages this led to the burning of witches and the Inquisition. Due to the persistence of this taboo in modern times, an individual who inadvertently makes contact with these realms will meet with little or no understanding or support. Such contact often happens as a result of a trauma that thins the filmy screen and leads to a shocking encounter with forces of which most contemporary human beings know little or nothing. For the unlucky individual who enters within without sufficient preparation, the result is likely to be madness.

The story of John Custance, as told by psychiatrist Edward Podvoll in his book *The Seduction of Madness*, provides a sense of the inner forces that one encounters when the structure of the surface self becomes ruptured by a trauma of some kind.

~~~~~~

During World War II, Custance was engaged in intelligence work for the British government. Working long hours under intense pressure, he became increasingly high-strung, irritable, and depressed, and eventually suffered a severe breakdown. For the next twenty years, he

---

a. The cosmic, subtle physical, vital, and mental energies.

experienced repeating cycles of mania and depression.[a]

Believing he could control his "madness," he practiced giving free reign to his mind in order to help bring on the manic states. "I was carrying out a rather dangerous experiment... of letting myself go into mania with a view to seeing if I could control it. I found I could, but only with some difficulty and strain."[10] He became so fascinated by these experiences, particularly during the manic periods, that he began to record them in a series of journals and books.

During his manic states, Custance experienced an unusual intensification of his sensory perceptions. There was an increased clarity of vision and hearing, enabling him to distinguish far more qualities of sound than in his ordinary state. He developed a much finer discrimination between different smells and tastes. Even his body underwent a kind of metamorphosis, with his voice becoming deeper and richer, his body developing an extraordinary looseness and suppleness. Custance also became aware of what he described as channels of energy, which, when fully unobstructed, led to ecstatic and ultimately overwhelming sensations.

Writing of his experience at the highest pitch of mania, he describes feeling forced

> through the crust of normal consciousness and into illimitable unexplored caverns of the soul[b] in which hidden springs of being were somehow revealed in thoughts, fantasies and feelings[11]...The world is transforming itself around me as I write; it is coming alive, and all the Powers of actuality, the spirits of the past, the gods and goddesses, yes and the devils too, tell me to let them have their way.[12]

Of the eight most severe manic episodes Custance experienced, five were followed by months of suicidal depression as intensely negative as the mania was positive. When he felt the manic state beginning to wane, he recognized this meant the onset of a crushing period of depression.

---

a. What is now referred to as "bipolar disorder."

b. It seems likely that by "soul," Custance was not referring to the true soul, but a vital-mental formation within the inner realm of consciousness.

Podvoll explains that

> almost all psychotic occurrences of whatever species
> (organic, chemical, situational) can be seen to be infused by
> manic consciousness at their onset or as they recycle. This
> consciousness is usually reported to have a dreamlike qual-
> ity. Some people who have experienced this state call it the
> "dream time," the "dream world," or the "dream machine."
> The sense of time, space, cause and effect; the availabil-
> ity of memory images, the way external perceptions are
> woven into the ongoing scenario, the shifting of experience
> between subject and object, the play with words and puns;
> the electrical sense of power and magic, and above all the
> sense of conviction in the reality of what is in front of one's
> eyes—are all marks of both manic and dream consciousness.
> It could be said that manic consciousness borrows, or per-
> haps commandeers, the mechanics of dreaming.[13]

Elaborating, Podvoll writes that

> mania is marked by the activation of dream states of con-
> sciousness within the apparent state of wakeful activity.[a] Such
> dream states become mixed with moment-to-moment sen-
> sations. And in mania, thoughts and images intensified by
> the heightened senses are made abnormally vivid, compelling,
> and "often so overpowering that they cause marked physi-
> cal sensations."[14] This mixture of dream state and heightened
> wakefulness allows underlying urges or instincts the freedom
> to express themselves…The resulting state of mind is thus
> experienced as magical and beyond conventional patterns and
> constraints. Its possibilities appear limitless.[15]

---

a. The inner consciousness is not "state-specific," as is clear from Podvoll's
description. One can be completely aware of the inner realm while in the waking or dream states.

From the yogic perspective, looking at Custance's description together with Podvoll's explanation, it is clear that what he experienced was an opening to the powerful forces of the inner realm. In the inner realm, the consciousness is in more direct contact with the physical world, leading to a powerful intensification of sensory experience. Custance spoke of "channels of energy," which appear to be similar to what the yogis call *nadis,* currents of subtle energy running throughout the body.[a] His reference to nonphysical beings would most likely be taken by the average contemporary individual to be signs of a diseased mind. However, if science begins to make use of yogic methodology to explore subjective experience, the objective[b] existence of such beings may eventually be confirmed.

Custance's experience helps us understand why the ancient explorers of the inner worlds warned against pursuing such exploration without proper preparation or right motive. Unlike the experience of the Soul consciousness, which is always calm and luminous, the inner worlds—intermediate between the Soul and the surface nature—are subject to ego, and thus, distortion. In fact, the distortions with which we're familiar in our surface nature can be more exaggerated and powerful in this more vivid realm of consciousness. This is why a precipitous entry into the inner realm can be so dangerous, leading to states of disorientation and imbalance. The best safeguard against such egoic distortion is to have a calm, deep, and steadfast openness to the influence of the true Soul.

THE LIMITATIONS OF THE THINKING MIND

At the present time, our alienation from the inner consciousness has become extreme, and our experience of the world has become greatly impoverished as a result. Another consequence of our overreliance on

---

a. In Chinese medicine these are referred to as "meridians." The differing descriptions in Chinese and Indian texts do not necessarily point to contradictions. Rather, they illustrate the subtle, pliable, and ever-changing nature of the inner realms.

b. Or, if one prefers, "intersubjective."

the outer, analytic mind has been a lack of harmony among the different aspects of our consciousness. In Sri Aurobindo's words:

> The Life is at war with the body; it attempts to force it to sat-
> isfy life's desires, impulses, satisfactions and demands from its
> limited capacity what could only be possible to an immortal
> and divine body; and the body, enslaved and tyrannised over,
> suffers and is in constant dumb revolt against the demands
> made upon it by the Life. The Mind is at war with both: some-
> times it helps the Life against the Body, sometimes restrains
> the vital urge and seeks to protect the corporeal frame from
> life's desires, passions and over-driving energies; it also seeks
> to possess the Life and turn its energy to the mind's own
> ends, and the Life too finds itself enslaved and misused and is
> in frequent insurrection against the ignorant half-wise tyrant
> seated above it. This is the war of our members which the
> mind cannot satisfactorily resolve because it has to deal with
> a problem insoluble to it, the aspiration of an immortal being
> in a mortal life and body.[16]

In recent times the dividing tendency of the thinking mind has
come to have still greater influence, with a resulting increase in conflict and alienation from our deeper selves. Several centuries ago, Galileo and Descartes applied mathematics to the investigation of matter,
analyzing it into ever-smaller component parts. In the past century,
individuals in other disciplines began using measurement to understand and gain control over their respective fields of endeavor. Applied
to economics, the love of measurement has led to the misuse of "cost-
benefit analysis"—weighing the material pros and cons of financial
decisions without taking into account the human consequences. In
biology, this habit of "divide and conquer" has reduced living creatures
to a collection of parts, leaving the nature of the living organism a
mystery. In psychology it threatens to reduce us to a series of quantifiable brain and other biochemical processes.

This analytic mode of thought, in turn, has had a great impact on those who have employed it to the exclusion of other ways of knowing. In a particularly poignant account of this, Charles Darwin writes in his autobiography:

> Up to the age of thirty, or beyond it, poetry of many kinds... gave me great pleasure...I have also said that formerly pictures gave me considerable and music very great delight. But now for many years I cannot endure to read a line of poetry...I have also lost almost any taste for pictures or music...My mind seems to have become a kind of machine for grinding general laws out of large collections of fact, but why this should have caused the atrophy of that part of the brain alone, on which the higher tastes depend, I cannot conceive...The loss of these tastes is a loss of happiness, and may possibly be injurious to the intellect, and more probably to the moral character, by enfeebling the emotional part of our nature.[17]

As the analytic tendency of mind has come to affect greater numbers of people, it has led to widespread feelings of loneliness and isolation. Describing this trend, Jean Gebser writes:

> Compelled to emphasize his [separate and distinct individuality] ever more strongly... man faces the world in hostile confrontation...Isolation is visible everywhere, isolation of individuals, of entire nations and continents.[18]

Focusing on the understanding and conquest of the material world, the analytic mind has ended up analyzing away mind, consciousness, and spirit. Beyond that, we seem to have lost our moorings with respect to matter as well. The process that began with dividing up the physical world did not stop until the very atom was split, revealing a strange, incomprehensible world.

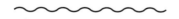

The emergence of the thinking mind heralded a new phase of evolution, the awakening of the universe to self-consciousness. Complex thought has enabled human beings to create great civilizations, beautiful works of art, and machines of immense utility and staggering complexity. Because of their capacity for self-reflection, humans can choose to direct their lives toward the achievement of noble aims, working for causes beyond their own narrow self-interest. They can aspire to create a world in which beauty and harmony prevail. Ultimately, the gift of self-consciousness has made them capable of awakening to the Infinite.

However, neither the most discriminating analysis nor the most integrated mental synthesis will suffice to resolve the problems that stem from the essential limitations of the mind. No matter how it attempts to put together what it has divided into parts, the mind can never arrive at the unified vision that alone can ultimately resolve the problems facing humanity. The action of the mind deals

> with wholes that form part of a greater whole, and these subordinate wholes again are broken up into parts which are also treated as wholes...Mind may divide, multiply, add, subtract, but it cannot get beyond the limits of this mathematics. If it goes beyond and tries to conceive a real whole, it loses itself in a foreign element; it falls from its own firm ground into the ocean of the intangible, into the abysms of the infinite...Mind cannot possess the infinite, it can only suffer it or be possessed by it; it can only lie blissfully helpless under the luminous shadow of the Real cast down on it from planes of existence beyond its reach.[19]

Sitting on the wooden bench in her father's backyard, Sharon is staring at the bottle of pills in her hand. She feels frozen—unable to move, barely able to think. Her thoughts go to her car parked in front of the house…maybe she'll drive up to the mountains to that secluded forest several miles past Clarissa's house… the note… she has to write a note…

"Sharon." It takes a moment before she registers the sound of her brother's voice. Catching her breath, her hand tightens around the bottle. She doesn't respond. Willie approaches the bench. As he sits down, he sees the pills in her hand, waits for a moment, then softly repeats, "Sharon?" As she struggles to find her voice, her body starts to tremble and she begins to cry. Willie gently places his hand on her shoulder. Slowly, Sharon pulls herself together and begins to speak.

"I always thought if I just kept going, I'd be able to figure it all out. I don't know why nothing was ever enough. I loved the people in the neighborhood who came by the store every day. I loved helping those women set up their own businesses… I don't know, maybe I shouldn't have given up medicine… Nothing is making sense anymore. I just can't go on pretending…

Sharon stops talking, and they sit quietly, watching the fish playing just below the surface of the pond. Her attention is drawn to the sound of leaves rustling in the wind. For the moment, she feels safe with her brother sitting by her side. She looks over to the large oak tree on her left and recognizes that her mind has become calm. As her heart softens, she feels something stirring inside and becomes aware of a kind of presence, something strange yet familiar…

PART III

THE KNOWER OF THE FIELD

OVERVIEW

Up until this point we've been speaking mostly about the evolution of the Field of Conscious-Energy. Now we turn to the Knower of the Field. In chapter 12 we tell the story of the evolving Soul—the individual Knower, the "I AM" we are in truth in the depths of our being. In chapter 13, we look at how the "ego" is constructed—the false identity we mistakenly take ourselves to be.

Cultivating Inner Silence

There is a background for everything. Every movement moves upon something.

And that something is a Silence which upholds everything including your own mental activity. All the thoughts and mental movements come and go, against a base that is ever stable. That is Silence...

Suspend for a moment your thought-activity and you'll become conscious of this presence.

...Think of this Silence again and again and try to become aware of it. By a steady digging in of this idea in your consciousness, this fact will become a reality to you—not merely for the mind but for the rest of the being.

Into this Silence you must learn to relax yourself.

Instead of trying to get at it, simply relax, call and let yourself lie in the folds of the Silence.

That will slowly come over you and claim you.[1]

—Kapali Sastry, paraphrasing Sri Aurobindo

> Consciousness is... the fundamental thing in existence—It is the energy, the motion, the movement of consciousness that creates the universe and all that is in it... [Consciousness] can subjectively formulate itself as a physical, a vital, a mental, a psychic consciousness—all these are present ... but as they are all mixed up together in the external consciousness with their real status behind in the inner being, one can only become fully aware of them by releasing the original limiting stress of the consciousness which makes us live in our external being and become awake and centred within... If [the consciousness] goes inside, puts its centralising stress there, then it knows itself as the inner being or, still deeper, as the psychic being... Then we can become aware of the large and rich and inexhaustible kingdom within.[1]
>
> —Sri Aurobindo

CHAPTER 12

The Soul and the Psychic Being: The Knower "Within" the Field

The true soul[a] secret in us...burns in the temple of the inmost heart behind the thick screen of an ignorant mind, life and body... the flame of the Godhead always alight within us. It is a flame born out of the Divine and,

---

a. As Sri Aurobindo defines it, the individual Soul—the Knower within the Field—"is a spark of the Divine Spirit which supports the individual nature." Over the course of evolution, it develops a "soul individuality [the psychic being] which grows from life to life, using the evolving mind, vital and body as its instruments." The term "psychic being" is derived from the Greek word "psyche,"

luminous inhabitant of the Ignorance, grows in it till it is able to turn it towards the Knowledge. It is the concealed Witness and Control, the hidden Guide, the Daemon of Socrates, the inner light or inner voice of the mystic. It is that which endures and is imperishable in us from birth to birth, untouched by death, decay or corruption, an indestructible spark of the Divine.[2]

—Sri Aurobindo

In the beginning, the Soul—the Knower within the Field—was asleep, completely absorbed in Its movements of Conscious-Energy. Over billions of years of evolution the Soul gradually awakened, becoming increasingly able to step back from those movements and become aware of them. Eventually human beings emerged with the capacity for self-awareness, making it possible for the Soul to finally awaken fully. While it is the Light of the Soul that illumines our every thought, feeling, and sensation, to the extent our attention continues to be absorbed in the surface movements, we remain unaware of the Source of illumination by which we experience them:

> We must go inwards if we would find [the source of the Light of Consciousness]. Like salmon in the breeding season we must ascend that River…as an arrow we must shoot ourselves against the current to the Source from which it springs. There and there only shall we find the Bliss that throbs at the heart of being, the Bliss that is the World's desire and whose reflections in the forms that come and go, lend the attractiveness to our desires.

> When that Point is reached a wonderful sight is seen. The Waters of Light that we have traced back, narrowing and narrowing to their Source, are seen to widen out again on the

and has nothing to do with what is commonly referred to as "psychic" powers. Following Sri Aurobindo's usage, we sometimes use the word "soul" to refer to the psychic being. The meaning should be clear in context.

other side into a great Ocean of calm and living Light whose blue waters shine with a radiance never before beheld.[3]

Finding this Infinite Consciousness in the depths of our being, we can taste the Delight that moves the planets and the stars, and makes up the ground on which we walk as well as the cells and organs of our bodies:

> Softly the waters rise and fall in ceaseless rhythm and with each wave a throb of bliss pulses through the watching Soul, so that, forgetting all, it longs to plunge for ever in their cool depths.

> It is the eternal Summer Sea, the Sea whose waters wash for ever the inner shores of being. A channel leading to it is to be found in the heart of every living creature and all these separate channels lead to the same Sea, one and all-pervading, in whose Waters all sense of separateness is lost. Therefore we are bidden to seek the Way in our own hearts for only there shall we find it.

> As it bursts upon our view we realize that it is That for which all our life we have been seeking. Nor has our search been confined to this one life alone. Spurred on by a dim memory of having known it long ago, we have wandered on and on through life after life in a darkness so great that we have almost forgotten that this Sea of Light existed. Always it has lured us on over the next range of hills and always when we got there the view disclosed has been of a country similar to the ones we have been wandering through so long. Only when we realize that the blue light that makes those far hills so magical comes from a Light that shines within our eyes do we call a halt to our endless wanderings, and, turning back upon ourselves, enter the Stream that leads us to the Sea.[4]

In all ages there have been testimonials to this experience of the Soul, the Unborn, Infinite Being who is seeing through our eyes, hearing through our ears in this and every moment. And the experience is not confined to the yoga tradition of India. It is found in spiritual traditions the world over. Seventeenth-century French Christian monk Brother Lawrence, known for the "practice of the presence of God," described it as a feeling of boundless love filling the air as he moved through the world. Llewellyn Vaughan-Lee, a contemporary Sufi teacher,[a] writes of something similar:

> Sometimes I feel this love during the day, and the heart is so happy knowing that He is near. Then joy suffuses everything and there is a sense of sunlight everywhere. Not just the heart, but the whole body feels the joy of the sacred. There is a deep happiness that has nothing to do with external circumstances, and even difficult outer situations do not infringe upon this inner joy. Wherever I walk, each breath carries the beauty of an early summer day.[5]

THE EVOLUTION OF THE SOUL

> Your life on this earth is a divine poem that you are translating into earthly language.[6]
>
> —Sri Aurobindo

The Soul, as described by Sri Aurobindo, is a "spark" of the Divine Consciousness residing in the heart of all things. Infinite, boundless, eternal, the source of all joy and bliss, the Soul is our personal, intimate connection to the Divine Presence. Manifesting simply as a diffuse spark in matter and plants, it slowly becomes more

---

a. Sufism is a mystical sect of Islam.

organized, more complex in animals, and still more fully defined in human beings as the psychic being "which changes, grows, develops from life to life."[7] In most human beings the psychic being is hidden behind the dense intermingling of physical, vital, and mental energies, influencing the outer personality as best it can through a thick web of thoughts, feelings, and desires.

The soul willingly forgets its Oneness with the Infinite in order to undertake the evolutionary journey. It accepts its temporary limitations for the sake of participation in the cosmic game of hide-and-seek, for the pure joy of self-discovery. However, always possessed of a dim remembrance of its unbroken connection to the Divine, it aspires for reunion:

> [The aspiration for reunion] is not limited to human beings...Look at the flowers and trees. When the sun sets and all becomes silent, sit down for a moment and put yourself into communion with Nature: you will feel rising from the earth, from below the roots of the trees and mounting upward and coursing through their fibers up to the highest outstretching branches, the aspiration of an intense love and longing, a longing for something that brings light and gives happiness, for the light that is gone and they wish to have back again. There is a yearning so pure and intense that if you can feel the movement in the trees, your own being too will go up in an ardent prayer for the peace and light and love that are unmanifested here.[8]

As long as the consciousness of the Soul is hidden from the surface, it cannot fully participate in this game. When self-consciousness emerges in humans, the awakening of the Soul becomes possible for the first time. However, most individuals, limited to their surface consciousness, remain unaware of the promptings of the Soul from within. And, even when some of the Soul's Light does make its way to the surface, it easily becomes distorted:

> [T]he soul is at first but a spark and then a little flame of
> godhead burning in the midst of a great darkness; for the
> most part it is veiled in its inner sanctum and to reveal itself
> it has to call on the mind, the life-force and the physical con-
> sciousness and persuade them, as best they can, to express it;
> ordinarily, it succeeds at most in suffusing their outwardness
> with its inner light and modifying with its purifying fine-
> ness their dark obscurities or their coarser mixture.[9]

Restless, unsettled, ever dissatisfied, the human being tries but
cannot find fulfillment outside himself. Whatever temporary satisfaction he achieves soon fades as he discovers, once again, this is not what
he was looking for. Sri Aurobindo describes this unsettled state as
"a hurtling field of joy and grief, love and hatred, hopes, disappoint-
ments, gratitude, revenge and all the stupendous play of passion which
is the drama of life in the world." Because these intense feelings are so
compelling and feel so much a part of us, we tend to mistake them for
promptings of the Soul:

> But the real soul...which for the most part we see little of
> and only a small minority in mankind has developed, is an
> instrument of pure love, joy and the luminous reaching out
> to fusion and unity with God and our fellow-creatures.[10]

The drive to fulfill our surface desires, the pull of our unconscious
evolutionary past, the wish to maintain a separate personality—all
make it difficult to fully awaken and discover our true nature. But
despite these difficulties, we can have intimations of the Soul. In fact,
we do all the time if we know where to look, if we "stay awake" to the
clues that are ever around and within us.

INTIMATIONS

I have felt

A presence that disturbs me with the joy

Of elevated thoughts; a sense sublime

Of something far more deeply interfused,

Whose dwelling is the light of setting suns,

And the round ocean and the living air,

And the blue sky, and in the mind of man;

A motion and a spirit, that impels

All thinking things, all objects of all thought,

And rolls through all things.[11]

—William Wordsworth

"Stay awake," Jesus told his disciples, because the spirit may visit when we are least aware. In the midst of the seemingly mundane, there are moments when the light of our Soul may shine brightly enough to catch our attention—if we are sufficiently awake. Rushing to meet a deadline, we pass a coworker whose face is laced with pain. Moved by some nameless force within, we pause—perhaps uncharacteristically—and allow ourselves to be touched by their hurt, and in the process a previously unknown depth of feeling rises to the surface.

Walking down a dark city street strewn with empty coffee cups, half-smoked cigarettes, and other discarded remnants of the workday, we feel uneasy, our hearts heavy. Turning the corner, we're struck by the outline of a building previously unnoticed. Its strange symmetry and subtle curves touch us deeply, and, without realizing it, we stop to take in the scene more fully while others pass us by. Our mind grows quiet, something inside us resonates with something in the simple elegance of the design. Slowly, mysteriously, our hearts open and a feeling of nostalgia steals over us.

What is the source of this "sense sublime of something far more deeply interfused, whose dwelling is the light of setting suns"?

Somehow, in spite of the conditioning to which we are relentlessly subject in a consumer society, we continue to have moments that remind us of something inside we find difficult to forget and hard to explain away. The Portuguese have a beautiful word for this special kind of nostalgia, this homesickness for the majesty and sweetness of our innermost depths—*saudade* (so-dah'de), a deep longing or ardent desire. Sufism, the mystic tradition of Islam, gives us a clue to the origin of this nostalgia when it declares, "That which you are looking for is that which is looking."

Perhaps our sophisticated modern mind objects to the suggestion of a deeper reality. If there is a "Soul" of some kind, why can't we see or touch it? Given the widespread absence of any direct experience of this deeper reality, religions call upon their followers to have a mental faith in the existence of the soul. Yet even in those who consider themselves to be ardent believers, this faith often coexists with an undercurrent of doubt. In the yoga tradition, the word *shraddha*—usually translated as "faith"—actually conveys something more than mere mental or even emotional "belief." Beyond a belief of the mind or a feeling of the heart, *shraddha* refers to those glimmers of light that reach the surface consciousness from the depths of our being—"the gleam sent before by the yet unrisen sun."[12] These direct intimations of the Soul can serve as a reference point and guide. All of the more limited forms of faith are intimations of this deeper *shraddha*.

Even in its more dilute forms, faith can have a powerful effect on virtually every aspect of our lives. In medicine, for example, a mental faith—what psychologists refer to as "expectation"—underlies the potency of the placebo effect. Though an apparently inert substance, the placebo has been shown to exert a definitive healing effect. Within mainstream medicine, its healing power is considered by some to be evidence of the power of the mind to affect the body. As Alan Wallace observes, "If the placebo effect could be reduced to some physical substance or mechanism, the production of that biological phenomenon would be a multi-billion dollar industry."[13]

But we don't need a tablet or injection to harness the power of faith.

Our attention, when intensely focused by a clear intent or aim, is sufficient to effect far-reaching changes in the mind, body, and emotions. Scientists have determined that through the power of the mind alone, it is possible to reduce the symptoms of, or actually cure, a wide variety of both psychological and physical illnesses, including depression, anxiety, asthma, and arthritis. Psychologists like Martin Seligman speak of "learned optimism"—which might be considered a secular translation of "faith"—as an essential factor in psychological health. Dr. Herbert Benson, who coined the term "relaxation response," found what he calls the "faith factor" to be an essential element in all mind-body healing.

While a vital or mental faith in the possibility of healing has been shown to yield powerful results, from the perspective of yoga psychology, it is the deeper faith or *shraddha* of the Soul that has "the power to move mountains." Nineteenth-century psychologists like William James, open to the philosophies of both East and West, spoke of a power of volition emanating from a source deeper than that of the surface consciousness. James's own philosophy of pragmatism was strongly influenced by yogic tenets, such as the one embodied in this verse from the *Bhagavad Gita:* "Whatever is a man's faith, that he is" (and, as Sri Aurobindo elaborates, "Whatever he has the faith to see as possible in himself and strive for, that he can create and become"). [14]

In contemporary society, desire has become the main motivating force behind individual and societal action. In such an environment, the notion of *shraddha* or faith as the reflection of a deeper soul knowledge becomes the object of deep skepticism—if not outright scorn. Or it may become a guise through which desire asserts itself. When Abraham Lincoln appealed to the "better angels of our nature," he was attempting to direct our attention to something deeper than the Freudian conscience, or "superego." According to yoga psychology,

> [I]t is [the Soul] which is the true original Conscience in us deeper than the constructed and conventional conscience of the moralist, for it is this which points always towards Truth and Right and Beauty, towards Love and Harmony and all that is a divine possibility in us, and persists till these things become the major need of our nature. [15]

It is because we have so long followed the siren call of desire[a] that we have almost entirely lost touch with this deeper Conscience within. The yoga tradition has always taught the necessity of stilling the din of desire in order to hear the softer voice of the Soul. Much as an auto mechanic can learn to hear the slightest knock in an engine that would be imperceptible to the untrained ear, so can we learn to hear even the softest murmur of the innermost consciousness, the wordless promptings of the Soul making their way to the surface. As the power of inner quietude grows, a faculty develops that can, in any situation, discern the path most in harmony with our innermost being.

For a long time, however, it is easy to mistake our desires for something deeper, coming as they so often do with the compelling force of the vital consciousness, and having, as they do, their ultimate origin in the Soul. In Sri Aurobindo's words,

> Where the [soul] personality is weak, crude or ill-developed... even though the mind may be forceful and brilliant, the heart... strong and masterful, the life-force dominant and successful, ... the outer desire-soul... reigns and we mistake... its desires and yearnings for true soul-stuff.[16]

There is much talk these days of the "soul"—the soul of business, the soul of law, "care of the soul." But is it the true Soul or what Sri Aurobindo has called the "outer desire soul"? For all too many of us, behind the explicit aspiration to "let Thy Will be done" is the implicit demand, "if only Thou wouldst let *my* will be done."

In order to develop sufficient discernment to be able to rely safely on the promptings of our inner voice, it is necessary to leave the surface awareness and plunge even more deeply within than the inner consciousness. Having sufficiently calmed the surface waves of thought, feeling, and sensation, we can enter into that sacred domain for which,

---

a. Urged on, to a great extent, by relentless advertising that pervades our lives as well as leaders who tell us it is our patriotic duty to keep shopping during times of national crisis.

often without realizing it, we so deeply long. Calming the clamor of the surface, and stilling the subtler stirrings of the inner consciousness, we can follow the thread of our longing and restlessness "to the Source from which it springs."[17]

GOING WITHIN

> To find the soul you must withdraw from the surface, silence your mind as far as possible, and enter deep into the core of your heart beyond all sensations and thoughts. You must draw back from the surface, withdraw into the deep and enter... go down and down... into a pit deep, silent, immobile...There you see something warm, quiet, of a rich substance, very still and very full, and exceedingly soft—that is the soul. And if you continue and are conscious... there comes a feeling of plenitude, something full, with unfathomable depths. You feel that if you entered there, many secrets would be revealed; it's like the reflection of something eternal on a calm, peaceful surface of water. Time doesn't exist anymore. You have the impression of having always been and of being for eternity.[18]

Fortified by our awakening faith in a greater reality, we can begin to focus all our attention on listening for the still, small voice of the Soul. We can become like the lone wayfarer wandering through the forest, suddenly captivated by the notes of a distant melody wafting softly through the trees. Stopping to listen, the body and mind are unified, effortlessly poised in one-pointed attentiveness to the beauty of a far-off song. When our yearning for the soul arises as spontaneously and becomes as all-consuming as that of the wayfarer for his song, we naturally, joyfully focus on what has been the true object of our yearning all along.

The Tree at the End of the Earth

Sitting next to Willie on the bench, the feeling of that "strange yet familiar presence" becomes more intense. Feeling uneasy, Sharon's mind becomes active trying to analyze what is happening to her. Willie, sensing the shift in the atmosphere, seeing the intent look on his sister's face, tells her to just let it be, not to worry about trying to figure it out. They sit in silence, together becoming aware of something filling the air, surrounding and embracing them.

As her mind grows still quieter, Sharon's attention is drawn to a leaf falling from the large oak tree to her left. Thoughts about what is happening continue to arise in her mind, but, ignoring them, the feeling of a pervading presence continues to grow. A warm feeling of delight, like an inner smile, grows deep within her.

Some days later, searching for words to convey her experience, Sharon said it was as though she had been sitting next to "the tree at the end of the earth." For a long time afterward, it was in recalling this experience beside the tree that she was able to recapture—if only for brief interludes—a sense of peace and contentment. With the emergence of this deeper consciousness, Sharon would be able to begin to harmonize and integrate the many conflicting parts of herself, a process that would ultimately take not just one life but many lifetimes.

Rebirth: Across the Gap of Death

> The body of Benjamin Franklin, printer (like the cover of an old book, its contents torn out and stripped of its lettering and gilding), lies here, food for worms: but the work shall not be lost, it will (as he believed) appear once more in a new and more elegant edition... revised and corrected by the author. [19]
>
> —Epitaph of Benjamin Franklin (Self-composed)

> [The Soul, the] inmost entity... puts forward a psychic personality [the psychic being], which changes, grows, develops

> from life to life; for this is the traveler between birth and
> death and between death and birth, our [surface personality
> is] only its manifold and changing vesture.[20]
>
> —Sri Aurobindo

According to Sri Aurobindo, the purpose of rebirth is the evolution of consciousness. This evolution is not just for the sake of awakening the Soul to its true nature, but for expressing its infinite and unique qualities. Over the course of many lifetimes, the growing psychic being strengthens its connection to the Divine Soul behind, making it possible for the essential soul nature to be communicated more directly to the outer personality. In moments of special intensity, we may become aware of an inexplicable attraction or affinity, drawing us toward some goal of which we are—on the surface—entirely unconscious. These may be intimations of our true Divine Nature, summoning us to some work that is aligned with our deeper purpose. In those whose psychic being is more awake, such intimations may emerge spontaneously, or may be summoned by the touch of a synchronous outer event.

Lama Govinda was a German man who spent many years studying Buddhism in Tibet. In the course of his life he received several striking confirmations that the work to which he had been drawn was an expression of his Soul that transcended the surface personality of his current lifetime. As a child he had written a story describing his spiritual beliefs and experiences—a story he thought one day to expand into a mystic novel. Years later as a young man, he read that story to an archaeologist friend who suggested he look at the work of a writer who, more than a century earlier, had started a similar novel that was left unfinished due to the writer's early demise. Intrigued, Lama Govinda sought out this author's works and found that not only were the ideas and characteristic phrases of the author uncannily similar to his own, but certain passages were literally identical. He also discovered that the writer had died of the same disease that had brought Lama Govinda to the sanatorium where he met his archaeologist friend.[a]

---

a. For the skeptical reader, we include in Appendix A (Science and Yoga) some information regarding rigorous scientific research on rebirth.

Around the same time, he attended a gathering where he was introduced to a man who happened to be writing a biography of the deceased author. The man stared at Lama Govinda in shock because of the striking resemblance he bore to the only existing portrait of the author. More significantly, the earlier author had outlined a spiritual vision of the universe—an outline that precisely mirrored a plan Lama Govinda, as a youth, had drawn up for his present life's work. He had realized the plan was too large in scope to be fulfilled in a single lifetime and had contented himself with addressing those subjects to which he felt most drawn by training or temperament. Lama Govinda later wrote that being able to pursue his work in the context of many lifetimes filled him with such peace and confidence that he was able to concentrate unhurriedly on the task of the moment, trusting that whatever was left undone would be continued in lives to come.

Lama Govinda had been living out his Soul's calling across lifetimes but had been unaware of it until, as an adult, he encountered the series of "coincidences" initiated by reading his story to a friend. While traveling in Burma in the 1930s, he met an eight-year-old boy who had awakened to the continuity of his Soul's work at the age of four. Lama Govinda described seeing the little boy preach: "It was an astonishing sight to see a small boy speaking with the ease and self-assurance of a practiced speaker, his face radiant with happiness and his voice clear and melodious like a bell... it was a joy to hear this voice, that seemed to come straight from the depth of his heart like the song of a bird."[21] Lama Govinda later met with the boy's father, who told him this story.[22]

One day, on the way to a local fair, he and his two sons met up with a man who offered sugarcane to the children. The younger boy eagerly took the candy, but four-year-old Maung Tun Kyaing told him, in a rather authoritative tone, not to eat it until he had offered a blessing of gratitude. As he uttered his admonition, a memory suddenly awakened and he directed his father to lift him to his shoulders so that he could give a sermon to the people on the virtues of giving. Considering this a childish whim, his father good-naturedly did as he was told. Much to his surprise, his little son began to speak with an eloquence and wisdom way beyond his years. Crowds gathered to hear him preach, but Maung Tun Kyaing was unfazed. Upon completing his sermon, he turned to his father and said, "Come...let us go to my [monastery]."[23]

The boy gave directions to a nearby monastery—one he had never visited—and was taken there by his father. When the senior abbot came to meet them, the boy, rather than bowing as he had been taught, greeted the monk as an equal. The abbot said to him:

> "Don't you know [I am the head of this monastery]?"
>
> "Certainly I know!" said the boy without the slightest hesitation. And when the [abbot] looked at him in surprise the boy mentioned [the abbott's] name.
>
> "How do you know? Did somebody tell you?"
>
> "No," said the boy. "Don't you remember me? I was your teacher, U Pandeissa."
>
> The abbot was taken aback, but in order to test him he asked the boy, "If that is so, what was my name before I entered the Order? If you know it you may whisper it into my ear."
>
> The boy did so. And when the Abbott heard his name, which nobody knew except those who had grown old with him and had known him intimately, he fell at the boy's feet, touched the ground with his forehead, and exclaimed with tears in his eyes: "Now I know, you are indeed my teacher."[24]

Lama Govinda goes on to recount further tests that were given to Maung Tun Kyaing in order to make certain he was indeed who he claimed to be. The boy led the others through the monastery, pointing out the room where he had slept, his meditation room, and many details of his former daily routine. In addition, the boy was able to read and interpret the Buddhist scriptures, written in the ancient language Pali, despite having grown up in a home where nobody knew how to read or write.

After all these proofs, nobody doubted he was a rebirth of the former abbot. Subsequently, the four-year-old boy received numerous invitations to preach, and he spoke before groups of hundreds and thousands of people. When his family expressed concern that his health might be affected by his extensive preaching, he declared: "The Buddha spent innumerable lives in self-sacrificing deeds, striving to attain enlightenment. I too, therefore, should not spare any pains in striving after Buddhahood. Only by attaining the highest aim can I work for the benefit of all living beings."[25]

Soon news of the young boy's fame reached Sir Henry Butler, then governor of Burma, who wanted to determine for himself the veracity of the boy's story. After hearing only a little of the child's masterful exposition of the essential teachings of Buddhism, any doubts he may have had were quelled. It was obvious to the governor that the boy was expressing his own understanding and not simply reciting words he had been taught.

According to Lama Govinda, Maung Tun Kyaing

> spoke with such conviction and sincerity that Sir Henry was visibly moved and encouraged the boy to bring his message to all the people of Burma. "You should go from one end of the country to the other," he said, "and preach to high and low, even to the prisoners in the jails, because nobody could touch the heart of the people deeper than you. Even the hardest criminal would melt in the presence of such genuine faith and sincere good will."

> And thus it happened that even the gates of the jails were opened to Maung Tun Kyaing and wherever he went he inspired the people with new religious fervor, strengthening their convictions and filling them with fresh life.[26]

> Consciousness is... the fundamental thing in existence—it is the energy, the motion, the movement of consciousness that creates the universe and all that is in it... [It is the] external concentration or... limiting stress of the consciousness which makes us live in our external being.[1]
>
> —Sri Aurobindo

CHAPTER 13

Ego: The Mistaken Sense of Self

> The apparent freedom and self assertion of our [surface personality] to which we are so profoundly attached, conceal a most pitiable subjection to a thousand suggestions, impulsions, [and] forces...[2] When the human ego...realizes that its will is a tool, its wisdom ignorance and childishness, its power an infant's groping, its virtue a pretentious impurity and learns to trust itself to that which transcends it, that is its salvation.[3]
>
> —Sri Aurobindo

When we say "I," to what are we referring? We normally think "we" know who "we" are. "I" am sitting here, reading this book. "I" am walking there, to meet my friend. But behind, within and all around this little "I" lies the infinite, unbounded Self. This hidden "I" of our True Nature is all the time seeking to emerge into our awareness, into full self-expression. The force of its seeking is what impels us to travel to the ends of earth to satisfy our heart's desire. But the farther we travel, the greater does our dissatisfaction become. All the while, that which we seek is looking out through our eyes, patiently waiting for us to stop and turn within.

According to yoga psychology, when we turn within, we discover ourselves to be spiritual beings whose essential nature is infinitely calm and luminous. But how can we reconcile this assertion with our ordinary experience, with the everyday reality of dull routine, conflicted relationships, the insatiable craving for wealth and pleasure, random and deliberate acts of violence? If the true "Self," the Eternal Knower beyond space and time, is innately blissful, why is there so much heartache and pain, so much cruelty and insensitivity between people?

The fact that we—who are in truth infinite beings—mistakenly identify ourselves with finite movements of the physical, vital, and mental nature, is the root of all our problems and the cause of all evil and suffering. Yoga psychology refers to this mistaken act of identification as "ego."[a]

THE NATURE AND ORIGIN OF THE EGO

The ego is little more than an imaginary point around which a habitual stream of thoughts, feelings, and sensations is kept in orbit:

> This self we prize so dearly and to which we subordinate all
> is a mere emptiness, the empty heart of a whirlpool, a mathematical point which changes its position, not only from
> year to year, but even from hour to hour, as a man shifts
> from his "business" integration to that which is manifested
> at his home or his club.[4]

Out of all our sense impressions, we subconsciously select certain repeating patterns that we identify as "my body." The identification with this particular set of sense impressions could be called the "physical ego." Similarly, a "vital ego" is shaped through our identification with certain

---

a. The Sanskrit word for "ego" is *ahamkara* – literally, the "I-maker."

repeating emotional patterns, and a "mental ego" by virtue of our identification with habitual patterns of thought, memory, belief, and the like:

> In a certain sense we are nothing but a complex mass of
> mental, [vital] and physical habits held together by a few
> ruling ideas, desires and associations—an amalgam of many
> small self-repeating forces with a few major vibrations.[5]

The ego binds up the consciousness of the psychic being in the
play of the surface nature, creating a kind of mistaken identity. Imagine an actor who has forgotten he has an identity apart from the roles
he plays. He believes himself to be first Othello, then a struggling
salesman, an Irish gangster, then a Viking, but the one thing he fails
to recognize is that he is actually an actor playing a part. The actor lost
in these various identities represents the plight of the psychic being
wholly absorbed in the play of the surface personality.

The skeptic denying the existence of a deeper reality underlying
the surface ego is akin to the actor believing he has no existence apart
from the words and actions that define the character he is playing. It is
as if he felt, "When the play is over, I will disappear." The actor's roles
are no more than an empty shell until they are filled with his presence.
Similarly, the surface self is nothing apart from the psychic presence
that is all the time supporting it.

At the beginning of the evolutionary journey, what later evolves
into the psychic being[a] is no more than the merest spark, hidden in
the heart of matter. To the extent this psychic spark has the barest
degree of wakefulness, it is unconsciously identified with the surface movements of the physical conscious-energy. This identification
constitutes a rudimentary form of ego, albeit one completely lacking
in self-awareness.

The psychic spark is diffuse in matter, and over the course of billions
of years, slowly becomes more organized, more complex. Along with

---

a. At times, Sri Aurobindo uses the terms "Soul" and "psychic entity" inter-
changeably. The "psychic being" is the individualized expression of the soul.

this, the rudimentary ego develops, as physicist and Buddhist teacher Robin Cooper refers to it, a feeling of "centeredness."[6] However, it is not until the emergence of certain mammals and primates that something close to conscious individuality appears on the evolutionary scene.

By the time humans appear, the rudimentary ego has flowered into partial wakefulness. The psychic spark has developed into a psychic being and now has, for the first time, a vehicle through which it can, potentially, express its full nature. But the human consciousness remains divided, characterized by much obscurity, inertia, and unconsciousness. The psychic being, though more fully awake than it was at the beginning of the evolutionary journey, remains hidden deep within. As a consequence, it is the "ego" that human beings mistakenly take to be their "self."

Although the ego is a false identity, it serves several essential purposes. For one, in functioning as the screen that divides the surface personality from its Origin, it sustains the challenge that helps make the game of evolution so compelling. It also acts as a coordinating point around which the play of the surface physical, vital, and mental consciousness is organized, allowing for the development of a surface individuality. And finally, the suffering engendered by the sense of ego intensifies the aspiration of the psychic being to awaken. The ego[a] continues to carry out its various functions until the psychic being—the true individual—emerges fully, at which time the ego will no longer be needed.

PLAYING HIDE-AND-SEEK IN THE UNIVERSE

> In all is the one Self, the one Divine is all; all are in the Divine, all are the Divine and there is nothing else in the universe.[7]
>
> —Sri Aurobindo

---

a. It may seem here that we are referring to the "ego" as a solidly existing entity. A better word might be "egoing"—the activity of identifying one's true Being with a particular formation of the Field.

When the universe was born, the Knower "hid" Itself in order to engage in a cosmic game of "hide-and-seek"—what we know as evolution. The Divine hid Its true nature of Bliss behind a cosmic screen, giving rise to suffering; veiled Its Goodness, resulting in acts of apparent evil; concealed Its Infinite Intelligence, resulting in a universe of apparently random nonconscious energies.

What is the purpose of this cosmic game? Some have suggested that the purpose is nothing beyond the simple delight of playing the game.[a]

> But why this stamp of so many undivine elements and characters in the play of One whose nature must be supposed to be divine? To the suggestion that what we see worked out in the world is the thoughts of God, the retort can be made that God could well have had better thoughts and the best thought of all would have been to refrain from the creation of an unhappy and unintelligible universe.[8]

The Indian poet Rabindranath Tagore was once engaged in creating a story together with a young girl. At one point the story had him locked up in a room, and she challenged him to find a way out. Suggesting he might shout for help, she immediately cleared the area of anyone who would hear his cries. He suggested kicking in the door, to which she responded, "The door is made of steel." When he found a key to open the door, she immediately declared, "It will not fit the lock!"[9] Like Tagore's young child, the Divine created the challenges of the evolutionary journey in order to experience the joy of overcoming them. We—who are the Divine-in-hiding—have the opportunity to consciously and joyfully participate in the cosmic game of hide-and-seek, the adventure of evolution.

Yet, there is something that feels deeply irrational and heartless about seeing the unimaginable horrors of ethnic cleansing, and nuclear and biochemical warfare as an inevitable component of some kind of

---

a. The cosmic game is referred to in sanskrit as *lila*.

majestic evolutionary journey. We rebel against an apparently sadistic God who seems to allow, and still worse, take delight in the abysmal suffering of the creatures He creates. What we don't realize is that these reactions make sense only when we imagine God to be separate from and other than His creation. In spite of what we may consciously believe, most of us have a deeply ingrained subconscious habit that leads us to conceive of God (if we entertain the notion of "God" at all) in this way. If you think this doesn't apply to you, you might simply ask yourself whether you go about your day thinking of everything and everyone you see as a manifestation of the Divine.

If in each moment we were to see all things as God-in-disguise, the problem of evil and suffering would disappear, as there would no longer be a question of one being inflicting pain and suffering on another—there being only One Being. However, a new question would present itself: *Is God insane?* Is He some kind of perverse masochist, taking joy in self-inflicted torment? This latter question can arise only from within the perspective of the human ego—the small, limited self that recoils from any challenge that requires it to transcend itself. The Infinite with whom we are one in our deepest Being is the greatest and most fearless of adventurers, plunging willingly into the adventure of evolution, shrinking from nothing in the blissful game of rediscovering Himself in infinitely diverse forms of expression.

> The torment of the couch of pain and evil on which we are racked is his touch as much as happiness and sweetness and pleasure. It is only when we see with the eye of the complete union and feel this truth in the depths of our being that we can entirely discover behind that mask too the calm and beautiful face of the all-blissful Godhead and in this touch that tests our imperfection the touch of the friend and builder of the spirit in man. The discords of the worlds are God's discords and it is only by accepting and proceeding through them that we can arrive at the greater concords of his supreme harmony, the summits and thrilled vastnesses of his transcendent and his cosmic Ananda.[10]

However, even if our minds understand and our hearts can embrace the idea of a Divine adventure, it may still be difficult for us to actually feel the truth of it. Driven by self-regard—known in Buddhism as "self-cherishing"—we habitually react to things on the basis of desire and fear. If we were to step back from our identification with our desires and fears, we would be able to relate to people and events with less self-interest and greater equanimity. We might thus more readily experience the delight inherent in all things—even those that the ego finds repellent. Some get a glimpse of this capacity for equal delight when engaging with various forms of art.

The Indian aesthetic tradition speaks of the *rasa*, or sublime taste of the "sorrowful" and the "terrible"—even the "horrible" and "repellent"[a]—to describe the deeper experience of "the one Soul [who] sees harmony and beauty where we divided beings experience rather chaos and discord."[11] We may get a hint of this *rasa*, for example, when we are not so lost in the drama of a film or play that we can appreciate the beauty of pain and suffering within the larger context of the story. Even the most evil acts may be seen and appreciated as a necessary and ingenious foil for the hero's redemption. In the same spirit of equanimity with regard to the drama of "real life," the Indian saint Sri Ramakrishna, when asked the purpose of evil in the universe, is alleged to have replied "to thicken the plot."[12]

Paradoxically, it can be when we are most caught up in the drama of our life that something happens to let us see through the construction of the ego and gain a glimpse of our deeper Self. Throughout history, the intensity of war has provided one context in which this can happen.

The Glamour of War

Let me have a war, say I: It exceeds
Peace as far as day does night; It's spritely, waking, audible,
full of vent.

---

a. The *karuna* (sorrowful), *bhayanaka* (terrible), and *bibhatsa* (horrible) *rasas*.

Peace is a very apoplexy, lethargy, mull'd, deaf, sleepy,
Insensible; a getter of more bastard children than war is a
Destroyer of men.[13]

—William Shakespeare

In his book *War Is a Force That Gives Life Meaning*, Chris Hedges
tells the story of a young Serbian woman who had lived in an area
under constant shellfire and had known intimately the horrors of war.
When the war was over, she was determined to emigrate to Australia
and "marry a man who [had] never heard of this war and raise children who [would] be told nothing about it."[14] Yet, in spite of this, she
and her friends once spent an entire afternoon together lamenting
the days when they had been living in fear and hunger, the targets
of Serbian gunmen. Though they did not wish for the return of their
suffering, they reluctantly conceded that those days had in some ways
been the fullest of their lives, and by comparison, the present seemed
"sterile, futile, empty."[15]

Hedges, who spent a good part of his own life as a war correspon-
dent amidst the horrors of several wars, was familiar with this addic-
tion. As he explains it,

Peace had again exposed the void that the rush of war, of
battle, had filled...Once again they were, as perhaps we all
are, alone, no longer bound by that common sense of struggle, no longer given the opportunity to be noble, heroic, no
longer sure what life was about or what it meant...Many of
us, restless and unfulfilled, see no supreme worth in our lives.
We want more out of life, and war, at least, gives a sense that
we can rise above our smallness and divisiveness.[16]

There is little doubt that the experience of war is, for many, quite
literally shattering. From a yogic perspective, what gets shattered is the
internal screen that is created by the exclusive focus of our attention
on the surface of things. When that attention is jolted and the screen
is temporarily punctured by the violence of war, glimmers of a deeper

consciousness can peek through, infusing the mind and heart with a sense of greater vividness and aliveness in things. When people who have had such an experience return to peacetime life, the forces that originally created the screen work to recreate it. Though it may now be no thicker than it had been before the war, the intervening glimpses of something else, something greater, make life seem emptier and less fulfilling by comparison.

It is hard to grasp the precise nature of the screen separating us from the deeper reality, because it is something we begin to build from the day we are born,[a] and it is made up of a host of unconscious assumptions and expectations about ourselves and the world in which we live. We take ourselves to be solid and enduring and thus expect the world around us to be solid and enduring as well. However, during times of extreme upheaval, such as often occur during war, our assumptions are severely challenged, destabilizing the mental construction we hold of the world and ourselves. When this occurs, we may experience intense fear and suffering, proportionate in part, to the strength of our attachment to that construction. At the same time, the dismantling of our habitual mode of encountering the world may allow us to experience things with a richness previously unknown.

Sharon's sense of herself was shattered by her experience in Vietnam, allowing her, in the midst of violence and suffering, to be touched by a deeper reality. Returning home, she had no way to make sense of this, as nothing in her culture or surroundings reflected that deeper sensibility. She was no longer capable of engaging fully in the life story she had formulated in her childhood. She tried to construct a new story, one in harmony with her youthful ideals, but the wound had not healed and the story would not hold together. Though the inability to fully immerse herself in any story was exceedingly painful, from the perspective of her psychic being, it was also a gift. It prevented her from ignoring the intimations that led to an opening by means of which she experienced the presence of her Soul.

As long as we are identified with the surface nature, we take a par-

---

a. Actually, we bring it with us from countless past lifetimes.

ticular construction of thoughts, feelings, and sensations to be our true "self." We then become intensely attached to this false identity, reflecting as it does what we truly long for—the radiance of the Infinite Self. Mistaking this false construction for the real thing, we constantly engage in attempts to maintain it, often creating conflict within ourselves and between ourselves and others:

> The sense, the idea, the experience that I am a separately self-existent being in the universe, and the forming of consciousness…into the mould of that experience are the root of all suffering, ignorance and evil…The soul limited [in this way] feels itself no longer in unity and harmony with its Self, with God, with the universe, with all around it; but rather it finds itself at odds with the universe, in conflict and disaccord with other beings who are its other selves, but whom it treats as not-self; and so long as this disaccord and disagreement last, it cannot possess its world and it cannot enjoy the universal life, but is full of unease, fear, afflictions of all kinds, in a painful struggle to preserve and increase itself and possess its surroundings.[17]

STEPPING OFF "THE END OF THE EARTH"

As Sharon became caught up in her new roles—competent businesswoman, charismatic politician—the tension intensified between her surface "self" and the deeper Self she had glimpsed in Vietnam. Once glimpsed, the experience of that deeper Reality had remained partially unveiled in her. But she had no way of understanding that the experience did not depend on an external situation—neither the violence of war nor the intensity of her business or political career. As long as she continued to search for deeper meaning through external experiences, the inner tension continued to mount. Finally, it could no longer be ignored. Letting go of her drive to augment the false identity she had created, her consciousness was freed to attend to that "something deeper." And the fruit of that shift in attention was a glimpse of the Divine Presence within.

As long as Sharon was able to identify with her role as nurse, she had the strength to endure the terrors of war. After her identification with that role was shattered, she could no longer wholly identify herself with any role. All roles seemed to be little more than empty shells, devoid of meaning and purpose. When she was all but lost and on the verge of taking her life, Sharon stepped off "the end of the earth," away from that with which she had previously been identified. There, she encountered a reflection of the truth of her oneness with the Infinite. And, for a while at least, she experienced peace.

PART IV

AWAKENING TO THE KNOWER
AND TRANSFORMATION OF THE
FIELD

OVERVIEW

In chapter 14 we will look at karmic patterns—those movements of consciousness that block access to the wisdom, joy, and peace deep within us. In order to understand what creates and maintains these patterns, we will look in more detail at Sharon's life, understanding how the play of karma contributed to her experience and her suffering. To help readers identify karmic obstacles in their own life, we will look at several other examples of how karmic reactions are formed. In chapter 15 we look at the same process—the formation of karmic patterns—at the group level. We use examples from American history to illustrate how karmic patterns intensify the conflict between the desires of the group ego and the aspiration of the group soul.

In chapters 16 and 17 we look at the means by which the energy of karmic patterns is transformed, becoming an expression of the deeper aspiration of the soul. In each of these chapters we begin by exploring the role of the thinking mind in preparing for this process. We then see how it is the awakened Soul that makes it possible to begin the transformation of the physical, vital, and mental nature from a limited to a full and clear expression of our true Divine Nature. In chapter 16, we focus on this process at the individual level. We look in chapter 17 at several examples at the societal level where we see hints that this process of transformation has begun to occur.

Having explored the awakening of the psychic being (the individual Knower "in" the Field), we look briefly in chapter 18 at the process of awakening to the Knower beyond space and time. We then touch on the awakening of the supramental or Truth-consciousness—a grade of consciousness within the Field of Conscious-Energy that is altogether beyond the mind. To help get a glimpse of the nature of this consciousness, we look at the faculty of intuition, understanding it to be—when it is genuine—a reflection of that greater supramental consciousness. In the case of each awakening, we look at the transformation of the nature it makes possible.

In the last section of chapter 18 we rely entirely on statements from others regarding supramental awakening and transformation because we are unable to say anything about it ourselves.

Cultivating Inner Silence

There is a background for everything. Every movement moves upon something.

And that something is a Silence which upholds everything including your own mental activity. All the thoughts and mental movements come and go, against a base that is ever stable. That is Silence...

Suspend for a moment your thought-activity and you'll become conscious of this presence.

...Think of this Silence again and again and try to become aware of it. By a steady digging in of this idea in your consciousness, this fact will become a reality to you—not merely for the mind but for the rest of the being.

Into this Silence you must learn to relax yourself.

Instead of trying to get at it, simply relax, call and let yourself lie in the folds of the Silence.

That will slowly come over you and claim you.[1]

—Kapali Sastry, paraphrasing Sri Aurobindo

> Consciousness is... the fundamental thing in existence—it is the energy, the motion, the movement of consciousness that creates the universe and all that is in it... [It is the] external concentration or... limiting stress of the consciousness which makes us live in our external being... It is this stress of consciousness that makes all the difference. That is why one has to concentrate the consciousness in heart or mind in order to go within... It is the disposition of the consciousness that determines everything, makes one... bound or free.[1]
>
> —Sri Aurobindo

CHAPTER 14

The Play of Karma in the Individual

THAT BY WHICH WE FALL IS THAT BY WHICH WE RISE

For much of her life, Sharon was intensely driven—by her ambition, by her desire to help, to serve, and to heal. But in the course of facing and surmounting a series of daunting obstacles, her mind and heart had gradually softened. And in the crucial moments after nearly deciding to take her own life, Sharon became more permeable to something altogether beyond the ambitions, desires, and fears that had previously motivated her.

What is the driving force in our lives? What keeps us going in the face of enormous obstacles? What is it in us that prevents us from waking up to our true nature? And how do these inner obstacles contribute to our ultimate awakening?

We've seen throughout the course of cosmic evolution that the growing psychic being is ever aspiring to awaken, to become free from its absorption in the surface play, and to fully express its true nature. We've seen how the psychic consciousness becomes caught, wrongly taking itself to be limited to a particular physical, vital, and mental formation. However, we haven't yet looked in detail at the process by which this limitation takes place and is maintained.

The Soul consents to the cosmic game of hide-and-seek, choosing to "lose" a part of itself in order to rediscover the fullness of itself in infinitely new and creative ways. But the game is not completely random or directionless. There are what might be called "rules" to the game of evolution. It is, in part, the purpose of these rules to keep the psychic being, the individual Knower, lost in the Field for many lifetimes. In the yoga tradition, the force that keeps us lost, the process by which desire and attachment bind the Soul to the limited surface personality, is known as karma.

Paradoxically, according to the rules of the cosmic game, the same force that keeps the psychic being lost in the Field also assures that it will ultimately awaken. In the words of the *Kulanarva Tantra*, "that by which we fall is that by which we rise." The very desires and attachments that bind us to a finite identity can, when turned within, become aligned with the Force that sets us free.

KARMA AND THE FORCES THAT MOVE US

> Ultimately karma is not a law but a many-sided dynamic truth of all action and life, the organic movement of the infinite; it follows and takes up many potential lines of the spirit…many waves and streams of combining and disputing world-forces; the long and multiform way of the progression of the individual and cosmic soul[a] in Nature.[2]
>
> —Sri Aurobindo

---

a. The cosmic soul is the Divine as the one Knower *(Paramatman)* of the universe.

Overview

"Karma," a Sanskrit word sometimes translated simply as "action," is often thought to be a purely mechanical process of cause and effect. With regard to matter, it was expressed by Sir Isaac Newton as the law which states, "For every action there is an equal and opposite reaction." According to popular notions of karma, the consequences of our actions are often understood to come about by an equally mechanical process of cause and effect: "My home was washed away by a flood. I must have done something very bad in the past that caused this to happen."

In the yogic tradition, the understanding of karma is more subtle and complex than this popular formulation. It is based on the understanding that all exists as one inseparable whole: "[A]ll is a continuous chain in which every link is bound indissolubly to the past infinity of numberless links."[3] With every action we take—whether inner or outer—an energy is set in motion, directed toward a certain result or set of results. To the extent we act out of a sense of separation—that is, when we act on the basis of the ego or separate self—we set up a tension in the fabric of oneness, which then seeks a restoration of balance and equilibrium.

In the yoga tradition this is sometimes thought of as "karmic debt." Each time we act out of ego, it is as if we have wrongly appropriated some portion of the totality for ourselves. This "loan" then must be "repaid." Because we are ignorant of the debt we are incurring, we continue unwittingly to "borrow" from the whole; that is to say, we egotistically take some part of the physical, vital, or mental field of conscious-energy to be part of our separate "self" rather than an insep-arable part of one unbroken Reality.

Over the course of many lifetimes, our debt accumulates a great deal of interest. Difficult or painful experiences—our house burning down, a friend deserting us—are like debt collectors knocking at our door, reminding us of what we owe. At first they knock gently, but the more we ignore them, the more aggressive they are forced to become to get our attention—we get sick, go mad, die a painful death.[a] But

---

a. This of course is an exaggeration for the sake of illustrating one aspect of the karmic process, which is infinitely more complex than anything that can be set

karma is not a linear or mechanical process. The karmic "debt collectors" have the well-being of the whole at heart, and in their infinite wisdom deliver the karmic consequences of our actions at times and in ways we will most benefit from them.

The Workings of Karma in the Surface Consciousness

Let's look at a mundane example of how the karmic process works, then explore its larger implications. David is taking his daily walk in the park near where he lives. It's dusk, and he is appreciating the cool breeze and the subtle colors of the sky. As he passes by a particularly lush garden, he notices, with some irritation, that someone has dropped a candy wrapper by the side of the path.

David's feeling of irritation is premised on experiencing himself as separate from, and in conflict with, the person he assumes has carelessly dropped the wrapper. This feeling of irritation leaves an impression in his consciousness associated with the memory of the event. We'll call this impression the "direct effect" on his psyche of his reaction to the wrapper. The energy of the impression carries a certain momentum, making it more likely that David will react with irritation in similar kinds of situations in the future. This energy, generated by actions performed out of a sense of separation, is the energy or momentum of karma.

Is karma generated only by negative reactions? Suppose David were walking along, noticed the candy wrapper, stooped to pick it up, and walked on, hardly registering any conscious feeling other than a slight sense of pleasure. To the extent he was taking himself to be an individual separate from the environment, the wrapper or the person who dropped it, the experience would still create a karmic impression. That is, an action taken on the basis of-perceived separation would reinforce his sense of himself as separate, and make it more likely that his future actions will also arise out of a sense of ego.

If we could observe David's mind as he continues walking along the

---

out in a verbal explanation. Coming across a phrase in a book or seeing a particularly inspiring work of art, one may experience a spontaneous inner awakening, "canceling" in a brief moment a large portion of karmic debt.

path that evening, we would see it constantly reacting to various stimuli as pleasant, unpleasant, or neutral, depending on the extent to which he perceives them as supportive or potentially threatening to his "self." This process of reaction goes on in most of us almost all the time, usually beneath the level of conscious awareness. It takes place on the physical, vital, and mental levels simultaneously. For example, David's feeling of irritation is inseparable from his mental judgment regarding the person whom he assumed was responsible for dropping the candy wrapper. It is also associated with some degree of physiological change. Whatever subsequent thoughts or feelings David may have will in turn be shaped by his current mental, vital, and physical state.

Over time, as we react in similar ways across different situations, the karmic impressions build up, making it increasingly likely we will repeat the same reactions in the future. Our behavioral, emotional, and mental patterns become more fixed, causing our reactions to become more predictable. These various reactive patterns together make up what we take to be our "self" or personality, which is actually little more than a constantly shifting interaction of mental, emotional, and physiological habit patterns.

As the various impressions accumulate, they act as filters through which we experience our self and the world, coloring all aspects of our knowing, willing, and feeling. As our consciousness becomes increasingly preoccupied with the fixed patterns of the surface nature, our connection to deeper dimensions is gradually occluded. The deeper meaning and purpose of life is obscured, and we come to rely increasingly on superficial external stimulation to make us feel alive.

Even when we struggle to get free of the burden of these karmic patterns, we find ourselves repeatedly trapped in the well-worn grooves of old physical, vital, and mental habits. What makes it so difficult to rise above these patterns?

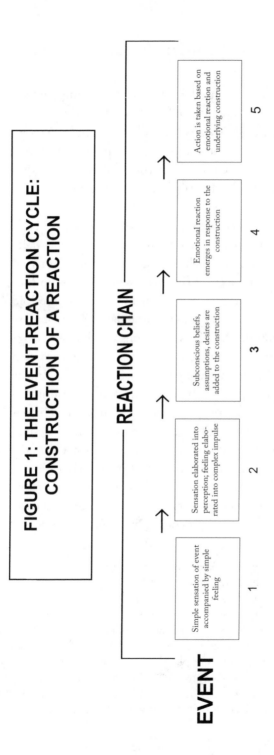

FIGURE 1: THE EVENT-REACTION CYCLE: CONSTRUCTION OF A REACTION

EVENT

REACTION CHAIN

1. Simple sensation of event accompanied by simple feeling

2. Sensation elaborated into perception; feeling elaborated into complex impulse

3. Subconscious beliefs, assumptions, desires are added to the construction

4. Emotional reaction emerges in response to the construction

5. Action is taken based on emotional reaction and underlying construction

Reacting mindlessly in this fashion, we deepen the karmic impression, making it more likely we will react mechanically in the same way in the future.

The Play of Karma and the Individual and Collective Subconscient

Every karmic impression created by thoughts, feelings, or sensations arising on the basis of a separate self is deposited in a region of consciousness that Sri Aurobindo calls the "subconscient."[a] We have previously described the physical consciousness as being dull and mechanical, but in comparison to the subconscient, the physical is vibrantly awake and wildly unpredictable. As described by Sri Aurobindo:

> The subconscient is below the waking physical consciousness—it is an automatic, obscure, incoherent, half-unconscious realm...[which] retains the impressions of all our past experiences...[These impressions] rise up into our waking consciousness as a mechanical repetition of old thoughts, old mental, vital and physical habits or an obscure stimulus to sensations, actions, emotions which do not originate in or from our conscious thought or will and are even often opposed to its perceptions, choice or dictates. In the subconscient there is an obscure mind full of obstinate... associations, fixed notions, habitual reactions formed by our past, an obscure vital full of the seeds of habitual desires, sensations and nervous reactions, a most obscure material which governs much that has to do with the condition of the body...[C]hronic or repeated illnesses are indeed mainly due to the subconscient and its obstinate memory and habit of repetition...It is...why people say character cannot be

---

a. Sri Aurobindo coined the term "subconscient" to refer to a region of consciousness more distant from our surface consciousness than either the physical or vital consciousness. We're using the word "subconscious" in a general sense to refer to any level of consciousness below the ordinary waking state. This would include much of what goes on in our mind as well as everything "below" the mind (vital, physical, and subconscient). For example, the initial process of sensing and perceiving is almost entirely subconscious. Anything arising out of the physical or vital consciousness—which precedes the mental functions of sensing and perceiving—is thoroughly "mentalized" long before it reaches our conscious mind.

changed, the cause also of the constant return of things one
hoped to have got rid of for ever.[4]

The influence of the subconscient is further compounded by the fact
that our individual consciousness is not separate from the consciousness of the world. We are therefore affected by what might be called
a "cultural subconscient" as well as a pool of subconscient impressions
accumulated by our plant, animal, and human ancestors over billions
of years of evolution. Suppose that David, walking in the early evening along a secluded portion of the path, is startled by a sound in the
wooded area to his left. His body tenses in fear as images of what may
have caused the sound rapidly pass through his mind. Even after he
realizes that it was simply the sound of a squirrel jumping from one
tree to another, he continues to feel a slight tinge of anxiety.

David's reaction of fear is in part shaped by his own past experiences of actual or perceived danger. In addition, he is subject to the
cultural subconscient that holds images, gleaned from the media and
other sources, of dangerous things that happen in secluded areas of city
parks. Further, our ancestral subconscient comes into play, which holds
billions of years of karmic impressions related to predators ambushing
their prey.

The Play of Karma and the Inner Consciousness

There is yet another powerful factor that keeps us bound in the web
of karma. Our individual consciousness is in communication with
movements of consciousness throughout the world in each moment,
through subtle physical, vital, and mental fields of conscious-energy.
So we are all the time participating in the karmic process of action and
reaction taking place in these subtle fields of the inner realm.

David may not, in his surface consciousness, be aware of the person who dropped the candy wrapper. However, in the inner realm,
through the subtle fields of conscious-energy, he is in direct contact
with that person. But that is just the beginning. David is someone who
has thought a great deal about environmental concerns. As such, he

has developed many strong feelings and well-developed beliefs about the careful use of our natural resources and the importance of appreciating and maintaining the beauty of the natural environment.

The subtle waves of vital and mental consciousness generated by his response of irritation to the candy wrapper create a karmic connection to the countless other individuals who share his concerns and sense of aesthetic beauty. They also create a karmic connection to those who mindlessly deface the environment, as well as to the workers who manufactured the candy wrapper, the truckers who transported the materials to make it, the business responsible for marketing it, the trees that went into the paper, the rain that nourished the trees, the sun that makes life possible, and ultimately to everything in the universe—and beyond.

By virtue of this inner connection, the energy engendered by David's momentary reaction to the wrapper will, in some way, have an impact on everything with which he is connected. And whatever is touched by this energy will in turn generate a response, sending out waves of subtle-physical, vital, or mental energy that will eventually, in some form, come back to him. We'll call this returning energy the "indirect effect" of karmic action. The subsequent impact on him will not in itself cause David to incur further personal karma. He will incur further karma only to the extent that he reacts to these indirect effects (most likely on a subconscious level) from an egoistic perspective.

With every mental, vital, or physical action we take on the basis of ego, we weave a dense web made up of various interacting and conflicting lines of physical, vital, and mental karma. Contributing to this web is the entire set of our reactions past and present, the culture in which we live, our inner interactions with others, and our past biological inheritance. How did this complex karmic process arise and how did it evolve?

KARMA AND THE EVOLUTION OF CONSCIOUSNESS

In some way incomprehensible to the ordinary human mind, the karmic process of action and reaction occurs even in the earth, the stone, the subatomic particle. Yogis who have an opening to the inner consciousness are capable of perceiving directly the conscious-energy manifesting in and as matter. They describe the response of this conscious-energy to impacts from the environment as being extremely minute or limited. The material object, in turn, is modified only to a small degree by its reaction. Despite the limitations of both the response and the accompanying inner modification, it is by means of this essential process of action and reaction that material forms grew in complexity—that is, molecules evolved out of the interaction among atoms.

Because so little consciousness had evolved to the surface, this process of increasing complexity at the material level was extremely slow, taking billions of years. With the emergence of the vital and mental consciousness in plants and animals, the karmic process picked up speed, becoming more complex. However, the way the karmic process works to further evolution[5] is essentially the same in matter, plants, animals, and humans.

For example, an animal is presented with challenges from the environment. To the extent the surface consciousness of the animal is unable to meet the challenge, more of the hidden consciousness is called forth. With more capacity for knowing, willing, and feeling now evolved, the animal has a greater capacity to respond to the demands of its environment. Each response leaves an impression in the subconscient. As consciousness evolves to the surface, there is more freedom to respond, and the reaction becomes more intense. This leaves behind stronger impressions, adding momentum to the karmic process.

At some point, when the animal's particular level of consciousness is no longer sufficient to meet its environmental challenges, a heightening of consciousness takes place, manifesting physically as a genetic mutation that gives rise to a more complex form. There is thus simultaneously an increase in the complexity of both consciousness and form. When mammals first emerged, for example, there was both an increase in the complexity of knowing, willing, and feeling and a parallel increase in the complexity of brain structure.[a]

[a.] We realize that this description of the evolutionary process is contrary to the prevailing neo-Darwinian view that sees consciousness as, at best, a secondary survival mechanism and, at worst, a useless epiphenomenon. We are trying to

In all forms—atom, plant, animal, and human—the Soul "behind" is ever aspiring to awaken and manifest more of its latent capacity for knowing, willing, and feeling. However, neither the atom nor the animal has evolved a conscious self and therefore cannot contribute consciously to this process. Prior to the human level, because there is no conscious self and therefore no conscious individual will, karma does not accrue to the individual. Rather than being deposited in an individual subconscient, karmic impressions are collected in the subconscient of the species.

In human beings, with the full awakening of the thinking mind, a conscious self—and along with it, the individual will—emerge. Richly diverse lines of physical, vital, and mental karma now accrue to the individual over many lifetimes lived out in diverse environments, encountering a wide variety of experiences. With the birth of self-consciousness, humans potentially have the capacity to recognize the consequences of their actions. To the extent they realize this capacity, they are responsible for their karma and can consciously participate in their own evolution.

Behind the individual will of the human being, the Soul continues to aspire for awakening and full expression. But experiencing himself as a separate individual, the human being directs the energy of the Soul's aspiration—which in his unenlightened surface consciousness takes the form of desire—toward things of the world. He seeks to enlarge himself, not through developing his consciousness, but through the accumulation of things, the search for ever-greater pleasure, wealth, power, fame, relationships, and knowledge. Having obtained the object of his desire, the human being remains dissatisfied, because the energy behind desire is the "hunger of an infinite being,"[6] which can only be

---

present here our understanding of how, from the yogic perspective, the karmic process works to further evolution.

We realize also that the way we're describing this process makes it sound as if there were a "consciousness" behind the form, separate from the form, and that directs the form to change in response to an environmental challenge. This process might be better expressed by speaking of the "mammal-developing-a-complex-brain-structure-in-response-to-environmental-challenges." In other words, the whole phenomenon is nothing other than the appearance of the evolving consciousness to our human senses.

satisfied by the Infinite.

Through the ongoing quest for the fulfillment of desire, karmic ties binding us to others grow ever more complex, linking all in one inextricable karmic web. As long as the energy of desire is turned outward, oriented toward external fulfillment, the karmic web continues to grow thicker. The endless chain of action and reaction increases the sense of burden and limitation, intensifying the aspiration of the soul to awaken.

To the extent an individual's reactions are negative—that is, out of harmony with his environment—the karmic consequence is that he will be more likely to act in negative ways. This makes it more likely his future acts will be in conflict with his environment, further intensifying his sense of separation. When his reactions are positive—more congruent with the needs of the whole—karmic momentum is generated that makes it easier for him to respond harmoniously in the future. However, both negative and positive reactions that arise out of a sense of separation ultimately create further karmic bonds. The soul cannot fully awaken until it rises above both negative and positive reactions by eliminating all sense of separation, thus becoming altogether free from the bondage of karma.

Though the web we weave is thick and the law of consequences inexorable, the way in which karmic seeds bear fruit is infinitely flexible. They can ripen in infinite ways and within vastly variable time frames. Rather than a mechanical linear process, or a means of reward and punishment, the ripening of karma occurs according to what will be most favorable to the awakening of the individual, and ultimately to the whole of humanity.

How does it happen that the consequences of a day laborer's actions in eighteenth-century France will ripen in just the right way and just the right time so as to fulfill not only his own karma but that of the architect in nineteenth-century San Francisco and the dancer in twentieth-century Kyoto? Within the consciousness of the One Divine Being, the web of karma is one coherent whole in one eternal present moment; the infinite Artist in His infinite capacity for knowing, willing, and feeling, sees to it that every note of His superorchestra is, ever in right relation to every other note, in an endlessly creative outpouring of Delight.

THE PLAY OF KARMA IN OUR MOMENT-TO-MOMENT EXPERIENCE

> [Supporting the four functions of mind], [t]here are secret operations in us, in our subconscient and superconscient... but of these we are not aware in our surface being and therefore for us they do not exist. If we knew of them, our whole conscious functioning would be changed.[7]
>
> —Sri Aurobindo

We've looked at the way the karmic process is generated in the individual, and how it evolved over time. By looking again at an individual human being and zeroing in on the more minute dynamics of a reaction, we can see more clearly how the karmic knot is tied. This will also give us clues as to how karmic knots[a] can be untied. In the process of looking more closely at a single reaction, we will see that in a sense, the entire range of consciousness—and in fact, the entire spectrum of space and time—participate in each and every moment of experience.

Before looking at how karmic knots are formed, we need to carefully examine a deeply ingrained habit—that of blaming our reactions on external events. If David had been asked why he became irritated, he might well have said something to the effect, "People who thoughtlessly destroy the environment have no consideration for other people, and that makes me angry." Thus David sees the external situation (a thoughtless, inconsiderate person) as the cause of his anger, feeling no responsibility himself for that reaction.

However, the simple awareness of the candy wrapper did not in itself impel him to become irritated. What if, when he first came upon the wrapper, he somehow realized that he was the one who had accidentally dropped it there earlier? He might in that case have had little or no conscious reaction and may instead have simply bent over, picked

---

a. These karmic knots are a major component of the barrier dividing the surface awareness from the infinite depths and heights of consciousness.

it up, and thrown it away.

But suppose his initial assumption was correct—a thoughtless, inconsiderate person had carelessly dropped the wrapper. Even this *in itself* would not have constituted a cause of anger. If David were someone who didn't care about littering or the state of the environment, he would most likely have had little if any reaction at all. So without his desire for a clean environment he would have had no cause for irritation.

But David did care about the environment. And, let's grant that his evaluation of the person who discarded the wrapper was a valid one. Together, these are *still not sufficient* to compel him to respond with anger. The underlying cause of his anger was his *own internal attachment* to his desire for people to act in harmony with his beliefs. The event of seeing the wrapper was thus only the occasion rather than the cause of his reaction.

Taking with us this understanding that the primary cause of our reactions is always internal rather than external, let's look in much finer detail at the karmic process.[a]

The Reaction of the Surface Consciousness and the Contribution of the Personal Subconscient

Sharon is walking down the street near her father's house. Off in the distance she catches sight of a truck moving in her direction. Absentmindedly, she remains focused on the truck as it comes closer. At a certain point she becomes aware that there is something vaguely familiar about it. Before she consciously recognizes it as an army vehicle, she feels her body begin to tense up, accompanied by some vague emotional discomfort. It has been some time since Sharon had a flashback or even thought much about her war experience. She is surprised by the intensity of emotion, the mixture of fear, sadness, and anger that she feels as the truck passes by.

---

a. This understanding of the way our attitudes shape our reactions forms the basis for cognitive-behavioral therapy, which in recent years has been greatly influenced by ideas and practices from the yoga tradition.

What happened in that moment Sharon first saw the truck? Was it the truck that caused her to react as she did? When she first caught sight of it, she was not consciously aware of any reaction. But already, a subconscient impression from her previous experience had been triggered. A subconscious dread of the familiar feelings associated with that impression, and a subconscious wish to ward them off, created some degree of physiological tension and emotional discomfort that barely emerged into her surface awareness.

The Contribution of the Cultural Subconscient

In addition to her personal association to the truck carrying dead bodies in Vietnam, what other subconscious impressions helped trigger Sharon's physical and vital reactions? These are impossible to enumerate in full, since the influences on any given moment of experience include everything we've experienced in our current lifetime and beyond. However, it is possible to identify some of the major karmic patterns associated with any particular reaction.

For Sharon, the cultural influences involved in being an African-American woman who grew up in a poor, crime-ridden neighborhood contributed to her sense of her self and helped shape the kind of mental, vital, and physical responses she would have. It is not uncommon, growing up in such circumstances, to develop both a sense of physical and psychological vulnerability along with the corresponding toughness one needs to confront the daily sense of threat.

The neighborhood where Sharon grew up fostered in her an intense desire to change her environment, to create a sense of community where people would feel safe and nurtured. But there are many ways one might respond to these circumstances. What in Sharon's personal karma led her to respond in this particular way?

For one thing, her experience of growing up in a close-knit, deeply supportive family helped foster in her the belief that it was possible to create a sense of community. Each time as a teenager she acted out of that belief—creating youth programs, running for student office—she strengthened the karmic impression that nurtured her faith in the possibility that things could be better. In addition, she may have brought with her, as karmic tendencies from previous lifetimes, a strong idealistic bent and passionate desire to help create more supportive circumstances in peoples' lives.

Bringing these karmic imprints to her experience in Vietnam made it, in some respects, even more shocking to be confronted with such an overwhelming degree of disease, suffering, and death. The truck filled with dead bodies, arriving daily in the medical compound, came to symbolize for her everything she had wished to fight against, and in the face of which she now felt so completely helpless. Each time that truck arrived, her feelings of helplessness and hopelessness intensified, building a karmic momentum that would make it more likely for her to have that reaction in the future.

These extremely intense energies of desire and fear, which had accumulated throughout her childhood, culminated in one particular moment—the moment when she saw the truck arrive in the compound and simultaneously heard a round of gunfire that impelled her to dive to the ground to avoid being hit. The image of that moment and the feelings attached to it were seared into her mind, heart, and body. The energy stored in this karmic impression had such an immense trajectory that, more than a quarter century later, walking down the street near her father's house, the distant sight of an army truck could trigger a powerful reaction of tension and discomfort.[8]

Every memory, every image of the truck loaded with dead bodies that had ever arisen in Sharon's mind since her time in Vietnam, was also triggered that day walking down the street. In addition, the sense of futility she felt since returning from the war, which had come to be associated with those painful wartime images, was also triggered—the pervasive feeling that nothing could restore the lost sense of meaning and purpose she had once felt—not her work as a nurse, not the business she started, not the service she attempted to render her community as a councilwoman. Along with this sense of futility, there arose a wave of nausea associated with the shame she felt at having used her charm and charisma to attain a certain measure of power and status.

All these feelings were intimately bound up in Sharon's reaction that moment she saw the army vehicle coming toward her.

The karmic web affecting our every moment of experience is unimaginably dense and complex. In addition to all the imprints of our personal past, and the direct influence of the various cultures in which we partake, we also carry deep within us the heritage of billions of years of biological evolution. Our physical consciousness bears the imprint of its origins at the birth of the universe. Similarly, all levels of the vital consciousness carry with them the karmic imprints of our myriad biological ancestors. Thus the physical and vital consciousness of the very cells of Sharon's body responded to the sight of the truck in some ways not unlike those of an animal fleeing from its predator in the far distant evolutionary past. But there is still more.

The Contribution of the Inner Consciousness

Beneath the unfolding of the four functions of the surface mental consciousness are a vast array of subconscient mental, vital, and physical impressions that contributed to shaping Sharon's reaction. There is yet another, still greater realm of consciousness affecting this moment of her experience. Corresponding to the four mental functions of the surface consciousness, there is the greater capacity of the inner subliminal consciousness for sensing, perceiving, understanding, and volition. There are more powerful layers of vital and subtle physical consciousness behind the surface as well.

This subtle, inner consciousness is affecting us all the time, though we are rarely aware of it:

> Each man has his own personal consciousness entrenched in his body and gets into touch with his surroundings only through his body and senses and the mind using the senses. Yet all the time the universal forces are pouring into him without his knowing it. He is aware only of thoughts, feelings, etc., that rise to the surface and these he takes for his own.[9]

Though Sharon's reaction to the sight of the army truck coming toward her was in part shaped by her past experiences, her every thought, feeling, and sensation was also affected by these mental, vital, and subtle physical waves of conscious-energy:

> Thoughts come from outside, from the universal Mind or universal Nature, sometimes formed and distinct, sometimes unformed and then they are given shape somewhere in us. The principal business of our mind is either a response of acceptance or a refusal to these thought-waves (as also vital waves, subtle physical energy waves).[10]

For example, as Sharon caught sight of the army vehicle, someone else walking down that street may also have noticed it and reacted with fear. Unconsciously picking up on this energy may have intensified her own reaction of fear. Through this inner realm of consciousness, Sharon is still connected to everyone with whom she has been in contact—her family, and the people she knew as a child, in Vietnam, in business, and in politics:

> There is a constant mental, vital, subtle-physical interchange going on between all who meet…of which they are themselves unaware… for the most part it is subtly and invisibly that this interchange takes place; for it acts indirectly, touching the subliminal [i.e., inner] parts and through them the outer nature.[11]

Thus, the fears and desires of those she has known also affected, in some way, every aspect of her reaction in that moment.

THE CONFLICT BETWEEN KARMIC MOMENTUM AND THE SOUL'S ASPIRATION

Each moment of experience is the intersection of the past, present, and future, the convergence of the inner and outer. Behind the working of the physical, vital, and mental fields of conscious-energy—surface and subliminal—is the Soul. Sharon is connected to the culture-at-large in part through the vaster inner domain of the inner consciousness. But in a still deeper way, her Soul—the true Self in the depths of her being—is connected to the Soul of her culture.

Sharon's desire to be of service to her community, her faith in the potential of people around her, were in part instilled in her by the strength of the love and support she received from her family. But beyond her family's influence, her Soul—from birth, or even "before" birth—may have aspired to use this particular body, heart, and mind as instruments for the manifestation of Its latent capacity for love and service. Her individual Soul's unique purpose[a] may have sought to express itself through the creation of circumstances that could help bring people together in community and foster in them the capacity to express more fully their own deeper nature.

Throughout her adult life the energy of her Soul's aspiration was repeatedly diverted toward the fulfillment of her ego's desires and ambitions, and further distorted by fear and anger. She experienced this diversion as a driving, relentless force, prodding her to be success-ful, at times by attempting to control and manipulate others. The gen-tle aspiration of her Soul was always behind the ambition and driven energy, but it was only after a nearly complete breakdown of her sur-face personality that the thick, karmic knots loosened sufficiently for her to begin to awaken to that deeper reality.

Sharon struggled for most of her life with this conflict between the aspiration of her Soul and the diversion of her Soul's energies toward satisfaction of the desires of her ego. While the conflict is a universal one, the particular form it took in Sharon is in part reflective of a struggle at the core of the American Soul. The resonance of her own Soul's conflict with that of America is perhaps what drew her psychic being to take birth in this country. "Sharon" was born into the American culture, at least in part, because the larger drama of the country's soul-purpose could provide a context and a mirror for her

---

a. In Sanskrit, the word *swabhava* is used to refer to the soul's true nature and unique purpose.

own struggle. In turn, to the extent she is able to resolve the conflict in herself, she will be able to contribute to its resolution in the larger consciousness of the culture of which she is a part.

We'll see in the next chapter how this karmic conflict plays out on the collective scale, in the "being" and "personality" of the American nation.

CHAPTER 15

Collective Karma:
The Conflict between Soul and Ego in the Life of America

> My concern is not whether God is on our side; my greatest
> concern is to be on God's side.[1]
>
> —Abraham Lincoln

THE HIDDEN SPIRITUAL TRADITION IN AMERICA

Eugene Taylor, historian of psychology and psychiatry at Harvard University, in his book *Shadow Culture*, refers to a tradition of folk psychology which he describes as "an inwardly oriented psychology of spiritual consciousness that has been an integral part of American culture from its very inception."[2] This "folk tradition" has been concerned with the exploration of "different states of interior consciousness" and is "spiritual insofar as its function is the evolution and transformation of personality."[3] Although for much of American history this folk psychology has been spurned by the mainstream culture, in the last half century it has emerged "out of the shadow"[4] into the light, as evidenced by increasingly widespread interest in meditation and other ways of transforming consciousness.

Taylor proposes that this tradition of folk psychology represents a fundamental spiritual impulse native to the American Soul. He describes the tradition as fundamentally optimistic, eclectic, and pragmatic in nature, involving a "blending of science and religion, spirit and matter, mind and body."[5] And it is an impulse that reverberates throughout the American character—expressing itself as a seeking for freedom from outer authority, the freedom to pursue individual inner experience and express it within one's community.

The yearning for freedom of religious expression and experience has been a driving force in American culture since the founding of the colonies. Religious scholars identify two periods in American history, known as the Great Awakenings, when this yearning became particularly intense. During these times, large numbers of people became involved in a search for immediate inner or spiritual experience, in the process experimenting with new forms of religious ritual. This experimentation took place within the dominant Christian culture. Taylor identifies two subsequent periods of intense spiritual seeking, in which an Asian influence became more prominent.

The first Great Awakening took place in the early eighteenth century. It was characterized by experimentation with religious practices that induced "trance states... [of] joyful exuberance and spiritual happiness."[6] Having been previously forbidden, such states were now "fully sanctioned"[7] by governing church bodies. One might speculate that the movement of consciousness behind the sense of joy and freedom may also have been behind the energy and momentum that fueled the Revolutionary War, and may also have nourished the spirit behind the drafting of the Constitution.

The second Great Awakening took place a century later in the 1820s, during which time religious revivals—some lasting for months and involving hundreds of thousands of people—proliferated on the American frontier. Along with a flowering of unusual inner experiences, many spiritual communities were established at that time, experimenting with new forms of governance and economics that reflected deeper spiritual ideals.

Taylor identifies a third Great Awakening as having taking place in the late nineteenth century, a period when there was a strong influx of Asian-inspired spiritual practices and much questioning of traditional religious forms. Indian meditation techniques were utilized in the psychotherapy of the time, and mind-body healing grew in popularity. Transcendentalist writers like Emerson and Thoreau wrote essays that inspired people to seek new forms of spiritual experience and expression.

The fourth Awakening, which Taylor sees as taking place at the current time, stems from a renewed interest during the 1950s and 60s in various Asian spiritual traditions—from Taoism to Tibetan Buddhism. True to the impulse present during the earliest settlement of the American colonies, today's spiritual seekers are experimenting with forms that go beyond the traditions of either East or West.

EMPIRE VS. DEMOCRACY: EGOIC SELF-AGGRANDIZEMENT VS. SPIRITUAL SELF-DETERMINATION

It is striking—and no coincidence—that America[a] now faces the prospect of military action in many of the same lands where generations of colonial British soldiers went on campaigns... where, by the nineteenth century, ancient imperial authority... was crumbling, and Western armies had to quell the resulting disorder... Afghanistan and other troubled lands today cry out for the sort of enlightened foreign administration once provided by self-confident Englishmen in jodhpurs and pith helmets.[8]

—Max Boot, *The Case for American Empire*, 2001

Arrogant, full of self-esteem and the drunkenness of their pride, these misguided souls delude themselves, persist in false and obstinate aims and pursue the fixed impure resolution of their longings. They imagine that desire and enjoyment are... the aim of life... [and] are the prey of a devouring, a measurelessly unceasing... anxiety till the moment of their death. Bound by a hundred bonds, devoured by wrath and lust, unweariedly occupied in amassing unjust gains... they think, "Today I have gained this object of desire, tomorrow I shall have that other; today I have so much wealth, more I

---

a. The observations in this section regarding American karma are offered in a nonpartisan spirit. Over the course of American history, both egoic and soul-inspired actions can be seen across the political spectrum. The degree to which any particular individual or administration expresses one or the other is for the reader to determine.

will get tomorrow. I have killed this my enemy, the rest too
I will kill. I am a lord and king of men, I am perfect, accomplished, strong, happy, fortunate, a privileged enjoyer of the
world; I am wealthy, I am of high birth; who is there like
unto me? I will sacrifice, I will give [alms], I will enjoy." [9]

—The *Bhagavad Gita*, circa 400 B.C.E.–400 C.E.

Taylor's view of the underlying spiritual significance of the Great
Awakenings is not the common one. Religious studies scholar Karen
Armstrong, presenting the more prevalent view, sees them as times
of "frenzied religiosity."[10] According to Armstrong, it was a period
of great societal change, which led many colonists to seek solace in
intense religious experience, sometimes taking the form of "born-
again conversions."[11] People in revival meetings "fainted, wept, and
shrieked; the churches shook with the cries of those who imagined
themselves saved and the groans of the unfortunate who were convinced they were damned."[12] Commenting on the dangers of experimentation with such altered states of consciousness, she writes, "Once
faith was conceived as irrational, and the inbuilt constraints of the best
conservative spirituality were jettisoned, people could fall prey to all
manner of delusions."[13]

There seems to be quite a disparity between Armstrong's picture
of "frenzied religiosity" and Taylor's image of "joyful exuberance and
spiritual happiness." Armstrong does suggest, however, that the experience of the First Great Awakening helped pave the way for greater
participation in the coming battle for American independence. "The
ecstatic experience left any American who would be quite unable to
relate to the [highly intellectual]... ideals of the revolutionary leaders,
with the memory of a blissful state of freedom. The word 'liberty' was
used a great deal to describe the joy of conversion, and a liberation
from the pain and sorrow of normal life."[14]

From the perspective of yoga psychology, it makes sense that
the deeper spiritual impulse Taylor describes would have easily been
diverted by the desires and needs of the surface vital consciousness and
significantly distorted by the undisciplined physical and vital mind. As

Armstrong noted, "all manner of delusions" may result when an individual opens himself to the intense energies of the inner realm without sufficient preparation. In fact, Taylor is quite aware that the "shadow culture" of "folk psychology" has been a complex mixture made up of many different qualities and grades of consciousness. The yoga tradition has taught for thousands of years that it is crucial to develop a rigorous and astute sense of discernment if one is to navigate safely the domains of consciousness beyond the ordinary waking state.

One of the greatest impediments to the development of a calm, clear discernment is the uncritical belief in one's own purity and innocence. As the great theologian Reinhold Neibuhr writes, "Nations, as individuals, who are completely innocent in their own esteem are insufferable in their human contacts."[15] Neibuhr was someone who recognized both the deeper spiritual impulse in American culture as well as the delusions and temptations to which the human being may easily fall prey. Wishing to bring attention to the delusions so that they do not subvert the spiritual impulse, he wrote in 1952, "From the earliest days of its history to the present moment, there is a deep layer of messianic consciousness in the mind of America…[coupled with a widespread] inability to comprehend the depth of evil to which individuals and communities may sink, particularly when they try to play the role of God to history."[16] Rather than "claiming God too simply as the sanctifier of whatever we most fervently desire," Neibuhr appeals to us to hold "a sense of modesty about the virtue, wisdom and power available to us… [and] a sense of contrition about the common human frailties and foibles which lie at the foundation of both the enemy's demonry and our vanities."[17] To the extent this discerning awareness has been wanting over the course of American history, the culture (i.e., the collective personality of the nation) has accumulated a very heavy karmic debt.

While the spiritual impulse is always mixed to some extent with ego and desire, the tendency for it to be co-opted by the forces of self-interest is especially great during wartime. Looking back on the comments of American leaders during various wars, it is not always so easy to discern where and in what way the deeper impulse has been distorted. For example, in 1917, President Woodrow Wilson, exhorting the

American public to enter the fray of World War I, said in an address to the nation, "The world must be made safe for democracy."[18] On its face, this statement alone could be either an expression of American imperialism or a genuine desire to spread freedom. Wilson continues, "Its peace must be planted upon the tested foundation of political liberty. We have no selfish ends to serve. We desire no conquest, no dominion... We are but one of the champions of the rights of mankind. We shall be satisfied when those rights have been made as secure as the faith and the freedom of nations can make them."[19] As noble and selfless as these declarations appear to be, it is hard to know whether they are as innocent as they sound.

There are other wartime proclamations in which it is more apparent that spiritual claims may in part have been a guise for egoistic pride and self-interest. During the Civil War, the Reverend George S. Phillips spoke to Union troops, exhorting them to see themselves as fulfilling a greater mission, one that would "only be accomplished when the last despot should be dethroned, the last chain of oppression broken, the dignity and equality of redeemed humanity everywhere acknowledged, republican government everywhere established, and the American flag should wave over every land and encircle the world with its majestic folds."[20] Even here, one might excuse the reverend's excessively messianic language as an unusually intense but genuine passion for the liberty of all mankind. It seems more likely, however, that his vision of the American flag encircling the globe reflected, at least in part, a desire for American domination and control.

An absence of innocence and humility in the following words is unmistakable. They are the words of Sen. Albert J. Beveridge in an 1898 speech to the Union League Club, in which he objected to suggestions for bringing home American troops from the Philippines. Beveridge proclaimed that a retreat

> would be a betrayal of a trust as sacred as humanity... And so, thank God the Republic never retreats... American manhood today contains the master administrators of the world, and they go forth for the healing of the nations. They go forth in the cause of civilization. They go forth for the betterment

of man. They go forth, and the word on their lips is Christ and his peace, not conquest and its pillage. They go forth to prepare the peoples, through decades and maybe centuries of patient effort, for the great gift of American institutions.[21]

If any doubt remains as to the intention behind Beveridge's piety, consider his response to the assertion that the American involvement in the Philippines was an imperialist venture that violated the spirit of the Declaration of Independence: "[The Declaration of Independence] applies only to people capable of self-government...[not to] the Malay children of barbarism." And he further argues that the invasion had its roots in something "deeper even than any question of constitutional power... [God Himself] has marked the American people as His chosen nation to finally lead in the regeneration of the world."[22]

Underlying the birth of the American experiment, there was a profound spiritual impulse, however much it may or may not have been conscious in the minds of the Founding Fathers. At the same time, due to the nature of the human psyche at this stage of evolution, there were also tendencies toward self-interest, greed, and power-seeking of all kinds.

To the extent America as a nation has repeatedly acted on each of these impulses (spiritual and egoic), the momentum engendered by both types of action has intensified, bringing us to a point of karmic reckoning. On the one hand, the deeper spiritual impulse has grown—not only in America but throughout the world, such that we now have the possibility of a global spiritual awakening. On the other hand, if we continue to be lost in the karmic momentum of ego and self-interest, adamantly asserting innocence of any wrongdoing, we may perish. In his work, *The Irony of American History*, Reinhold Neibuhr writes:

> If we should perish, the ruthlessness of the foe would be only the secondary cause of the disaster. The primary cause would be that the strength of a giant nation was directed by eyes too blind to see all the hazards of the struggle; and the blindness would be induced not by some accident of nature or history but by hatred and vainglory.[23]

ABRAHAM LINCOLN: NAVIGATING THE CONFLICT BETWEEN THE SOUL'S ASPIRATION AND THE DESIRES OF THE EGO

Perhaps few individuals in American history have risen to the challenge of spiritual discernment to the degree exemplified by Abraham Lincoln, the sixteenth president of the United States. Neibuhr, expressing his belief in Lincoln's capacity for genuine humility and discernment, wrote the following commentary on his second inaugural address: "The combination of moral resoluteness about the immediate issues, with a religious awareness of another dimension of meaning and judgment, must be regarded as almost a perfect model of the difficult but not impossible task of remaining loyal and responsible toward the moral treasures of a free society on the one hand, while yet having some religious vantage point over the struggle."[24]

At the point he delivered his second inaugural address, Lincoln was feeling the weight of his responsibility to win the Civil War and bring the country back from the brink of dissolution. In spite of this, he chose to challenge the claim of religious righteousness that would have conferred upon him authority to accomplish the task as well as the highest justification for his resolve. And he dared others to do the same:

> Neither party expected for the war the magnitude or the duration which it has already attained... Each looked for an easier triumph, and a result less fundamental and astounding. Both read the same Bible and pray to the same God, and each invokes His aid against the other. It may seem strange that any men should dare to ask a just God's assistance in wringing their bread from the sweat of other men's faces, but let us judge not, that we be not judged. The prayers of both could not be answered. That of neither has been answered fully. The Almighty has His own purposes.[25]

Lincoln, commenting afterward on how his address had been received, said:

> I believe it is not immediately popular. Men are not flattered by being shown that there has been a difference of purpose

between the Almighty and them. To deny it, however, in this case, is to deny that there is a God governing the world. It is a truth which I thought needed to be told; and as whatever of humiliation there is in it, falls most directly on myself, I thought others might afford for me to tell it.[26]

Acknowledging his imperfection as an instrument of the God he aspired to serve, and exercising a rare discernment between the true and distorted spiritual impulse of the nation, Lincoln concluded his inaugural address with these words:

With malice toward none; with charity for all; with firmness in the right, as God gives us to see the right, let us strive on to finish the work we are in; to bind up the nation's wounds; to care for him who shall have borne the battle, and for his widow, and his orphan—to do all which may achieve and cherish a just, and a lasting peace, among ourselves, and with all nations.[27]

The Infinite Stillness of the Knower and the Ever-Present Possibility of Freedom

For much of her life, Sharon's attention was absorbed in the habitual movements of her physical, vital, and mental consciousness, almost completely obscuring the deeper realm of the Spirit. However, having been subject during the Vietnam War to a slow, painful erosion of the ties to her surface consciousness, her self-construct was sufficiently thinned to allow the deeper longing of her Soul to begin to influence her surface awareness.

This awakening was impeded by the various karmic tendencies she developed. Her habit of acting and reacting continually in the same egoic way was so strong it was almost irresistible. However, the access to her inner consciousness that had stayed with Sharon since the war—however minute—was enough to drive her to try to resolve the tension between the desires of her surface nature and the aspiration of her Soul to awaken. Facing the choice as to whether to live or die, she felt, for a brief moment, the Presence of the Divine. In the weeks and months that followed, as her inner discernment grew, she came to recognize she had a choice as to how and where to direct her attention.

This same choice is one the world now faces on the collective level. We have received a number of karmic blows, each of which has given us an opportunity to wake up and take note.[a] It remains to be seen whether it will take a crisis of still greater magnitude before we awaken to a sufficient degree and in sufficient numbers to begin bringing a deeper sensibility to our day-to-day actions and decisions. In each and every moment, no matter how thick the karmic web in which we may be embroiled, there is the possibility of withdrawing our attention from the clamoring of the Field, of turning it inward toward the Stillness and Silence of the Soul, the Infinite Knower, and in turn allowing the power of the Spirit to infuse our lives.

Looking once again at the moment when Sharon saw the army truck approaching on the street near her father's house, we see that prior to her conscious reaction there was a vast array of impressions that contributed to shaping the reaction—those from her own past experiences in this lifetime and previous lives, those from the vast conscious-energies of the inner realm, and going back even farther, from the biological conditioning over billions of years of evolution. But we can look still deeper. Prior to the initial sensation—before there was even the first glimmer of awareness of "Sharon" here and "truck" there; prior to all movements of the Field; prior to and supporting the entire range of Conscious-Energy—there is an infinite Consciousness in which the whole always exists as one. Awakening to That, everything changes, and we are free.

> Before the untiring persistence of your effort [towards the awakening of the psychic being], an inner door will suddenly open and you will emerge into a dazzling splendor

---

a. And, of course, this is true on a global level as well.

that will bring you the certitude of immortality, the concrete experience that you have always lived and always shall live, that external forms alone perish and that these forms are, in relation to what you are in reality, like clothes that are thrown away when worn out. Then you will stand erect, freed from all chains, and instead of advancing laboriously under the weight of circumstances imposed upon you by Nature, which you had to endure and bear if you did not want to be crushed by them, you will be able to walk on, straight and firm, conscious of your destiny, master of your life.[28]

—Mirra Alfassa

> Consciousness is… the fundamental thing in existence—it is the energy, the motion, the movement of consciousness that creates the universe and all that is in it…[301] [As the psychic being awakens], it takes up its greater function as the guide and ruler of the nature... As a final result the whole conscious being is made perfectly apt for spiritual experience of every kind, turned towards spiritual truth of thought, feeling, sense, action…[1]

—Sri Aurobindo

CHAPTER 16

Psychic Awakening and the Transformation of the Individual

> As the crust of the outer nature cracks, as the walls of inner separation break down, the inner light gets through, the inner fire burns in the heart… the soul begins to unveil itself… A guidance, a governance begins from within which exposes every movement to the light of Truth… All is purified, set right, the whole nature harmonized, modulated in the psychic key, put in spiritual order.[2]

—Sri Aurobindo

When we quiet the noise of the surface consciousness, it is possible to go within and enter the vast realm of the inner consciousness, a subtler region of the Field of Conscious-Energy. We can also go still deeper and awaken to the psychic being—the individual Knower. That in itself, however, does not necessarily result in a change of the nature, the individual Field of physical, vital, and mental consciousness. It is possible, though, if one aspires to do so, to bring about a fundamental transformation of the nature following the awakening of the psychic being.

SELF-CONTROL: MILITARY MUSIC OR QUANTUM JAZZ?

Karmic Momentum

The yogis say that at any moment it is possible to step out of the chain of karma into the freedom of the Infinite Consciousness. If this is true, why is it so difficult for us to change? Sometimes, our attention is so thoroughly absorbed in our thoughts and feelings and outer events that we simply ignore the signs that some kind of change is needed. An extreme instance of this kind of inattention took place during the Manhattan Project, the government-sponsored effort during World War II to produce the first atom bomb.

At one point, the physicists working on the project calculated there was a small possibility that testing the bomb would initiate a chain reaction that would explode the atmosphere—resulting in the end of all life on earth, and possibly even the destruction of the planet itself. There was some discussion about discontinuing the project, but according to several of the scientists involved, they were so absorbed in their calculations that the reality of the potential consequences did not seem quite real to them. As one of the physicists put it, "We were like automatons, programmed to do one thing, and we did it."[3]

Even when we know we need to change, often, we are so caught up in the momentum of desire, we find we are incapable of shifting direction. Freeman Dyson, one of the physicists involved in the Manhattan Project, described in an interview conducted many years after the end of the war the thrill the scientists had felt while grappling with the enormous intellectual challenge of producing the bomb:

> I have felt it myself, the glitter of nuclear weapons. It is irresistible if you come to them as a scientist and feel it's there in your hands to release this energy that fuels the stars, to let

limited state of harmony. This is because in our ordinary waking state, action is taken on the basis of separation—"I" am separate from that upon which "I" am acting. From this surface vantage point, no matter how ardently we wish to achieve integration, our fundamental perception remains that of a "mind," "body," and "environment" separate from each other. Lacking direct awareness of the connection between our self and the greater Reality of which we are a part, we have a very limited capacity to effect real and lasting change.

Change from the Inside Out

When we open to the deeper, inner consciousness, we gain the capacity to bring about more far-reaching change, because in the inner realm we are in more direct contact with the whole. In 1971, in a series of experiments conducted at the Menninger Foundation in Topeka, Kansas, Swami Rama was able to demonstrate this power of change initiated from within. He demonstrated the ability to generate delta waves—brain waves that normally occur only in the state of deepest sleep—when he was fully awake. In addition, he was able to intentionally "produce and maintain [various] brain wave patterns on demand"[6] with a level of precision that amazed researchers.

It is not possible to retain wakefulness and generate delta waves as long as one's consciousness is confined to the ordinary limited surface awareness. Swami Rama did not control his brain waves by means of the ordinary limited "self." Even if he had described his experience by saying "I" shifted my consciousness, it would not have been the same "I" as that with which we normally identify. The way he brought about the change in his brain waves was not the way we ordinarily think of controlling our bodies—by an effort of our separate, egoic will. By means of a gentle withdrawal of attention from the surface, Swami Rama was able to "surf" the ocean of consciousness, allowing different waves to emerge and subside. This movement of consciousness is what manifested in the laboratory as different brain wave patterns.

There is a way of "control" that is still deeper than that which can be initiated from the inner realm. Biologist Mae Wan-Ho gives intimations of this deeper way in her description of a state of integration that she refers to as "quantum coherence"—a state that involves simultaneous, nonlocal connections between all parts of an organism. She extends this notion of coherence to the interconnection between the organism and its environment, and has even suggested that the entire universe may exist in a profound state of quantum coherence.

Describing the nature of coherence in terms of a musical performance, she writes:

> To get a feeling for [the coordination of activities involved in the workings of an] organism, imagine an immense super-orchestra, with instruments spanning the… spectrum of dimensions from molecular piccolos of 10^{-9} (one billionth) meter up to a bassoon or a bass viol of a meter or more, performing over a musical range of seventy-two octaves… [T]his super-orchestra never ceases to play out our individual songlines, with a certain recurring rhythm and beat, but in endless variations … Always, there is something new, something made up as it goes along. It can change … as the situation demands, spontaneously and without hesitation. What this super-orchestra plays is the most exquisite jazz, jazz being to classical music what quantum is to classical physics. One might call it quantum jazz. There is a certain structure, but the real art is in the endless improvisations, where each and every player, however small, enjoys maximum freedom of expression, while maintaining perfectly in step and in tune with the whole. There is no leader or conductor, and the music is written as it is played.[7]

From the perspective of yoga psychology, Mae Wan-Ho's description points to the capacity of the awakened soul to "see" in one all-encompassing and joyous gaze the whole Divine Reality in whom, as St. Paul said, "we live and move and have our being."[a]

If fundamental change requires such a profound state of consciousness, is there any hope for those of us who find it challenging to

a. We're not asserting (or denying) here that Mae Wan-Ho is directly describing a spiritual experience. We offer this beautiful passage as an intimation of something deeper than the ordinary surface consciousness.

quiet our minds for more than a few seconds? In fact, it is possible to begin wherever we are. By looking calmly at what is happening in this very moment, we can learn to refine our attention and thus initiate a process of bringing about change in a profoundly new way.

Preparing for the Process of Transformation: Using the Thinking Mind to Sort Out the Tangles of the Surface Nature

> All that we are is the result of what we have thought: it is founded on our thoughts, it is made up of our thoughts. If a man speaks or acts with an evil thought, pain follows him, as the wheel follows the foot of the ox that draws the carriage.
>
> All that we are is the result of what we have thought: it is founded on our thoughts, it is made up of our thoughts. If a man speaks or acts with a pure thought, happiness follows him, like a shadow that never leaves him.[8]
>
> —The Buddha

Learning to direct our attention is at the heart of the process by which we can begin to free ourselves from the grip of desire and ego, and the karmic chain of action and reaction. By refining our attention, we can learn to perceive the subtler movements of our nature that keep us bound in the cycle of reactivity.

How exactly does attention facilitate change? Our ordinary consciousness is rather dull and inattentive. We are hardly aware of the thick web of subconscient impressions that affects every aspect of our physical, vital, and mental consciousness. We also subconsciously filter out a whole array of information that conflicts with our preconceptions and subconscious beliefs about our self and the world. And even that to which we do attend is generally distorted by our egoic preferences and desires:

On the surface we know only so much of our self as is formulated there and of even this only a portion... But there is also a distorting action which obscures and disfigures even this limited self-knowledge; our self-view is vitiated by the constant impact and intrusion of our... vital being, which seeks always to make the thinking mind its tool and servant: for our vital being is not concerned with self-knowledge but with self-affirmation, desire, ego. It is therefore constantly acting on mind to build for it a mental structure of apparent self that will serve these purposes; our mind is persuaded to present to us and to others a partly fictitious representative figure of ourselves which supports our self-affirmation, justifies our desires and actions, nourishes our ego. This vital intervention is not indeed always in the direction of self-justification and assertion; it turns sometimes towards self-depreciation and a morbid and exaggerated self-criticism: but this too is an ego-structure, a reverse or negative egoism, a poise or pose of the vital ego. For in this vital ego there is frequently a mixture of the charlatan and mountebank, the poser and actor; it is constantly taking up a role and playing it to itself and to others as its public. An organised self-deception is thus added to an organised self-ignorance; it is only by going within and seeing these things at their source that we can get out of this obscurity and tangle.[9]

According to psychologist Leslie Greenberg, the simple act of being attentive, without judgment, to what is happening in and around us each moment in itself initiates a process of change.[10] As attention to our present experience intensifies, it gives us the power to see through old reaction patterns and gain freedom from them.[a] It slows down the blur of experience, helping us see with greater clarity the strands of mental, vital, and physical consciousness that make up our experience.

Our habit of interpreting present experience through the lens of the past is in part what leads to the state of "organized self-ignorance"

---

a. Greenberg, using the language of cognitive science, refers to what we've been calling karmic impressions as cognitive or affective "schemas." From the perspective of

of which Sri Aurobindo speaks. By paying close attention to what is actually happening in the present, we allow in information that was previously unattended to. The simple act of incorporating new data— even without further effort on our part—can often be sufficient to begin to unravel some of our subconscious impressions and diminish the karmic momentum that fuels them.

To take a fairly common example, suppose you are experiencing some lower back pain. Ordinarily your conscious experience would be one of a general, undefined sense of physical "pain." You could instead choose to calmly direct your attention to the point in the back where the pain is most intense. If you were to observe very closely, you would see that the "pain" is not merely physical. Contributing to your experi- ence is a vital reaction, which, if put into words, might be expressed as, "This is bad, this shouldn't be, it has to change." Also contribut- ing to your pain construction are the subconscious mental impressions made up of memories of past pain, associations to others' back pain, future projections about how long it will take to go away, what might happen if the pain doesn't change, and so on. What you will find, if you look with sufficient calmness and clarity, is that the simple act of looking and distinguishing these components of your experience can in itself—with no conscious attempt on your part to "change" any- thing—significantly reduce the level of pain. Simply attending to the construction loosens the mental, vital, and physical threads that make up the pain experience, and is sufficient to begin to lessen the pain.

As Sri Aurobindo noted, in addition to this self-ignorance is an "organized self-deception." When our attention is guided by desire, we interpret everything through the lens of that desire. We subconsciously

---

yoga psychology, "schemas" are related to a relatively thin layer of the mental con- sciousness, one just beneath the surface awareness and relatively easily accessible to it. Cognitive science considers schemas to originate in what has been termed the "cognitive unconscious," which is thought to reside in brain processes that are inaccessible to conscious awareness. Karmic impressions, on the other hand, refer also to levels of consciousness far deeper, including the vital and physical consciousness (not our mentalized experience of them), and still deeper layers of the mental, vital, and physical subconscient. By means of highly refined yogic prac- tices, these deepest layers can become accessible to conscious awareness.

alter information to fit with our selfish needs and filter out anything that conflicts with them.

For example, suppose you are scheduled to play a game of softball with some friends, but you sort of know from past experience that because of the pain in your lower back, an afternoon of softball would leave you with worse pain that might last for several days. Nevertheless, your desire to play is so strong, you ignore this and go ahead with your plans. During the game one of your teammates remarks that you're moving a little awkwardly and asks if there's some kind of problem. Though on the fringe of your consciousness there's a vague awareness of physical discomfort, you're so focused on impressing your teammates with your physical prowess that you react with some irritation, dismissing his comment with a wave of your hand, "Nah, I'm fine."

You're so intent on proving you don't have a problem that you remain oblivious to the fact that the pain in your back is increasing throughout the game. The next morning you wake up in so much agony that you decide you can't go to work. Without realizing it, you exaggerate your incapacity, compelling your family to wait on you and attend to your needs. At some point, either as a result of your family's complaints or the intensity of the pain, you realize you need to do something to change the situation.

Normally at a point like this, we are so caught up in the cycle of action and reaction, any choice we make simply continues the cycle of reactivity. For example, rather than attending directly to the pain, you might try to override it and go to work anyway, only to create more pain. Or, still ignoring the cause of the pain, you might take a large dose of pain relievers and go through the day feeling dull and sleepy. However, at any point in this situation, there is a possibility of stepping out of the reaction chain altogether. If you are able to gain some measure of detachment, to look at yourself and the situation without judgment or self-criticism, you can, with sufficient attention, begin to dissipate some of the energy that fuels the chain of karma.

Deconstructing the Chain of Reaction

In previous chapters, we've looked at how the reaction chain gets built up in the moment, taking place too rapidly for us to see how our experience is constructed. Because of this, we are normally aware only of the initial event (the occasion for the reaction) and the end point of the reaction chain (our conscious reaction and subsequent behavior). It is possible to significantly reduce the intensity of the emotional reaction by refining our awareness of the elements of the reaction chain that lead up to it.

For example, if you had been slightly more attentive in the moment your teammate asked if you had a problem, you might have been aware of the feeling of irritation that preceded your response. You might not have realized why you were irritated, but given that extra measure of attention, you could have chosen to respond in a more gracious manner, perhaps thanking him for his concern.

If you were able to further refine your attention as the emotion was arising, you could have seen that preceding it were a host of desires as well as beliefs and assumptions about yourself and the situation that gave rise to the feeling of irritation: the belief that you needed to project an image of being tough; an assumption that people would think less of you if you appeared weak or vulnerable; the subconscious desire to push past the pain; and so on. The simple act of bringing attention to the thoughts, images, and desires that generated the feeling of irritation could, in itself, have been sufficient to significantly reduce the intensity of the feeling.

Refining the attention still further, you could see that, prior even to these subconscious desires, beliefs, and assumptions, there was the simple sensory awareness of the event (your teammate asking if you had a problem), accompanied by a primitive feeling of aversion to being asked. The capacity to see at this level of subtlety would have reduced the impact of the subconscious vital and mental impressions, leading then to a different emotional reaction and a greater choice as to how to respond.

Looking at the whole chain of reaction, we might see a pattern resembling the diagram which appears on the next page. It shows how we can direct our attention, successively, over time, to deconstruct the reaction, eventually becoming conscious of the initial feeling of attraction or aversion that sets the whole reaction chain in motion.

As we learn to step out of the reaction chain, we gradually become freer of the obscurations of ego, desire, and the many layers of subconscient

FIGURE 2: DECONSTRUCTION OF A REACTION
CREATING MORE CHOICE IN HOW YOU RESPOND

∞ = pause

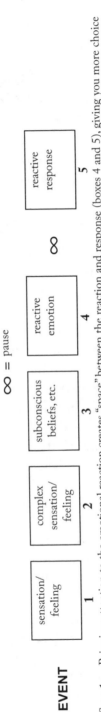

EVENT

Step 1: Bringing attention to the emotional reaction creates "space" between the reaction and response (boxes 4 and 5), giving you more choice as to how you will respond to the event.

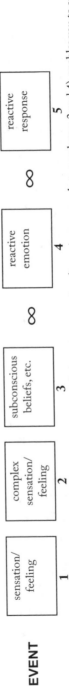

EVENT

Step 2: Bringing attention to the subconscious beliefs, etc., underlying your reaction (inserting a pause between boxes 3 and 4), enables you to see more clearly it is these, not the event, that are responsible for your reaction. This can diminish the intensity of the reaction and ultimately make it more possible for you to react differently.

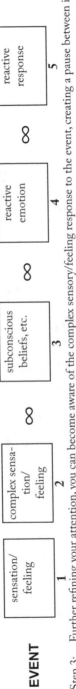

EVENT

Step 3: Further refining your attention, you can become aware of the complex sensory/feeling response to the event, creating a pause between it and the arising of subconscious beliefs, etc. (between boxes 2 and 3), thus further diminishing the intensity of the reaction.

It is possible to refine the attention still further and become aware of what gives rise to the initial simple sensation and feeling, and beyond that, to become aware of the "secret operations in us, in our subconscient and superconscient selves [which, when known, would change] our whole conscious functioning."* But this level of refinement requires a highly developed yogic consciousness.

The calm stillness of the Knower is always present behind the surface play of thought, feeling, and sensation, even in the midst of the most intense reactivity. To the extent you can be open to intimations of the inner peace and calm, it will be easier to insert these pauses in the reaction chain. Conversely, to the extent you are mindful enough to pause, you will become more receptive to intimations of the ever-present stillness of the Soul within.

Each time you bring a degree of mindfulness to the reactive movements of the surface nature, you do two things: a) you weaken the karmic impression fueling the reaction, and b) you create a new, positive** impression. Both make it easier to respond mindfully (i.e., with more freedom) in the future.

---

*Sri Aurobindo, *The Kena Upanishad*, p. 189.
**The word "positive" is not used here as a moral judgment. A karmic impression is "positive" to the extent it is more permeable to the inner Light.

impressions. As this occurs, our surface consciousness becomes clearer, and we begin to open to the influence of the deeper consciousness[a] as well as higher levels of consciousness above the thinking mind. Less obscured by desire, the inner vital and psychic being can open our heart, enabling us to be more responsive to others. Our mind, less bound by mental habits, becomes receptive to the wisdom of the more intuitive inner mental consciousness. Our body, less weighted down by the desires of the vital and mind, becomes more flexible and pliant, more deeply infused with the powerful energy of the subtle physical consciousness.

In recent years this act of refining attention has come to be identified with a particular technique of Buddhist meditation known as "mindfulness." This technique classically involves sitting in a particular position, at a particular time, sometimes using the breath as an object of concentration. There are also other mindfulness techniques that involve carefully observing the contents of one's consciousness while engaged in walking or other activities. In fact, there are virtually a limitless number of techniques and contemplative practices that can help support the development of attention. However, the process we're describing here is not essentially a "technique" or "method." Rather, what we are attempting to portray is a fundamental movement of consciousness, the act of stepping back and freeing up attention that underlies any process of transformation.

This process of refining attention can be a powerful means of bringing about substantial change in our bodies, hearts, and minds. However, from the perspective of yoga psychology, the process of attentional development described above is only the preliminary stage of a more comprehensive process that can lead to deeper and vaster dimensions of being and to the total transformation of the physical, vital, and mental consciousness.[b]

---

a. The inner mental, vital, and subtle physical consciousness and, still deeper, the psychic being.

b. Sri Aurobindo describes this process of attentional training in great detail in the first nine chapters (especially in chapters 6 and 7) of "The Yoga of Self-Perfection" in his book *The Synthesis of Yoga*.

Having described this process as one of directing attention, and having referred to it as involving "mindfulness," the reader may be led to think it is primarily a cognitive process. However, in the yoga tradition, the discipline of refining attention involves the heart at least as much as the mind. In fact, this process could just as well be referred to as "heartfulness." The freeing up of "mindful" and "heartful" attention has been shown to be applicable to a wide range of concerns and situations. In the field of health it has been shown to be beneficial in the treatment of asthma, arthritis, diabetes; back, head, and other kinds of pain; hypertension, and many other physical conditions. In the treatment of psychological disorders, it has been applied with success to anxiety, depression, attention-deficit/hyperactivity disorder, substance abuse, severe trauma, and even severe psychological illnesses such as bipolar disorder and various psychotic disorders. It has also been successfully used in many other fields, from prisoner rehabilitation to the training of Olympic athletes, business leaders, reporters, lawyers and others. This versatility supports the fact that what we are talking about is an all-pervasive movement of consciousness rather than a particular technique or some kind of all-too-simplistic panacea.

AWAKENING OF THE PSYCHIC BEING AND THE TRANSFORMATION OF THE NATURE

Yoga demands a constant inward remembrance of the one central liberating knowledge: In all is the one Self, the one Divine is all; all are in the Divine, all are the Divine and there is nothing else in the universe.[11]

—Sri Aurobindo

The whole problem of life is at root the problem of living in and as a divided consciousness, taking ourselves to be separate beings, apart from each other, the world, and the all-pervading Infinite. It would seem then, that in order to solve the problem, we would need simply to wake up to the truth of our Oneness. But is the whole point of evolution simply to wake up? When everyone has woken up, would the "game" of evolution be over? Or, is there a new, and quite different, game possible?

According to yoga psychology, once having awakened to the truth of who we are, it is possible to allow the true inner nature to gradually infuse and transform the outer personality.[a] Instead of it being "a hurtling field of joy and grief," a "stupendous play of passion," our personality can become a clear window through which something else may naturally emerge.

But we cannot do this by our own power. The mind can assist in the process of transformation by means of the kind of calm attentive mindfulness and heartfulness we described above. But even the deeper mind or heart cannot accomplish the transformation of the nature by themselves:

> A Divine power has to replace our limited energy so the instruments can be shaped into the divine image and filled with the force of a greater infinite energy; this will happen to the degree we can surrender our self to the guidance then to the direct action of that power; faith in [this Divine Power] is essential; faith is the great motor power of our being in our aspiration to perfection.[12]

Before the transformation can begin, we need to awaken the psychic being, the primary channel through which the Divine Power[b] can effect change in the physical, vital, and mental consciousness. To prepare ourselves for this awakening, we will need to have developed the capacity to step back from the surface noise of the mind.[c] There is no

---

a. Some Indian philosophers assert that liberation, not transformation, is the final goal of yoga. However, whether or not they consider it worthwhile, most do acknowledge that transformation is possible.

b. "Divine power" is a translation of the Sanskrit, *shakti*.

c. This should not be conceived of as being limited to a formal practice of sitting meditation. This is an inner stance to be maintained throughout the day, and to whatever extent possible, the night as well.

need at first to stop the chatter, simply to stop fueling the patterns with the energy of our attention:

> In the calm mind, it is the substance of the mental being that is still, so still that nothing disturbs it. If thoughts or activities come, they do not rise at all out of the mind, but they come from outside and cross the mind as a flight of birds crosses the sky in a windless air. It passes, disturbs nothing, leaving no trace. Even if a thousand images or the most violent events pass across it, the calm stillness remains as if the very texture of the mind were a substance of eternal and indestructible peace. A mind that has achieved this calmness can begin to act, even intensely and powerfully, but it will keep its fundamental stillness.[13]

As the surface noise begins to soften and the inner consciousness awakens, there is an intensification of the psychic being's aspiration to awaken. At a certain intensity of attention, the sense of a separate self temporarily dissolves and there arises a feeling of self and other moving together as one. Quarterback John Brodie describes moments during a game when "time seems to slow way down... as if I have all the time in the world to watch the receivers run their patterns and yet I know the defensive line is coming at me just as fast as ever... [T]he whole thing seems like a movie or dance in slow motion."[14] Based on accounts of pro football player Pat Toomay, Larry Dossey describes moments such as these in the lives of various professional athletes—moments "when everything functions perfectly—knowing the flow of a play before it develops, where the ball carrier will run, where the ball will be thrown before it is released. In baseball, the ball and bat become one, the batter can't miss; for the pitcher, the curve ball breaks perfectly, the fast ball is alive, and hitters are retired in effortless sequence, for the basketball player the ball and the net form an arc of oneness from the moment of the ball's release."[15]

The experience of these athletes, while no doubt extraordinary, does not constitute an awakening of the psychic being, nor even a direct entry into the inner consciousness. Rather, it is an example of the surface consciousness being touched by the influence of the inner realm and perhaps, still deeper, the psychic being. It is only when such intimations are accompanied by an all-pervading aspiration, one that persists through day and night, steadfast and unyielding in the face of any disturbance or challenge, that a true reversal of consciousness can take place, allowing the full light of the psychic being to come to the surface:

As Tibetan Buddhist nun Tenzin Palmo describes her own experience of the Soul's[a] awakening:

> One has to become completely absorbed, then the [awakening] will occur. The awareness naturally drops from the head to the heart—and when that happens the heart opens and there is no 'I'. And that is the relief. When one can learn to live from that center rather than up in the head, whatever one does is spontaneous and appropriate. It also immediately releases a great flow of energy because it is not at all obstructed as it usually is by our own intervention. One becomes more joyful and light, in both senses of the word, because it's going back to the source.[16]

Thus, by allowing the action of the surface mind to continue, but taking no interest in it, an awareness grows of the ever-present Silence behind the action of the mind. In that silence is a Force to which we can surrender.[b] To the extent we remain quiet, opening ourselves, this Force can continue to work for a transformation of the mind, the vital and the physical body.

---

a. We are aware that Buddhism is thought to deny the existence of the Soul. It is our understanding that this denial relates specifically to the assertion of some kind of separate, inherently existing entity—which is not what the word "Soul"—as used here—points to. A "Buddhist" understanding of "Soul" might be expressed as "the Buddha nature within—a (not inherently self-existent) focus of the Infinite, Ineffable, Unthinkable, and Immeasurable."

b. In fact, from a deeper perspective, even the surrender is "done" by the Force, not by our small self.

BEGINNING THE PROCESS OF TRANSFORMING THE SURFACE NATURE

At this point, though we continue to use the word "she" to refer to Sharon, it is no longer the same "she" as before; the whole foundation of her identity has shifted. How can we use words to describe this new and utterly different sense of who "she" now realizes herself to be? In the following passage, the Indian sage Ramana Maharshi attempts to convey the distinction between this deeper consciousness—that of the Infinite Knower—and the separative egoic consciousness. He does so in response to someone having said, "I have come here from far away":

[T]hat is not the truth. Where is a "coming" or "going" or any movement whatever, for the one, all-pervading Spirit [the Infinite Knower] which you really are? You are where you have always been. It is your body that moved or was conveyed from place to place till it reached [here]. This is the simple truth, but to a person who considers himself a [separately existing] subject living in an objective world, it appears as something altogether visionary.[17]

It will be helpful to keep the sense of this experience in mind as we look at the process of transformation.

Sharon had had several glimpses of the Divine Presence, but for some time they remained special experiences apart from her day-to-day life. She had no knowledge of "meditation" practice, and didn't realize it might be possible to cultivate the experience of this Presence. For a while she drifted from one odd job to another, wondering what it was she was really supposed to be doing. Though still feeling some intense pain, the sense of hopelessness had waned. She spent a good deal of time reflecting back on her life, her ideals, her many regrets, her sense of dislocation since the war.

Several years after her initial experience of the "tree at the end of the earth," she returns to visit her father. It has now been several months since she's had one of those calm moments of Presence.

~~~~~~~~~~

Sitting on the bench in the backyard of her father's house, Sharon gazes out at the pond, reflecting on the course of her life. Looking back at the many ways she had driven herself to succeed, she feels the sting of unsatisfied desire and thwarted ambition bringing a dull pain to her gut. Though she still doesn't know what she is supposed to be doing, she feels strongly that whatever it is, she has to engage with it in a new way, without having to prove herself, without being driven. As she continues to reflect on this, her mind grows slightly more agitated. Aware of the growing tension, she realizes that, once again, she is trying to figure it all out. Seeing this, her mind slows down.

She returns her attention to the water and the red hibiscus flowers beside the pond. A calm begins to descend; she starts to feel the familiar Presence, more substantial and powerful than in the past. It slowly gathers strength in and around her. She knows by now there's no point in trying to analyze it. She doesn't understand it, can't understand it, but she can just be present and let the experience unfold.

She feels her attention being gently drawn back to painful memories from the past—she sees Bobby sipping water from the cup she held in her hand, and the notice several years later of his death in a drive-by shooting. Familiar images arise of the truck with dead bodies, followed by the faces of people she had used to ascend the ladder of success. Though these images are accompanied by familiar waves of pain and anguish, in some way she can't understand, her experience of the pain is different. However intense each wave may be, it doesn't in any way affect the stillness she feels behind. As these images continue to flow through awareness, the sense of who "she" is shifts in subtle but definite ways.

While this is taking place, Sharon becomes aware of a kind of "Force" that has been guiding her attention, showing her the thoughts, beliefs, memories, feelings, and images of herself that went into constructing her experience of the events of her life, that continue to come together to form what she has taken to be her "self," and which until the last few years were all she had known of herself and the world.

Slowly, with the guidance of this gentle but powerful Force, Sharon sees the various threads that have woven the fabric of her life. She "sees," as if part of a single tapestry, the generations that preceded her birth, her ancestors who were brought over on slave ships from Africa. She understands the connection between her birth as a black woman in mid-twentieth century America, the difficulties she struggled to overcome, and the ways in which she tried to overcome them. She can feel in each phase of her life—leading youth groups, tending wounded soldiers in Vietnam, working in business and politics—the tension between her deeper aspiration and the desires of her surface nature. Watching as the flow of her life unfolds before her inner eye, she feels the tension reaching a kind of crescendo and begins to perceive a poignant beauty in the choreography of her life

Once again, Sharon is shown, with searing intensity, the utter desolation and sense of emptiness that followed her war experience. Her awareness piercing still further below the surface, she understands how it was the desire to escape from despair that drove her from one pursuit to another, seeking but never finding relief. And still deeper, she begins to feel, underlying the emptiness, the Grace that prevented her from finding solace in anything less than that deepest sense of calm and simplicity she had come to know beside the "tree at the end of the earth." She understands how the suffering served to wear down her egoic pride, helping to make her consciousness more flexible and pliant; how it prepared her for the experience that day by the pond in her father's backyard, and allowed her to let go of her desire to analyze and capture the experience with her mind. She sees that each and every experience of her life has been an expression of a greater whole.

Her awareness becoming more global, taking in her life in a single glance, Sharon recognizes that this guidance, this loving Presence, was there all along, guiding her through the vicissitudes of her life. But it had been obscured, unable to shine through the thick screen of her surface nature. Nevertheless, her psychic being had been there as a formative presence at every moment—from early infancy through the idealism of her adolescence; amidst the horrors of war, the pressured years as a successful entrepreneur, and the years she was haunted by memories of dying soldiers and a deepening sense of life's futility.

Full of wonder, her mind quiet, her heart soft and open, her body suffused with a flowing energy, she observes with quiet delight as an image emerges suggestive of some work she might do. This image arises without any feeling of effort, ambition, or striving on her part, inviting her participation without insistence, without demand. She feels as if she is truly awake for the first time in her life. Involuntarily she lets out a sigh, and finds herself laughing at the simplicity of it all.

The image of what she is to do is still vague, uncertain. But it doesn't matter. Sharon feels almost no concern at this moment about her future. She sees it will be a different kind of adventure from any she has yet experienced. All that matters to her at this moment is to remain open to this process, to bathe in the simple delight of this gentle untangling of knots, this opening of her mind, her heart and her body to the Force of the Divine Presence. She smiles and looks over at the sparrow that has just alighted on the lowest branch of the tree.

Chapter 17

Psychic Awakening and the Transformation of Society

> Without a global revolution in the sphere of human consciousness, nothing will change for the better.[1]
>
> —Vaclav Havel, playwright, former president of
> Czechoslovakia

> We must accept that today's problems were created by our thoughts and actions; peace, human development and environmental sustainability must begin in our own minds and deeds. The world cannot change without a transformation in human consciousness.[2]
>
> —Oscar Arias Sanchez, from a talk on the need for
> A Declaration of Human Obligations

In grappling with the decision of whether or not to take her life, Sharon began to undergo a process of awakening. Something in her surface consciousness relaxed its grip, and a ray of light from the psychic being shone through. After some months she gained sufficient equanimity and insight to be able to look back over her life and see how every experience had been part of one seamless whole, each helping her to grow and awaken. Even her greatest suffering had challenged her to develop greater physical, vital, and mental capacities. It forced her to draw on the deeper resources of her inner consciousness and Soul, and ultimately to open to a Force beyond herself. Through this opening to a larger Force, her awakening Soul could begin the process of reshaping and transforming the instruments of her physical, vital, and mental consciousness.

In our lives, it is often through the encounter with challenging circumstances that our consciousness evolves. Similarly, in the broader process of evolution, the challenges from the environment help the sleeping Soul awaken and bring forth greater capacities.

At the human stage, with the emergence of the thinking mind, a conscious collaboration in this process of evolution was made possible. As human beings, we can choose to turn our attention inward and begin to sort out the often conflicting strands of the surface physical, vital, and mental consciousness, thus dismantling the filmy screen that separates us from a deeper, vaster inner awareness. Stepping back from the karmic web in which we've been caught, we can bring our attention still deeper, and awaken as the infinite conscious-beings that we are in truth. Having thus awakened, surrendering to a Force greater than ourselves, we can allow it to infuse our lives, and the instruments of mind, heart, and body, with the qualities of the Divine nature.

The same process of awakening and transformation can occur at the collective level as well. Over millions of years of human evolution, the thinking mind has grown more complex, and with that development, civilization has grown to a level of complexity that is now beyond the capacity of the thinking mind to encompass. If humanity is to survive and continue to grow, a way needs to be found to collectively turn our attention inward, to see the karmic patterns we weave as peoples and as nations, to awaken to our various "group-souls," and create an opening for the power of a Force beyond the mind to transform us and the world in which we live.

TURNING WITHIN TO TRANSFORM THE WORLD?

Given the real, tangible problems that threaten to annihilate us, what is the basis for the assertion that our survival depends on some kind of intangible inner change? Consider the following:

> Imagine you were handed a magic wand. With the first wave of the wand, you could end hunger, provide abundant clothing, shelter, and other material goods for everyone on

earth. All political constitutions would be instantly rewritten to allow for both maximum liberty and equality, all laws amended for the greater good, all business and medical institutions reshaped entirely to be a means of service rather than individual gain. In short, all institutions and structures would be completely transformed with one wave of your magic wand. How long would it take before the individuals living in such a world would begin to reshape that world according to their own desires—changing the laws, institutions, etc. to serve their own ends, with some amassing material goods at the expense of others?

Now imagine a different wave of the magic wand. This time, all outer institutions, structures, laws, etc. remain exactly the same. However, even as your hand lifts for this wave of the wand, the hearts of all people begin to be filled with love and compassion, their minds illumined by intuitive wisdom, their vision imbued with the ability to see the Divine Essence in all. How long might it take before such people would spontaneously create a world endowed with beauty, one dedicated to the material well-being and spiritual unfoldment of all beings?

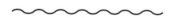

If we take inner change to be fundamental, then efforts toward implementing external change can be seen from a deeper perspective. We can still work for the equitable provision of material goods, just laws, and political institutions. At the same time, however, we can recognize that the purpose of these changes is not primarily to assure the survival and comfort of our fellow human beings, but rather to create conditions that would be most conducive to the awakening and flowering of the Soul—individual and collective. We can further recognize that, as the Soul of humanity continues to awaken, it will naturally bring about a greater transformation of the world than anything our minds can imagine.

To say this sounds overly optimistic or a bit naïve may seem to some a gross understatement. In the past twenty-four hours, more than forty-five thousand people have died of starvation, and another 13 million tons of toxic chemicals have been poured into the atmosphere.[3] More than 3 billion people in the world subsist on the equivalent of less than one U.S. dollar per day, and a majority of the earth's population does not have access to basic health care. To make things worse, we have the material resources to rectify this. According to the 1998 United Nations Human Development Report, it would require approximately $65 billion a year to provide universal access to such basic services as education, health care, and safe water for the entire population of the planet—about the same amount of money spent in Europe each year on cigarettes and on perfume in Europe and the United States combined.[4]

We're not suggesting that everyone stop smoking or using perfume, nor that a weekend workshop in yoga psychology would provide an immediate resolution to these problems. Evolution takes place over billions of years. However, with the emergence of increasingly complex grades of consciousness, the evolutionary process appears to be speeding up. Most people would agree—whatever their philosophical bent—that in the past century the pace of change has quickened dramatically. A small but growing number of observers of the global scene contend we are in the midst of a cultural and spiritual awakening that is unfolding on a scale of decades rather than centuries. There are individuals and groups throughout the world who, in line with these emerging possibilities, are actively creating businesses, developing legal and political structures, organizing communities, and engaging in other activities that are helping to bring about a cultural, and perhaps even spiritual renaissance.

AWAKENING OUT OF THE CULTURAL TRANCE

The whispered resolve of the individual becomes the roar
of collective action. Its righteous sound reverberates in the

structures and institutions of a new society. Its voice is steady and its message is clear: we can act with compassion; we can be more humane; we can live in peace.[5]

—Oscar Arias Sanchez

The following suggestions regarding parallels between the psychology of the individual and society are of course gross oversimplifications. This association of different realms of society—economic, political, and cultural—with specific movements of consciousness is a very broad generalization, meant only for purposes of illustration. In actuality, all levels and grades of consciousness are involved, to some extent, in all activities. Ultimately, it is possible to discern the complex intermixture of conscious-energies associated with any particular activity only through the faculty of yogic vision, which can directly perceive the various energies at play from moment to moment.

There are many parallels between the psychology of the individual and the psychology of a society. The individual psyche is made up of a complex mixture of physical, vital, and mental consciousness. It has various layers—the surface, inner, and inmost soul consciousness, with the subconscient below and superconscient[a] above. Similarly, these various grades and layers make up the consciousness of societies. There is what might be called the "soul" of a family, a community, an organization, or a nation. There is also a collective ego—the limited and distorted expression of the Soul on each of these scales. There are parallels at the individual and social level with regard to development, awakening, and transformation as well. For both the individual and the group, the "game" of evolution involves an interplay between the aspiration of the soul to awaken and the various karmic knots that present challenges

a. Just as the term "subconscient" refers to levels of consciousness below the level of our waking awareness, "superconscient" refers to levels above. These are both relative terms—for example, for a plant, the mental is superconscient.

to that aspiration. In both cases the process of transformation happens through allowing our individual and collective actions—physical, vital, and mental—to be initiated from within by the Soul, and ultimately by a Force beyond.[a]

The collective process of awakening and transformation may become clearer if we consider the various aspects of collective endeavor as analogous to various aspects of the surface consciousness of an individual. In any particular domain of society, the nature of the activity involved tends to mobilize particular types of consciousness. For example, business involves the production and distribution of goods and services. To the extent its focus is on material goods and the needs and desires of the consumers those goods are designed to satisfy, the group consciousness of the business tends to be focused at the level of the physical and lower vital consciousness. Politics and government involve leadership as well as the writing and administering of laws and public policy. While these no doubt require complex mental activity, they tend to keep the energy of consciousness focused at the level of the central and higher vital—related, respectively, to power and relationships. Cultural endeavor—in its manifestation as art, music, philosophy, science, and so on—involves the creation of complex symbols expressing inner and outer vital and mental feelings and ideas, and this tends to mobilize the deeper and higher aspects of the mental and vital consciousness.

In the individual, before the psychic being is awakened and takes over leadership of the mental, vital, and physical consciousness, it is the thinking mind that can best maintain harmony among them. Similarly, in a society, before the soul of a group awakens, it is the "thinking mind" of the culture that is its best means of harmonizing the various aspects of the collective consciousness. To the extent the state—as an instrument of the distorted[b] vital consciousness—

---

a. Ordinarily when people refer to the soul of a nation, or the consciousness of a culture, they intend it to be taken metaphorically. From the perspective of yoga psychology, there are actually collective "fields" of consciousness that have an existence and integrity of their own, beyond the combined consciousness of the individuals who make up the group at any given moment in time.

b. That is, egoic.

dominates business and culture, they cannot fulfill their appropriate functions. The flow of goods and services is impeded, becoming subordinated to the ambitions of those in power. And culture becomes merely a tool of political propaganda.

When business dominates government and culture, the laws and policies of the state are no longer geared toward serving the needs of the nation, but rather to facilitating the acquisition of wealth, usually for a select few. Culture then degenerates into entertainment that is exploited for financial gain. If culture dominates, rather than serving to harmonize the relationship between itself, government, and business, it can lead to a loss of grounding in the physical and vital spheres such that both business and the state may seriously falter. When it performs its rightful role as the integrating force of society, then culture can work together with government and business as an instrument of the deeper and higher aspirations of a people.

However, culture can perform its true function only to the extent that it is free from the distorting influence of ego and desire. In their essay, "Global Civil Society," David Korten, Vandana Shiva, and Nicanor Perlas distinguish between "falsified" and "authentic" culture. What they call a falsified culture is what we referred to earlier as the "consensus reality"—the worldview inculcated into us at such an early age that we are generally unaware of the degree to which we view everything through its filter.

In yoga psychology terms, falsified culture—much like the surface personality of an individual, which is dominated by ego and desire—is one dominated by the desires, attachments, beliefs, and fears of the collective ego. As Korten et al. point out, in the contemporary world, this culture is shaped and sustained to a large extent by the self-interest of powerful corporate and political entities, and is thus dominated by commercial, materialistic values.

From the yogic perspective, authentic culture would be an expression of the consciousness of the thinking mind acting in harmony with the vital and physical consciousness. At a deeper level, authentic culture would be an expression of the Soul and infused with the soul-qualities of wisdom, joy, and compassion. Korten, Shiva, and Perlas believe that we are now witnessing both an increased awareness of the destructive influence of the falsified culture and an intensification of the collective aspiration for authentic culture. They see this aspiration manifesting in a number of ways, including efforts to bring greater awareness to patterns of consumption and a growing desire to prioritize inner over outer goals.

As a means of supporting this process of awakening, Korten, Shiva, and Perlas describe the creation of what they call "zones of freedom":

> A zone of freedom may be as simple as a local study group. It might be a farmer's market, a school to develop inquiring minds, or a course on voluntary simplicity... No matter how small or isolated such initiatives may originally be, each creates a protected space in which diversity, experimentation, and learning can flourish to create the building blocks of a new mainstream culture, politics, and economy.[6]

Such zones of freedom can be linked up

> to create ever-expanding social spaces in which the emergent processes of cultural, political and economic innovation can flourish. As zones of freedom expand and merge, they contribute to the process of liberation from the cultural trance... by offering ever more visible manifestations of [alternative, more harmonious and creative possibilities].[7]

Over the past quarter century, there have been a series of large-scale social surveys identifying a widespread shift in values reflective of this awakening cultural consciousness. For example, the 1990–91 World Values Survey, covering 70 percent of the world's population, discerned a "postmodern shift" toward a "greater search for inner meaning and development; subordination of economic growth to environmental sustainability; cultural pluralism [and] greater freedom for women."[8] More recent surveys have shown a similar shift in values, with a distinction being made between those focused primarily on changing society and those interested in combining social change with spiritual awakening.[9] In yoga psychology terms, the first group reflects an awareness of the need to bring greater harmony to the workings of the collective surface mental, vital, and physical consciousness. The second reflects an awareness of the need to go deeper, to awaken the individual and collective Soul and allow Its Light to transform the surface nature. We will consider some examples of both, looking first at several zones of freedom where a greater harmonization seems to be emerging.

REFINING THE COLLECTIVE SURFACE CONSCIOUSNESS: TWO EXAMPLES OF ZONES OF FREEDOM

Ithaca HOURS: Making a Community While Making a Living

In 1989, community economist Paul Glover of Ithaca, New York, in the course of researching various local economic systems, encountered a form of currency that caught his interest. It was an "hour" note issued in the 1800s by British industrialist Robert Owens, intended for use by his workers when purchasing goods from his company store. Two years later, an alternative local economy was initiated in Ithaca when, in response to Glover's request, Gary Fine, a local massage therapist, agreed to accept payment in "Ithaca HOURS" in exchange for his services. Fourteen years later, over $50,000 in HOURS have been issued to over 1,000 participants. Ithaca HOURS are the first modern example of a local currency, and have since "inspired similar systems throughout the world."[10] The Ithaca program is "one of three monetary reform measures named as viable alternatives to [the] Bretton Woods system [at a] United Nations conference."[11]

One Ithaca "HOUR" is worth the equivalent of ten U.S. dollars, the average hourly wage in the region when the program was initiated in 1991. The aim of the HOURS currency is to strengthen the city's local economy. All who use HOURS are required to spend them locally, "thus building a network of inter-supporting local businesses."[12] HOURS can be used in exchange for a wide range of goods and services from plumbing, carpentry, and car repair to nursing, child care, and groceries. It is also possible to make rent and mortgage payments with HOURS, and they are accepted at local movie theaters, health clubs, farmer's markets, and restaurants.

Commenting on the value of this local currency, Glover writes:

> Federal dollars come to town, shake a few hands, then leave
> to buy rainforest lumber and to fight wars. Ithaca HOURS,
> by contrast, stay in our region to help us hire each other.
> While dollars make us increasingly dependent on multina-
> tional corporations and bankers, HOURS reinforce com-
> munity trade and expand commerce that is more responsive
> to our concern for ecology and social justice.[13]

In using the HOURS currency, Ithacans are also building a deeper sense of community. As Glover expresses it:

> We encounter each other as fellow Ithacans, rather than as
> winners and losers scrambling for dollars. As we do so, we
> help relieve the social desperation which has led to compul-
> sive shopping, wasted resources, and homelessness and hun-
> ger. We're making a community while making a living.[14]

The HOURS program demonstrates the potential power of awakening out of the general cultural trance, becoming conscious of the subconscious assumptions and beliefs that lead to compulsive, desire-driven activity. By the simple act of printing a local currency that supports the ethical values of their community, Ithacans have been able, to some degree, to free their consciousness during an act of currency exchange, from its habitual domination by the desire for possessions, and the craving for comfort and security. They have created the possibility for a more refined mental consciousness to bring the vital and physical consciousness of the community into harmony with its ethical concerns.

Let's look at the Ithaca HOURS experiment in the context of

was unmistakable: They were happy. They rose before dawn, worked hard and productively, ate simply but well, and were peaceful."[17]

The story of Gonzalo and Cecilia Bernal and their son Juan David, offers a beautiful illustration of the deep sense of camaraderie that prevails amongst Gaviotans. Juan David was born with a brain lesion, resulting in damage to his left eye and ear. He walked with a pronounced limp and had little use of his left arm. Even simple physical activities were difficult for him. When at age ten he was given a bicycle, he was unable to ride it despite repeated attempts. A doctor's assessment that he would never be able to ride one left him feeling miserable. At a certain point the Bernals felt they needed to leave Gaviotas in order to have access to more sophisticated medical rehabilitation facilities for their son.

Once ensconced in the suburbs of Bogotá, the Bernals missed life in the community terribly. Describing the difficulties their son faced in his new environment, Weisman writes, "The cruelty he endured at school because of his limp and curled left arm would be unthinkable at Gaviotas, where the only friction he'd inspired among the children was over who got to babysit him next."[18] After several years away, the Bernals finally realized that life would ultimately be better for Juan David back in Gaviotas. When their son was thirteen years old, they decided to return. Two days after they were back, Gonzalo was talking with a friend outside a factory. He heard the shouts of children and looked up to catch sight of something that brought tears to his eyes. "The ecstatic boy with curly brown hair pedaling across the plain, leading the pack of cheering Gaviotas kids who had taught him how to ride was [Juan David]."[19]

Regarding the enormous potential value of what the community has to offer, Gaviotan founder Paolo Lugari comments:

> There are two hundred-fifty million hectares of savannas in South America alone. There's Africa. The tropical Orient. Places where there's space and sun and water. If we show the world how to plant in them sustainable forests, we can give people productive lives and maybe absorb enough carbon dioxide to stabilize global warming in the process. This is a gift we can give the world that's just as important as our sleeve pumps

and solar water purifiers. Everywhere else they're tearing down rain forests. We're showing how to put them back.[20]

Lugari has been intimately involved in the community from its inception. Asked what would happen when he is no longer there, he responded:

> The Gaviotas Foundation is what really runs things in Gaviotas now. The place runs much better when I am not there. There are lots of people involved in Gaviotas. Several generations of people work there now and will keep it going. Gaviotas is a state of mind, more than anything. It is not really so much a place. It's a way of living and thinking. It means not just thinking outside the box, but constant innovation and re-invention. For one problem there are ten solutions. In any crisis, there is an opportunity to try out any or all solutions.[21]

The Gaviotan community is a splendid example of a comprehensive experiment in which technology, the economy, and governing principles all function to support the ideals and aspirations of the residents, nurturing their inner growth and development. Living according to their ideals, relatively free from the domination of vital desire and the inertia of the physical consciousness, their imagination is set free. When the imagination, intellect, emotions, and body act in harmony, a greater flexibility and creativity is the natural result.[a] The abundant creativity manifest in both the technological inventions and in the everyday lives of Gaviotans testifies to the plasticity of their consciousness as well as their ability to generate an "authentic culture," one relatively free of the limiting karmic tendencies associated with the falsified culture of the consensus trance.

While the stated aims of the community do not include explicit mention of "spirituality," clearly, many qualities of the Soul shine

---

a. Neuroscientists speak of this as "neuroplasticity"—the capacity of the brain to create new synaptic connections.

through the life in Gaviotas: the beauty of the environment they created and even the machines they designed; the joy and peace that permeates their daily affairs; the powerful sense of fraternity among members of the community; the awareness of being part of a process that is larger than any individual resident. This is a lovely demonstration of the yogic understanding that when the aspiration of the Soul is no longer co-opted by the desires and greed of the untransformed surface consciousness, peace of mind and gentleness of heart are the natural result. The peace of mind and gentleness of heart that can flower when living in harmony with one's highest ideals is considered by yogis to be one of the essential prerequisites for spiritual awakening.

OPENING TO THE LIGHT OF THE COLLECTIVE SOUL: SOME EXAMPLES OF SPIRITUAL ZONES OF EVOLUTION

> [A] society which was even initially spiritualised would make the revealing and finding of the divine Self in man the supreme, even the guiding aim of all its activities, its education, its knowledge, its science, its ethics, its art, its economical and political structure... It would regard the peoples as group-souls, the Divinity concealed and to be self-discovered in its human collectivities, group-souls meant like the individual to grow according to their own nature and by that growth to help each other, to help the whole race in the one common work of humanity. And that work would be to find the divine Self in the individual and the collectivity and to realise spiritually, mentally, vitally, materially its greatest, largest, richest and deepest possibilities in the inner life of all and their outer action and nature. [22]
>
> —Sri Aurobindo, *The Human Cycle*

David Korten, Vandana Shiva, and Nicanor Perlas have observed that an increasing number of people are becoming aware of the materialistic values that shape the culture in which we live. They also describe a corresponding aspiration for the development of an authentic culture, one that would reflect our deeper human values. Beyond this, we can see signs of a still more profound awakening—the growing awareness of what might be called evolutionary consciousness—that is, the recognition that we are part of a larger, unfolding spiritual process. With this recognition, our engagement with the world undergoes a profound shift. Rather than struggling to create change, our task becomes one of attuning ourselves to that spiritual process, discerning as best we can the "music" we are called to play as instruments of the Divine "super-orchestra"[23] of the cosmos.

There are, throughout the world, a growing number of individuals and groups whose work reflects this awareness of their role in the larger evolutionary process. We'll look at several that draw on the yoga tradition of India for their core inspiration, but which are not confined to a particular religious tradition.

Sarvodaya: The Awakening of All

> We build the road and the road builds us.
>
> —Saying of the Sarvodaya Movement

The Sarvodaya Shramadana Movement of Sri Lanka was founded in 1958 by Dr. A. T. Ariyaratne. During that year, a group of Sri Lankan college teachers and high school students chose to spend their vacation living in a poor rural village in order to get firsthand knowledge of the conditions afflicting a significant portion of the country's population. The visitors set up a work camp and helped village residents "dig wells, build latrines, plant gardens, repair the school and build a place for 'religious worship.'"[24] The camp was a great success and became the model for what Ariyaratne later called the "*shramadana* camp." *Shramadana* means "the gifting or the voluntary sharing of one's labor and resources for the awakening of oneself and others."[25] Since 1958, over fifteen thousand villages in Sri Lanka have participated in *shramadana*

camps and become part of the national Sarvodaya movement. Dr. Ariyaratne adopted the word "Sarvodaya" from Mahatma Gandhi, trans-
lating it to mean "the awakening of all."[26]

The goals of the Sarvodaya movement are explicitly spiritual. Its
efforts toward economic and political development of poor rural villages
are ultimately intended to serve the more far-reaching goal of the evolution of consciousness. Describing the priorities of Sarvodaya, George
Bond, a longtime student of Buddhist activism in Sri Lanka, writes:

> Real development facilitates human awakening rather
> than increasing the GNP or the industrialization of
> the country... Rather than seeking economic growth,
> Sarvodaya seeks "right livelihood"... Right livelihood
> stresses harmony and the quality of life rather than
> ambition and working for profit only.[27]

The method of the movement has been to go into various villages and
organize a *shramadana* camp in which all residents participate—from
children under five to the village elders. They decide together what needs
to be done and work together on such activities as building roads, digging wells for clean water, planting trees, and creating schools and new
health facilities. During a work camp, they come together three times a
day, meditating on loving-kindness, singing songs, or dancing—all with
the aim of bringing out a deep spiritual awareness of working together
as one. Members of different religions—including Christians, Buddhists,
Muslims, and Hindus—all participate in these sacred activities.

For Sarvodaya, cultivating the "right modes of mind"[28] is considered every bit as important as selfless giving of one's labor. Adopt-
ing the ancient Indian practice of the *Brahma Viharas*,[a] they focus
on the meditative development of four particular states of mind: loving-kindness (cultivating a deep aspiration for a particular individual
or group of individuals to be free from fear, greed, sorrow, and other
causes of suffering); compassion (identifying with others' suffering as

a. Literally, "abiding in the Brahman," or abiding in the Consciousness of the
Infinite Knower.

if it were one's own); rejoicing in others' good fortune; and equanimity (the recognition that no one person is more special than another, that all are interconnected because ultimately there is no separate self). The goal is to build what Dr. Ariyaratne refers to as a "no poverty/no affluence"[29] society where the well-being of all is ensured and the ultimate goal is spiritual awakening.

Once an infrastructure has been set up to meet the basic needs of a village, village members can incorporate as a formal Sarvodaya Shramadana society. They can further choose to link up with other villages in clusters of ten, and if they choose, network at regional and national levels as well. Control always remains with the local village, but networking allows for a greater sharing of resources. The movement is currently focusing on incorporating modern technology, and to that end is developing telecenters that will link electronically the many thousands of Sarvodaya villages.

Sri Lanka has endured many years of violent civil war, and the Sarvodaya movement has had to make many accommodations. They have set up refugee camps to help Tamil separatists and created the People's Participatory Peace Program, which organizes peace seminars, conferences, peace camps and meditation walks. Over one hundred thousand people have taken part in mass meditation programs and walks, the longest walk spanning eighty-one miles between the sacred city of Kandy and the ancient sacred capital of Anuradhapura. On October 3, 2005, the movement "was awarded the United Nations' highest prize in the field of human settlement and shelter... [and] was recognized for its development work in villages with particular regard to its massive post-Tsunami reconstruction work."[30]

Though developed on the basis of Buddhist values, the Sarvodaya movement emphasizes the spiritual unity underlying all religions. Dr. Ariyaratne believes that

> what is most important... in religion is not its historical, political or ritualistic aspects. These are all secondary...what is most important is the essence of religion, which is spirituality... whatever one may call it, cosmic consciousness, or universal mindfulness.[31]

Ariyaratne frequently describes the goal of Sarvodaya as creating "a critical mass of spiritual consciousness"[32] that will eventually transform the world. As Bond describes Ariyaratne's view,

> transforming the consciousness of individuals and communities toward compassion and peace represents an essential step toward building a just and peaceful world.[33]

The Center for Contemplative Mind in Society

> We believe that [contemplative] practices offer insights that illuminate the central issues of our time, leading us to cultivate a wise, compassionate, meaningful life.[34]

The Center for Contemplative Mind in Society (CMS) is a nonprofit organization whose mission is to bring contemplative practice into mainstream institutional life. According to cofounder Mirabai Bush, CMS began in the mid-1990s "as a conversation about the relationship between contemplative practices and social change, and the relationship between individual and social transformation."[35] Over the past eight years CMS has established workshops, retreats, and long-term programs in such major institutions as Yale and Columbia Law Schools, the University of Massachusetts at Amherst, the Monsanto Corporation, and Searle Pharmaceuticals. According to Bush, CMS chose initially to target mainstream institutions because their values have such a profound and pervasive influence in our lives.

CMS has created programs to address the needs of individuals in a variety of fields—lawyers, prisoners, social activists, community organizers, and others. Their Social Justice Program brings contemplative practices to activists engaged in working to create outer change. By helping them to meet conflict and opposition with a quiet mind and open heart, the activists gain a new perspective, find a deeper source of motivation, and learn to create healthier working and living environments that reflect the deeper values of mindfulness and compassion.

The Law Program engages judges, lawyers, law professors, and students in ongoing dialogue and contemplative practice to help them "reconnect with their deepest values and intentions."[36] One of the outgrowths of this program has been support for the creation of the Network of Contemplative Prison Programs. CMS has also served as an adviser to people such as Chancellor David Scott, who is initiating a program on contemplative studies at the University of Massachusetts, Amherst.

Some social activists have expressed concern about the wisdom of incorporating contemplative practices in their work. In part, this stems from the fear that without anger, they will not have the motivation to work as vigorously for their cause. However, they're also concerned that the CMS project of teaching corporate executives to meditate may simply give them more peace of mind as they continue to pursue profit at the expense of the health and welfare of human beings and the environment.

In an interview published in *Tricycle* magazine, Mirabai Bush describes the conflict she faced in arranging the center's first retreat with the chemical company Monsanto:

> Monsanto was a big challenge for me personally, because I had spent the previous ten years working in sustainable agriculture with Mayan people in Guatemala. At that point [Monsanto's] main product was Round-Up, the largest-selling herbicide in the world. It had been used extensively in Guatemala, where the heart of my work was the recovery of land that had been destroyed by chemicals. I believed that Round-Up had contributed to destroying the land, to the hunger and poverty that the Mayan people were living in.[37]

In helping develop the Monsanto retreat, Bush saw her greatest challenge as letting go of her judgment without in any way forfeiting her own values.[a] After the retreat was over, Bush answered the

---

a. This does not mean, as we understand it, that she abandoned her capacity for ethical discernment. She did not change her assessment regarding the destructive effect of Monsanto's use of Round-Up in Guatemala. Nonjudgment, in this instance, refers to the capacity to balance exacting ethical discernment with an inner quietude while remaining open to the promptings of the Soul.

question as to whether they had done nothing more than help Monsanto employees lower their stress level and be more comfortable pursuing the same destructive behavior:

> When the practice is held in a safe space, and is taught with the best intention, insight, wisdom and compassion can increase. Over and over I've seen people have moments of awakening about their lives. It's not like, "Oh, Monsanto is making chemicals, I don't think that's good anymore."… It's people beginning to see that there is a process of awakening and they can begin to cultivate a different kind of awareness.[38]

Bush recounts an experience she had on the retreat while CMS teacher Steve Smith was conducting a loving-kindness meditation. The practice involves extending a deep feeling of kindness and goodwill, first to oneself, then expanding it outward, eventually including all living creatures. She observed that after several days of contemplative practice, the executives were open enough to be deeply affected by the meditation:

> We hadn't talked about sustainable agriculture or product mix; the executives hadn't explained why they thought Round-Up was good for the planet. I opened my eyes in the middle of the meditation as Steve was talking about these different species, and I looked around the room and saw tears rolling down the cheeks of many people there.[39]

The Samatha Project: A Manhattan Project for the Study of Consciousness

> At the beginning of the twenty-first century humanity is poised for a revolution in our understanding of consciousness, as the… modes of inquiry of the contemplative traditions of the world are integrated with the… methods of modern science.[40]

B. Alan Wallace is a scholar of comparative religion, teacher of Tibetan Buddhism, and translator for the Dalai Lama. Deeply influenced by a Christian upbringing yet strongly drawn to the natural sciences, as an adolescent Wallace felt compelled to find some way of bridging the apparently incompatible worldviews underlying science and religion. During his junior year abroad at the University of Göttingen, Wallace happened upon a book on Tibetan Buddhism that so moved him that he dropped all his courses to focus exclusively on learning the Tibetan language.

Further reading convinced him that within the wide diversity of world religions "there is a profound convergence at the deepest level of mystical experience, [one that points us toward] the most important reality human beings can realize."[41] Within a year he had sold all of his possessions that would not fit in his backpack and headed east to Dharmsala, India, home of the Dalai Lama and a Tibetan Buddhist spiritual community. He spent the next fourteen years immersed in the meditative and philosophical tradition of Tibet, including five years of solitary contemplative retreats in Tibetan monasteries in Switzerland.

Having found in Tibetan Buddhism a way to integrate spiritual practice with rigorous intellectual inquiry, Wallace now sought an integration of East and West. In 1984 he decided to return to the United States to pursue a degree in physics in order to gain a better understanding of the worldview represented by modern science. He later studied cognitive science and philosophy of mind, and completed a doctoral program in religious studies at Stanford University. "To be able to have all of these in one container, all of these in communication with each other, all enhancing and complementing each other—that's what I've sought since returning to [the West]."[42]

Based on his own contemplative experience and research he conducted with cognitive scientists on the effect of contemplative practice on the brain, body, and emotions, he was convinced of the enormous potential of such practice to effect a powerful and positive change in human nature.

> One way the contemplative traditions can be of benefit in this regard is to help us recognize that there are things that

we can do as individuals to address the various forms of suffering we experience. We can train the mind. We can develop
new habits. We can gain experiential insights… In so doing,
we can transform the mind in a way that is empowering and
ennobling to the human individual.[43]

However, in order to realize this potential, Wallace came to believe
that a large-scale research project on the nature of consciousness would
be required—one much like the Manhattan Project that developed the
atomic bomb during World War II. His vision is of "a concerted, collaborative effort on the part of professional cognitive scientists and
professional contemplatives, using their combined extraspective and
introspective skills to tackle the hard problem of consciousness."[44]

The Samatha Project is intended to be a small-scale model for such
a large-scale possibility. As a foundation for the project, Wallace helped
establish the Santa Barbara Institute for the Interdisciplinary Study
of Consciousness at the University of California, Santa Barbara. The
institute aims to conduct research that will explore the potentials of the
mind more fully than has ever before been done, using an integration
of scientific and contemplative methodologies. Research will focus on

> the cultivation of human flourishing and genuine happiness
> through exceptional mental health and balance, bringing
> the physical and psychological benefits of training aware-
> ness to ever-broader segments of the population and all
> areas of life.[45]

The Samatha Project was initiated in September 2006, with thirty
individuals beginning a one-year residential retreat during which, for
eight to ten hours each day, they will

> undergo a kind of "Olympic training" of the mind [that]
> will center on mindfulness of breath; settling the mind in its
> natural state; observing mental events without distraction or
> grasping; and resting the attention in pure awareness with
> no specific object of meditation.[46]

As part of the project, neuroscientists will use sophisticated brain scanning instruments to "find out which parts of the brain are activated when people enter into these states of refined attention."[47] State-of-the-art EEG research methodology will be used to measure brain wave activity. And cognitive psychologists will use complex psychological tests and measures to determine the level of attentional and emotional balance achieved by retreatants over the course of the retreat.

Whereas the training of Olympic athletes aims for physical excellence, the goal of the Samatha Project is the attainment of what Wallace calls "mental excellence."[48] Just as research conducted on athletes has provided valuable information on diet, exercise, and motivation that is relevant to the general population, Wallace anticipates that the findings of the Samatha Project will similarly yield broad insights that will prove useful in the treatment of a wide range of psychological disorders, both cognitive and emotional.

He further expects that ways will be discovered to help people refine and direct their attention that will be applicable in other areas, such as business, education, and interpersonal relationships, where attentional skills, mindfulness, and empathy all play an important role. While acknowledging that many claims regarding the efficacy of meditative techniques have been made in the past, Wallace suggests that, when subjected to intensely rigorous study, "it may turn out that there are potentials of consciousness that the contemplative traditions have been unveiling for centuries, for millennia, about which the modern scientific tradition knows nothing."[49]

Wallace foresees a number of potential long-term outcomes of the Samatha Project. He imagines that professionals in various fields (neuroscience, psychology, philosophy, etc.) will one day choose to undergo a postdoctoral program of intensive contemplative training. In addition, he anticipates the creation of a new vocation—the professional contemplative—who will devote years to sustained contemplative training, perhaps become a specialist in disciplines such as contemplative inquiry, the honing of attention, lucid dreaming, or cultivation of the heart, and who will be available to collaborate on research projects with natural scientists all over the world.

Reflecting on the larger context of such a training program, Wallace compares the present era to that of the sixth century B.C.E. when there were a series of cultural revolutions occurring around the same time in China, India, Greece, and elsewhere. He suggests we may now be entering into a new, global cultural revolution

> as we see the great traditions of the East and the West coming into contact with an attitude of mutual respect, mutual appreciation, and an eagerness to seek out the nature of reality with an open mind. We may be on the verge of a tremendous transition here. Not only could it unveil marvelous discoveries that will be of tremendous interest, great fascination, but it may also bring pragmatic benefits that may yield dividends for humanity as a whole. With the collaboration of the contemplative and the scientific, we may be moving towards a scientific revolution that will dwarf anything since Galileo.[50]

CREATING ZONES OF EVOLUTION WHEREVER WE ARE

The evolutionary process—the awakening of the Soul and the transformation of the Field—is occurring throughout the universe in each moment. Recognizing this, we don't need to travel to Sri Lanka or Santa Barbara to bring about change in our own community. How might one start working toward awakening and transformation at a collective level in a typical modern town or city filled with people living stressful, busy lives, who have little or no interest in contemplative practice?

The modern world is so focused on "doing" and achieving measurable practical results, we may feel that unless we are engaged in a vast Sarvodaya-like project, we will not be making an appreciable contribution to collective spiritual awakening. But each person has a unique role to play. Perhaps we are called to do no more than engage in inner practice, carrying whatever equanimity and insight we gain through that practice into our work and relationships. Perhaps no one will even know we have an interest in spirituality. Yet in some way we may not understand, we would be making a contribution to the whole.

For example, a friend or some people at work may one day ask us for a suggestion about dealing with pain or depression. Without the pride of being a "helper," we can share what we've learned from our inner practice, and this might make a difference for them. In addition, by staying receptive, attempting to tune in to the ongoing evolutionary process, we may get intimations of how we can further share our experience in ways we might not previously have considered.

Or, we may find ourselves taking a more formal role in bringing contemplative practice into a community. Along the lines of CMS, we may be invited into an institution, or a particular department within our current workplace, to introduce people to contemplative practice, giving them a sense of what it can bring into their work, their relationships with coworkers, and even into their lives as individuals.

We might find interested individuals in a particular department of a large institution—say, the oncology ward of a city hospital. Working with a few doctors, nurses, and other staff to develop classes, retreats, or an ongoing program, interest might be generated in other departments as well. If these are successful, the hospital might be interested in training the whole management staff so they can begin to bring similar programs into each of their respective departments. The fruits of such an endeavor might then be shared with other hospitals within the community, creating a new sense of collaboration and shared purpose. Going still further, classes and programs might be designed for different kinds of institutions, linking schools, businesses, the media, government agencies, places of worship, arts establishments, and others. If this kind of linking were to take place, a larger cultural shift might begin to occur throughout the community, awakening a sense among residents of participating in a collective evolutionary process.[a]

One might imagine a wide range of variability in the nature and progression of such zones of evolution. In many communities it may be that individuals interested in spiritual practice act simply as silent carriers of the flame of awakening. In what would likely be fewer communities, one might find a contagion of the Spirit, where a conscious

---

a. Though they might not specifically articulate their view of it as being part of a "collective evolutionary process"!

interlinking of various institutions might take off at a surprising rate.

Therapist and writer Arjuna Ardagh, over the course of a number of years, conducted more than 150 interviews with such prominent meditation teachers as Jack Kornfield, Ekhart Tolle and Joseph Goldstein.[51] All concur that a growing number of their students report having experienced an inner awakening of some kind. Such individuals are as likely to be executives in large corporations as they are volunteers for environmental advocacy groups. Often, after having had a taste of something deeper, these individuals find it hard to reconcile their emerging inner experience with a culture that does not reflect their aspiration or new values. Creating community-based contemplative resources—whether a small center offering classes or a community-wide initiative—could help people feel less alone and support their efforts to integrate their new sensibilities with the activities of their daily lives.

What might become possible when a number of people within a community develop an interest in working at a deeper level?

IMAGINING COLLECTIVE PRACTICE AT A DEEPER LEVEL: A SKETCH OF A TEN-DAY RETREAT

Imagine that a small business has spent several years integrating contemplative practice into its workplace. They've developed and refined their ability to identify the karmic knots that arise between them and to work through, in a relatively calm manner, the obstacles these knots present. The atmosphere has grown more harmonious, and the business has become more effective. Recognizing how valuable contemplative practice has been not only to their work together but to their individual lives beyond the workplace, a general feeling has grown among both management and staff that they would like to take some step that would help deepen their experience. They decide to arrange to have small groups of employees take time off for a ten-day contemplative retreat.

A small retreat center in a pastoral setting that caters to small contemplative groups provides an atmosphere of peace and calm. The swans and geese gliding gently over the surface of the lake outside the meeting room window add to the sense of tranquility. Retreatants spend the first two days in silence, establishing a stable inner calm.

On the third day a facilitator helps them bring to the surface some of the deeper karmic knots with which they've been dealing. Having had several years of contemplative practice in bringing an inner quiet to this process, they feel well-prepared to participate in this exercise, exploring difficult issues together with calm and equanimity.

In the course of the third and fourth days they learn to bring an increasingly intuitive awareness to these issues, seeing the layers of conscious and subconscient physical, vital, and mental energies that are entangled in the karmic knots. They see how their individual karmic patterns have been interwoven with those of the group as well as with those of the larger cultural matrix in which they live. As they begin to sense the greater subtle energies at play, remaining open to what emerges, their hearts soften.

As seems appropriate throughout the day, they engage in group dialogue interwoven with silent contemplation. Their facilitator skillfully guides them to remain attentive to the soft voice of the Soul and the deeper Silence behind while they interact and talk through their various issues.[52] Staying connected to the depths within, they begin to sense the deeper movements of the Soul that are seeking to emerge as well as the process by which these movements become distorted by desire, attachment, and ego. Staying connected to the Silence, they begin to become aware, as a group, of a greater Force sustaining and guiding them, filling the atmosphere with a palpable sense of peace.

During the final days of the retreat they begin to engage in more outer-directed activities—helping with meal preparation, gardening, and building projects for the retreat center. This will help make the transition back to their busy lives a gentler one, giving them the opportunity to practice maintaining inner Silence while being engaged in outer activity. On the last two evenings they develop support structures to help sustain the process of transformative dialogue they have begun. They work out ways to create a pause in the midst of their work and to conduct meetings in such a way that these times become further opportunities for awakening and transformation. They decide to set aside two days each month as partial retreats—what Zen teacher Thich Nhat Hanh calls "days of mindfulness." On these days they would take a half hour every few hours to meditate or dialogue, being mindful in the intervening times to stay inwardly connected, maintaining a sense of Presence as they speak, move, and work.

~~~~~~~~~

Suppose a few organizations in various locations were actually to embark upon some kind of transformational process. It might seem that it would take decades before any kind of substantial change could be felt at the national or international level. With the world in such dire need of change, what possibility of survival would there be if this slow, long-term process of transformation were our only hope?

TRANSFORMATION SEEN FROM THE INNER CONSCIOUSNESS

Living in a culture pervaded by the view from nowhere, it is difficult to avoid thinking that the only way to gauge the effect of spiritual practice on the outer world is in terms of changes we can see. Though scoffed at by modern rationalist thought, spiritual traditions the world over have known by means of direct perception that there are greater forces at play and greater changes taking place than those we can perceive with the outer mind and senses. We may think, for example, that wars are caused by disputes that occur over territory or oil, or by a hostile act one nation takes against another. But as Sri Krishna Prem writes:

> It is in the inner worlds of desire that wars originate, and from those inner worlds that they are maintained. What we see as wars upon this physical plane are but the shadows of those inner struggles, a ghastly phantom show, bodying forth events that have already taken place in the inner world, dead ash marking the destructive path of the forest fire, the troubled and unalterable wake of a ship whose prow

is cleaving the waters far ahead. In war or peace we live in a world of shadows cast by events that we term "future," because, unseen by us as they really happen, we only know them when we come across their wake upon this plane.[53]

According to yoga psychology, the changes we see in the outer world are only a reflection of changes that have been set in motion in the vaster realm of the inner consciousness. A powerful transformative Force is already at work on the subtle planes. More powerful even than the collective aspiration of humanity is the Will of the Silent Knower working through every heart, dynamically active in every atom of the universe. By aligning our individual aspiration with the Divine Will, we can collaborate with this inner process of transformation. In the words of Sri Aurobindo:

> [When we] realise in our experience the truth of the [statement in the *Isha Upanishad*], "What bewilderment can he have or what grief, when in all things he sees their oneness?" the whole world then appears to us in a changed aspect, as an ocean of beauty, good, light, bliss, exultant movement on a basis of eternal strength and peace... We become one in soul with all beings... and, having steadfastly this experience, are able by contact, by oneness, by the reaching out of love, to communicate it to others, so that we become a center of the radiation of this divine state... throughout our world.[54]

> Consciousness is... the fundamental thing in exis-
> tence— it is the energy, the motion, the movement of con-
> sciousness that creates the universe and all that is in it...
> Consciousness in us has drawn a lid...between the lower
> planes of mind, life, body supported by the psychic [being]
> and the higher planes which contain the spiritual kingdoms
> where the Self is always free and limitless, and it can break
> or open the lid or covering and ascend there and become
> the Self free and wide and luminous or else bring down the
> influence, reflection, finally even the presence and power of
> the higher consciousness into the lower nature.[1]
>
> —Sri Aurobindo, *Letters on Yoga*

CHAPTER 18

Spiritual and Supramental Awakening and Transformation: Tuning the Finite To Infinity

SPIRITUAL AWAKENING AND TRANSFORMATION

> The psychic life [one lived in full awareness of the soul] is
> immortal life, endless time, limitless space, ever-progressive
> change, unbroken continuity in the universe of forms. The
> spiritual consciousness, on the other hand, means to live the
> infinite and the eternal, to be projected beyond all creation,
> beyond time and space. To become conscious of your psychic
> being and to live a psychic life you must abolish all egoism;
> but to live a spiritual life you must no longer have an ego.[2]
>
> —Mirra Alfassa

We've described the awakening of the Soul, the Divine within, and the beginning of the transformation of the physical, vital, and mental nature that it can bring about. The full psychic transformation involves a complete change in the way the physical, vital, and mental consciousness function. Thoughts, feelings, and sensations are no longer referred to that imaginary point—the "ego"—which we had wrongly taken to be our "self." Rather, united with the Divine within, all the movements of our nature—every vibration of the Field—are felt to be infused with the Divine Consciousness.

Spiritual Awakening: Awakening To the Knower

As immense a change as this may be, there is an awakening and process of transformation yet beyond. While the psychic realization involves an awareness of that aspect of the Divine that ensouls the universe, it is possible to awaken to the Infinite Spirit that is beyond all time and space. The Buddhists refer to this as "primordial awareness." In the words of Evelyn Underhill, a writer on Christian mysticism, "This unmistakable experience has been achieved by the mystics of every religion; and when we read their statements, we know that all are speaking of the same thing."[3]

Sri Krishna Prem, describing the results of a sustained effort to pierce through the last remnants of ego, writes that:

> like a tree long bound by winter frosts bursting suddenly into glorious bloom, the arduous struggles of many lives will bear fruit and [the aspirant] will burst into the Light and attain ...contact with the Eternal, no longer sensed as a vague background, no longer even glimpsed fitfully through the inner door, but felt in actual contact, contact that will drench the soul in bliss. Gone is the sense of a separate finite self, with its individual gains and losses, its personal hopes and fears, and in its place comes the experience of the one [Infinite Spirit] abiding in all beings, of all beings as eddies in that all-pervading ocean of bliss.[4]

With the spiritual awakening, there is a new awareness of the timeless, spaceless reality beyond the universe, beyond all manifestation. And yet, one does not become aloof from the world. Quite the contrary—every least thing is now seen to be inseparable from that Reality.

As described by Evelyn Underhill, we come to recognize that

> [the] World of Becoming in all its richness and variety is... formed by Something other than, and utterly transcendent to, itself... [we] feel and know those two aspects of reality which we call... nature and spirit.[a] [We see that] this creation... with all its apparent collisions, cruelties, and waste, yet springs from an ardor, an immeasurable love... which generates it, upholds it, drives it... This love-driven world... within which the Divine Artist passionately and patiently expresses His infinite dream under finite forms—is held in another mightier embrace. The hunger and thirst of the heart is satisfied, and we receive indeed an assurance of ultimate Reality... It is... the seizing at last of Something which we have ever felt near us and enticing us: the unspeakably simple because completely inclusive solution of all the puzzles of life.[5]

The yogic tradition is often mistakenly taken to be advocating the loss of individuality. According to Buddhist writer John Blofeld, this mistake arises due to a misunderstanding of the relationship between the finite and the infinite. Many years ago Blofeld met with a Taoist sage living in a remote mountain region of China. In the course of his conversation, he cited the phrase "the dew-drop slips into the shining sea"—a phrase Sir Edwin Arnold had used to describe the Buddhist experience of losing oneself in an impersonal Nirvana. The sage replied,

> Your poet's simile is penetrating—exalted. And yet it does not capture the whole; for, when a lesser body of water enters a greater, though the two are thenceforth inseparable, the smaller constitutes but a fragment of the whole. But...

---

a. Or "Field" and "Knower of the Field."

when a finite being sheds the illusion of separate existence, he is not lost in the Tao like a dew-drop merging with the sea; by casting off his imaginary limitations, he becomes immeasurable... Plunge the finite into the infinite and, though only one remains, the finite, far from being diminished, takes on the stature of infinity... The mind of one who returns to the Source thereby becomes the Source.[6]

Spiritual Transformation: The Transformation of the Field

Neither the psychic nor the spiritual awakening in themselves necessarily involve a fundamental change in the Field of the mental, vital, or physical nature. Rather, both pertain to an awakening to the Knower. With the psychic awakening, one realizes the Knower in relationship to the universe; with the spiritual awakening, one knows one's true being to be rooted in the spaceless and timeless Infinite, the primordial awareness out of which the entire universe arises from moment to moment.

After awakening to the Knower, it is possible to bring about a transformation of the Field. With the psychic transformation, the ordinary human nature of physical, vital, and mental consciousness is totally changed. With the spiritual transformation, there is a vertical ascent, beyond the levels of the ordinary mind, that facilitates an even greater change of the nature.

According to Sri Aurobindo, once the psychic being has awakened and begun to transform the outer nature, a greater Divine Force begins to descend from levels of consciousness beyond the thinking mind, resulting in a still greater transformation of the mind, the vital, and the body. As the consciousness is transformed, it rises to progressively higher levels of what Sri Aurobindo calls the "spiritual mind."[a] With the ascent to each higher level, the power of the descending Force associated with that level increases, leading to a yet wider and more comprehensive transformation of each part of our nature. This force

works at the same time for perfection as well as liberation; it takes up the whole nature part by part and deals with it,

---

a. See Diagram #3 later in this chapter.

rejecting what has to be rejected, sublimating what has to be sublimated, creating what has to be created… It integrates, harmonises, establishes a new rhythm in the nature. It can bring down too a higher and yet higher force and range of the higher nature.[7]

Evelyn Underhill, describing the descent of this Force, writes:

You are thrilled by a mighty energy, uncontrolled by you, unsolicited by you: Its higher vitality is poured into your soul. You enter upon an experience for which all the terms of power, thought, motion, even of love, are inadequate: yet which contains within itself the only complete expression of all these things…Those ineffective, half-conscious attempts towards free action, clear apprehension, true union, which we dignify by the names of will, thought and love [willing, knowing, and feeling] are now seen matched by an Absolute Will, Thought and Love; instantly recognized by the contemplating spirit as the highest reality it yet has known, and evoking in it a passionate and a humble joy.[8]

Sri Aurobindo describes the transformed consciousness as having

the nature of infinity: it brings to us the abiding spiritual sense and awareness of the Infinite and Eternal with a great largeness of the nature and a breaking down of its limitations; immortality becomes no longer a belief or an experience but a normal self-awareness; the close presence of the Divine Being, his rule of the world and of our self and natural members, his force working in us and everywhere, the peace of the Infinite, the joy of the Infinite are now concrete and constant in the being; in all sights and forms one sees the Eternal, the Reality, in all sounds one hears it, in all touches feels it; there is nothing else but its forms and personalities and manifestations; the joy or adoration of the heart, the embrace of all existence, the unity of the spirit are abiding realities. The consciousness of the mental creature is turning or has been already turned wholly into the consciousness of the spiritual being.[9]

THE SUPRAMENTAL CONSCIOUSNESS: THE INTELLIGENCE EMBRACING AND PERVADING THE UNIVERSE

Once having awakened to the psychic being within and the Infinite Spirit beyond, the psychic and spiritual transformation of the nature having begun, a further evolution is still possible. Ascending beyond the summits of what Sri Aurobindo calls the "Spiritual Mind," one enters into the awareness of the Divine Intelligence that holds everything in its embrace, harmonizes and coordinates every part with every other. It is this supramental Truth-Consciousness[a] of which we see a limited reflection in physical matter as "laws of nature," in plants and animals as instinct, and in human beings as intuition.

This Divine Intelligence does not control the universe according to rigid, unyielding laws. In fact, what we call the "laws of nature" might more appropriately be considered "habits... for what Nature does is really done by the Spirit and can therefore be changed by the Spirit... [the Divine] is not subject to law but uses process...it is only the individual soul in a state of ignorance on which process seems to impose itself as law." Even in matter, the evolutionary process is not altogether predetermined. A degree of indeterminacy exists in the movements of atoms, reflecting their minute degree of awakened consciousness. The degree of unpredictability increases in the course of evolution, as the Knower gradually awakens within the Field of Conscious-Energy, revealing more of Its Infinite creativity.

In fact, the whole notion of a Divine Intelligence somehow controlling the universe is mistaken at the outset, as it implies a Divine Being that is in some way separate from the universe It controls. But the Truth-Consciousness is not a separate "Designer" God who, like a human craftsman, has created a purely physical universe apart from

---

a. Ṛita or Vijñana in Sanskrit. Both refer to the same plane of consciousness, but Ṛita emphasizes the aspect of Divine Harmony, while Vijñana stresses more the Divine Intelligence.

To our limited minds, the interplay between determinacy and indeterminacy in the universe manifests as mechanical law and meaningless chance. By means of intuition, it is possible to understand the relationship of law and chance in a different way. The word "chance" is derived from the Old French word *chéance,* meaning "the way things fall." This in turn comes from the Latin *cadentia,* which literally means "falling" but also carries a sense of rhythm, which is reflected in the English word "cadence," meaning a "balanced rhythmic flow" as in poetry or oratory. Going back still farther, the ancient Vedic sages saw the lawful patterns of the world as reflecting the harmony of the Divine Unity, manifesting in our world as the creative, rhythmic flow of experience. Viewed intuitively, the patterns of law and the spontaneity of "chance" contribute equally to the infinitely creative dance of evolution.

Himself. The Infinite Divine Consciousness is infinitely present at every point in His universe, with each point reflecting the totality in itself. Even to think in terms of separate "points" is an error.

Some spiritual writings use the metaphor of each object as a wave in the sea of the Divine Consciousness.

> But, in truth, these waves are each of them that sea, their diversities being those of frontal or superficial appearances caused by the sea's motion. As each object in the universe is really the whole universe in a different frontal appearance, so each individual soul is all [the Divine] regarding Itself and world from a center of cosmic consciousness.[10]

We're speaking here of a Consciousness so far beyond the mind, by what hubris might we hope to understand or even gain a glimpse of its nature? Since everything is the Divine—including every movement of our own consciousness—there is nothing in our experience that is not in some way a reflection—albeit limited—of His Conscious-Being. We have gained glimpses of the soul through intimations of Its Beauty amidst the simple events of our lives; and have seen even our basest desires to be distorted manifestations of the Soul's aspiration. By looking more closely at the faculty of intuition—the reflection of the Truth-Consciousness in the human mind—we may gain some distant sense of the Nature of the Divine Intelligence.

EXPLORING INTUITION: INTIMATIONS OF THE SUPRAMENTAL CONSCIOUSNESS

In yoga psychology, the word "intuition" refers ultimately to what Sri Aurobindo calls a "knowledge by identity"—a way of knowing that recognizes each and every thing as a manifestation of one's own Infinite Being, the One Divine that we are in truth:[a]

> In reality, all experience is in its secret nature knowledge by identity; but its true character is hidden from us because we have separated ourselves from the rest of the world by exclusion, by the distinction of our self as subject and everything else as object, and we are compelled to develop processes and organs by which we may again enter into communion with all that we have excluded.[11]

In the words of Sri Krishna Prem, intuition is "a power which depends upon the unity of the whole cosmos, upon the fact that any portion of the universe, even the smallest, reflects in its structure the pattern of the whole."[12] We are able to get a taste of this way of knowing even in our ordinary consciousness because "the structure of experience-levels far beyond our normal range is mirrored in that of this level, and the process of intuition is essentially a reading of what is remote by the contemplation of what is near."[13] To the extent that we

---

a. As noted earlier, in the tradition of yoga psychology, the same word may be used to refer to different levels of consciousness. Strictly speaking, Sri Aurobindo uses the phrase "knowledge by identity" to refer to the way of knowing native to the supramental or Truth-Consciousness. However, he uses the word "intuition" to describe the reflection of that way of knowing in the highest levels of the mind. He also at times uses "intuition" to describe its more limited reflection in the mental, vital, and physical consciousness. In this chapter the context should make clear the level to which we are referring.

are able to develop our capacity for intuitive knowledge, "the Cosmos is no longer seen as a chaos of separate selves and separate things but as one all-enfolding harmony."[14]

Even without deliberately developing our intuitive capacity, we may have spontaneous intimations of this greater harmony. In the experience of meaningful coincidences—referred to as "synchronicities" by psychiatrist Carl Jung—we may momentarily perceive the hidden connections between things.

Luke was browsing through a bookstore, and as he read the opening lines of one particular book, he knew it was something his friend Rachel would love to read. He mailed it to her, and not long afterward, received a call from her. She related to him that her mother had been visiting and just the day before had asked her what she wanted for her birthday. At first Rachel had told her mother she didn't want anything, then remembered there was a book she'd recently heard about that she really wanted to get. As she was telling her mother the name of the book, there was a knock at the door. When she opened the door, the postman handed her the package from Luke which contained the book she had asked for seconds earlier.

Laura had been longing to become pregnant for a number of years. One day there was a knock at her door. As she went to open it, her dogs, who never failed to bark loudly and persistently whenever anyone was at the door, on this occasion sat staring at it in total silence. Laura opened the door to find a man holding a bouquet of balloons, asking if she was the new mother. She told him he must have the wrong address, but he was quite insistent and only after repeating her statement to him several times did he reluctantly walk away. Within several days, Laura discovered that in fact she had become pregnant.[15]

Born in 1945, Aung San Suu Kyi was two years old when her father, General Aung San, a man who had spent his life fighting for Burmese independence, was assassinated. Burma achieved independence not long afterward, but 14 years later, General Ne Win seized power in a military coup, and ruled the country with an iron fist for more than 25 years.

Suu Kyi had spent most of her 20s and 30s living a quiet life outside Burma with her husband and two children. In March 1988, for the first time since Ne Win had taken power, students began demonstrating to demand an end to military rule. Several weeks later, Suu Kyi received a phone call informing her that her mother had suffered a severe stroke. Within days, she traveled to Burma from England, where she was living at the time, to care for her mother.

Four months later, General Ne Win suddenly and unexpectedly announced his decision to resign, calling for a referendum to determine Burma's future. The members of his party, however, opposed his request, and in response to massive uprisings, killed several thousand protestors.

In August, just five months after arriving in Burma, Aung San Suu Kyi announced that she had decided to join the struggle for democracy, saying, "This great struggle has arisen from the intense and deep desire of the people for a fully democratic parliamentary system. I could not, as my father's daughter, remain indifferent to all that was going on." She has remained in Burma ever since—most of the time under house arrest—and in 1991, was awarded the Nobel Peace Prize for her efforts.

By what turn of fate did circumstances conspire such that Suu Kyi was in Burma just when the desire for democracy had ripened into a movement in need of a leader—one imbued with the history of the country, capable of inspiring the confidence of an entire nation?

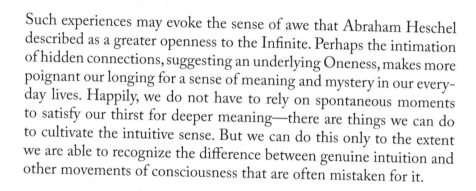

Such experiences may evoke the sense of awe that Abraham Heschel described as a greater openness to the Infinite. Perhaps the intimation of hidden connections, suggesting an underlying Oneness, makes more poignant our longing for a sense of meaning and mystery in our everyday lives. Happily, we do not have to rely on spontaneous moments to satisfy our thirst for deeper meaning—there are things we can do to cultivate the intuitive sense. But we can do this only to the extent we are able to recognize the difference between genuine intuition and other movements of consciousness that are often mistaken for it.

Distinguishing Intuition from More Limited Ways of Knowing

The consensus in contemporary psychology regarding the nature of intuition is that it is no more than a rapid process of reasoning that takes place outside of conscious awareness. Arthur Reber's *Dictionary of Psychology* defines intuition as "any knowledge or understanding which is largely based on unconscious factors related to one's feelings, values, background of experience, subliminal perceptions, etc. which operate outside the conscious, rational or analytical processes."[16] Yogis, aware of these various subconscious processes, consider intuition to be something entirely distinct. In order to help tease out the difference, we'll look at two examples of unusual cognitive skills.

1) Colonel H. S. Olcott recounts having witnessed a South Indian memory expert (known in India as an *ashtavadhani*) who simultaneously kept in mind and performed the following tasks and afterwards correctly repeated them all.:

1. Play a game of chess, without seeing the board;

2. Carry on a conversation on a variety of subjects;

3. Complete a Sanskrit verse for which he was given the first line;

4. Multiply a 5-figure number by a 4-figure number;

5. Add a sum of three columns, each of eight rows of figures;

6. Commit to memory a Sanskrit verse of sixteen words—the words being given to him out of order, and at the option of the tester;

7. Complete a "magic square" in which the sum of each horizontal and vertical row adds up to the same specified number;

8. Without seeing the chess-board, direct the movement of a knight so that it described the outline of a horse;

9. Complete a second "magic square" with a different number from that in number 7;

10. Keep count of the strokes of a bell rung by a gentleman who was present;

11. Commit to memory two sentences of Spanish, given in the same manner as the Sanskrit verses in number 6.[17]

2) Darold Treffert has collected many examples of the unusual feats performed by "savants." Savants are individuals who, despite generally limited cognitive abilities, display extraordinary skill in one particular area. Treffert describes one savant who had a working vocabulary of only 58 words, but who could provide the following information from memory:

1. the population of every city and town in the United States with more than 5,000 people;

2. the names, number of rooms and location of the 2,000 leading hotels in the US;

3. the distance from any city or town to the largest city in its state;

4. statistics concerning 3,000 mountains and rivers;

5. the dates and essential facts of more than 2,000 leading inventions and discoveries.[18]

What parts of the mind are being used in each of the above two instances? In the case of the memory expert, the physical and vital minds would have been used in picturing the chessboard or imaging the ringing bell. The thinking mind would have been employed for memorizing the words of various languages and for analyzing the magic square. As a well-trained expert, his reasoning processes were probably so well developed that a substantial portion of his thinking was likely carried out very rapidly on a subconscious level. And because he had cultivated profound levels of concentration, he quite possibly was able to pierce the "filmy screen" separating the outer and inner consciousness, giving him at least intermittent access to the subliminal memory that records and holds accurately all with which the conscious mind has been presented.

What role, if any, did intuition play here? Given that the memory expert may have had some opening to the inner consciousness—by nature more intuitive than the outer[a]—it is possible that he had access to a rapid intuitive grasp of meaningful connections. Thus, the *ashtavadhani* may have availed himself of various levels of consciousness, including the conscious mind, the subconscious, and the intuitive inner mind.

The savant, on the other hand, clearly did not use conscious reasoning, nor did he consciously cultivate deep states of concentration. One might be tempted to conclude that he relied totally on subconscious reasoning. However, given that savants may not always acquire their knowledge through ordinary means, it is possible that some of them make use of parapsychological means—in other words, direct inner sensing.

Since intuitive knowing is the basis of all knowledge, even the most mechanical, it would by necessity be involved even in the savant's capacity for recalling mundane facts. How might intuition contribute to this capacity? One possibility is that some kind of intuitive grasping of inherent connections between the various facts and figures may have been operating.

But what kind of meaningful connections could there be between population figures, hotel statistics, and the names of cities and towns? Looking solely from the perspective of the surface mind, these things

---

a. The inner consciousness, less bound to the external physical world than the surface consciousness, is more receptive to the influence of the higher planes where intuition functions more freely.

appear separate, disconnected, lacking in meaning. From the intuitive view, however, even the barest facts are manifestations of deeper realities, with every line, shape, and color reflecting some aspect of the Divine. To the yogic eye, awake to the subtle forms of the inner consciousness, the external shapes and forms that make up the physical world arise out of a deeper dimension of existence, in which color, number, shape, feeling, thinking, and willing are one unbroken whole. A savant, whose capacity for analytic thinking has not developed, may have some limited subconscious access to this deeper dimension of intuitive knowing.

In the above instances, we see either a way of knowing distinct from intuition or various limited reflections of intuitive knowing. The memory expert employed a variety of ways of knowing, including conscious and subconscious reasoning as well as a limited reflection of intuitive knowledge available to his inner mind. The savants appear to use primarily subconscious reasoning, but may also have some limited access to intuitive capacities that are reflected in the inner mind.

In the absence of some kind of conscious cultivation, the reliability of our intuition is at best haphazard—useful perhaps in helping generate insights, but in need of constant testing and confirmation by the intellect. Generally, whatever intuition does arise to the surface consciousness is unreliable, because it is distorted by desire and emotional bias. Is it possible to cultivate intuition to such an extent that it becomes a reliable instrument?

Cultivating Intuition

Nineteenth-century physicist Hermann von Helmholtz developed a theory regarding intuition and the creative process that is still considered to be valid.[a] He described the creative process as consisting of three stages, which he named saturation, incubation, and illumination. "Saturation" involves gathering information on a particular topic from a wide variety of sources and thinking intensely about it. In the phase

---

a. There are psychologists who are skeptical of the idea that creativity and intuition represent ways of knowing that are distinct from other kinds of thinking. The possibility that there is a real distinction is discussed in Appendix A, "Science and Yoga."

of "incubation," one leaves aside all conscious reflection, allowing subconscious processes to work. The stage of "illumination" is akin to the well-known "eureka" moment when a flash of insight emerges.[19]

The following is an example of how this three-stage process played out in a man's life over the course of seventeen years. In 1903, German physiologist Otto Loewi had the idea that nerve impulses might involve chemical rather than electrical transmission, but could not think of a way to prove it. Seventeen years later, in a moment when the noise of his conscious mind was attenuated, the solution to his problem came to him, ultimately resulting in his being awarded the 1936 Nobel Prize for Physiology and Medicine:

> The night before Easter Sunday of that year I awoke, turned on the light, and jotted down a few notes on a tiny slip of thin paper. Then I fell asleep again. It occurred to me at six in the morning that during the night I had written down something most important, but I was unable to decipher the scrawl. The next night, at three o' clock, the idea returned. It was the design of an experiment to determine whether or not the hypothesis of chemical transmission that I had uttered seventeen years ago was correct. I got up immediately, went to the laboratory and performed a simple experiment on a frog's heart according to the nocturnal design... Its results became the foundation of the theory of chemical transmission of the nervous impulse.[20]

Having initially "saturated" his mind with attempts to find a suitable experimental methodology, his question underwent a prolonged incubation resulting in the nocturnal moment of illumination seventeen years later. While Loewi did not set out to consciously cultivate an intuitive understanding, yogis say that it is possible through intense discipline to develop a steady, unbroken flow of intuitive knowledge.

An Exercise in Developing Intuitive Knowing

What makes it difficult for us to access our intuitive abilities? It is the same now-familiar culprits—overactivity of the surface intellect and the distorting influence of ego and desire. Thus, in order to cultivate our intuitive capacity, the first necessity is to develop the calm mind, one capable of quietly observing the play of thought. Having attained a certain measure of quietude, one may choose to engage in a contemplative exercise. One could begin by reflecting on a particular topic, making use of the imagination, the emotions, and the senses as well as a full range of critical and creative reasoning. This would be analogous to Helmholtz's "saturation" phase.

At some point during the reflection, if the mind is resting on a base of sufficient calm and the attention is sufficiently one-pointed, an insight or intuitive flash will arise. It is important to recognize this moment and to concentrate all one's energy on the arising insight, suspending all active thinking, remaining alert to the impulse of the intellect to grasp at or manipulate the intuitive perception. After a period of time, the capacity to remain concentrated on the intuition will flag and one can resume active thought.

This phase of the contemplative process combines Helmholtz's second and third phases, but it intensifies the incubation process by adding to it the heat of intense concentration. It also adds a sustained alertness to the arising of intuitive insights. Let's now consider an example of how such a contemplative exercise might unfold in practice.

CULTIVATING INTUITIVE AWARENESS

Imagine that having been intrigued by the possibility of dissolving the ego, the false sense of self, you wish to go beyond a mere intellectual understanding and gain some kind of intuitive insight. Engaging in the process described above, you might begin by inquiring into what contributes to the sense of "me" as an independent, clearly defined and separate being. What part does the body contribute to my overall sense of my self? What would happen if I lost my limbs? How can my identity depend on a body whose components are in a state of constant flux? What about my emotions? What if I were to become manic-depressive, subject to wild mood swings, would I still be "me"? Looking at my thoughts, if I were to lose my memory, or succumb to Alzheimer's disease and lose my ability to think, who would "I" be?

In the course of such reflections, remaining connected to the stillness "behind" the mind, I remain alert to the emergence of a visceral, intuitive sense of the nature of the ego, the sense of an independent, separate "self." If such an insight arises, I stop reflecting, and bring all my attention to that visceral sense of the illusive nature of the self I have taken myself to be. If my attention begins to wander or dissipate, I resume active reflection. I might now look at the interaction of the mental, vital, and physical consciousness, looking at the whole network of patterns created by sensing, feeling, and thinking. Can I find anywhere a solid unchanging "I" that the mind can define or grasp? Once again, if an intuitive sense of this arises, I stop active reflection and focus intently on the insight.

I may switch my focus, choosing an object such as a chair or desk, and again inquire, is there some hard, unchanging "thing" that constitutes the object? What would the object be apart from any awareness or experience of it? Continuing in this way, alternating between active reflection and quiet, focused contemplation, I may get a sense of the interdependent relationship between "self" and "world." An intuition may arise that my "self" as well as the objects that make up the "world" are a manifestation of some greater Reality, something beyond all conceptual frameworks, something Infinite, a Conscious-Energy pervading, containing all. Opening still further to this intuitive awareness, I may perceive some greater Force guiding my mind and feelings, deepening my consciousness, bringing it to a state of profound Silence.

The above is a contemplative exercise involving an alternation between periods of deliberate reflection and calm, focused attention. However, the same process can happen spontaneously. What is essential here is not a specific technique, but rather the basic movements of consciousness—a

deep concentration coupled with calm detachment, an attitude of receptivity to deeper or higher intuitive promptings, and an opening to a greater Force that can guide the consciousness to further development.

As described here, the development of intuition seems to require
solitude and physical immobility. However, this process can take place
just as readily while walking, interacting with others, or when engaged
in any other activity. The intense concentration that a basketball player
brings to his practice often results in a kind of body-intuition that
guides him to make the right movements on the court with effort-
lessness and spontaneous grace. Someone listening to the words of a
grieving friend may open to a kind of emotional intuition that brings
forward just the words the friend needs to hear at that moment. The
researcher, intensely focused on analyzing a particular hypothesis, can
stay attuned to the arising of an intuitive mental understanding that
can lead to further scientific breakthroughs.[a]

As these movements of consciousness are gradually perfected, several
things will begin to happen. The activity of discursive reasoning takes on
a more intuitive and global quality, and the intuitions that emerge gain
in acuteness of perception and discernment. Over time there develops
a greater integration of intellect and intuition. This affects not only the
mind but the vital and physical consciousness as well, because this newly
emerging way of knowing is, by nature, profoundly integral.

Eventually we awaken to the fact that behind all of our mental
functioning there has always been this essential intuitive way of knowing—a knowledge by identity. Prior to this we are cut off from it,
therefore our ordinary way of knowing is limited and distorted: We
(the subject) are separate from that which we attempt to know (the
object)—"I" am here, the "chair," a distinct object over there, exists

---

a. Each of these—the physical, emotional, and mental intuition—are limited
reflections of a more purely intuitive mind, on a plane of consciousness above the
thinking mind, which itself is a limited reflection of the still greater supramental
intuition. Sri Aurobindo considers what he refers to as the true Conscience to be
another, somewhat complex example of this kind of reflection. The psychic being,
itself receptive to a limited aspect of the intuitive knowing of the Supramental
consciousness, "sends out" rays of its Light to the surface, which manifests in us
(when not distorted by ego or desire) as the true Conscience.

independently of me. Therefore, I have to engage in a complex, arduous cognitive process with regard to the chair in order to gain what is at best a provisional, precarious, and limited understanding of it.

Rising above the thinking mind, the nature of knowing changes; we become progressively more conscious of the One Self in all. My consciousness no longer separate from the chair, I can understand it by entering into That Consciousness that holds both "me" and "chair" in its embrace. At this stage there is no longer a question of intuition alternating with reasoning, but rather a perfect integration of the two. Having awakened to the One Conscious-Being in all, we "know" everything by means of our essential oneness with it; we know it because in some sense we become, or recognize we essentially are it. There is an immediate knowing that grasps the nature of the object without recourse to the slow plodding process of the thinking mind. All the processes of reasoning and logic are effortlessly included in this greater intuitive knowing. The mind still has a role to play, but now only as an organizer, not as a source of knowledge.[a]

Now we are in a position to understand what Sri Aurobindo spoke of as "secret operations" beyond the mind which, if we knew them, would change our "whole conscious functioning." Underlying each of the four functions of mind is a greater way of knowing, based in the knowledge by identity. In our ordinary way of thinking, the functions of intellect and conscious will are attempting

> to do what can only be done with perfect spontaneity and mastery by something higher than mind. The intellect... form(s) a bridge by which the [human being] is trying to establish a conscious connection with the supramental and to prepare the embodied soul for the descent into it of a supramental action. In proportion as the intellectual action becomes associated with and dominated by a rudimentary supramental action [i.e., genuine intuitive knowledge]—and it is this which constitutes the phenomenon of genius—[the action of the intellect] becomes more and more easy, spontaneous, rapid and perfect.[21]

---

a. But this "reasoning" and "logic" are of the Supramental consciousness, not the mind. Whatever mental reason or logic plays a part is secondary.

FIGURE 3. THE EVENT-REACTION CYCLE IN THE CONTEXT OF THE KNOWER AND THE FIELD

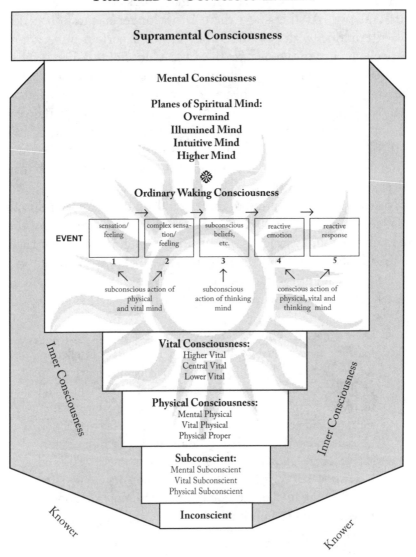

In Figure 3 we see the relationship between the reaction chain and the vast realms of consciousness outside our ordinary mind: "above" the mind, the planes of spiritual mind leading up to the supramental consciousness; "below" the mind, the vital and physical consciousness as well as the subconscient and inconscient; and "behind" the surface of our ordinary mind, the vast realm of the inner mental, vital, and subtle physical consciousness.

"Spiritual mind" is Sri Aurobindo's term for the intervening levels of consciousness between the thinking mind and the supramental consciousness. On these planes of consciousness, one is aware of the Divine in all and all in the Divine. Rising above the separative way of knowing characteristic of the mind, one opens progressively to the more intimate way of knowing of the higher mind, the still greater power of vision and direct seeing native to the illumined mind, the still more intimate knowledge by identity characterizing the intuitive mind, the unfolding of a still greater knowledge by identity in the overmind, and the perfect knowledge by identity of the supramental consciousness.

The "inconscient" is a region of being below the subconscient that seems to us totally unconscious. Sri Aurobindo uses the term inconscient to indicate it is actually an "involved consciousness." It is the inconscient out of which the material universe originally arose, and it contains in potential all the layers of consciousness that are eventually to manifest.

As long as we remain confined to the mental consciousness we are unaware of the various realms of consciousness "above," "below," and "behind" our ordinary awareness. Nevertheless, they are always there, contributing to the construction of the reaction chain.

The rays in the center of the diagram represent the light of the Soul (the individual Knower) coming through to the surface from the depths of the innermost consciousness. As long as we remain absorbed in the workings of the surface mental consciousness, we are unaware of this light as well as the process by which the Soul gets lost in and identified with a part of the Field. By inserting a pause between various links in the reaction chain, we can learn to disidentify from the karmic energies that make up the chain and begin to feel something of the calm stillness of the Soul, everpresent behind all movements of the Field. When we awaken sufficiently that our identity is no longer with the Field, but with the Knower of the Field, we can become receptive to the greater spiritual and supramental force, which has the power to "descend" into and transform even the deepest subconscient layers of our nature, progressively aligning us with the Knowing, Willing, and Feeling of the Infinite.

What is the nature—if it is possible in any way to hint at it—of this supramental consciousness? For this we turn to two great yogis whose words describing their own direct experience may evoke a sense of it.

SUPRAMENTAL AWAKENING

> For There everything is transparent, nothing dark, nothing resistant; every being is lucid to every other, in breadth and depth; light runs through light. And each of them contains all within itself, and at the same time sees all in every other, so that everywhere there is all, all is all, and each all, and infinite the glory.[22]
>
> —Plotinus, *Enneads* V, Tractate 8

> He who has known the [supramental Force], knows indeed that it is within all things. The vibrations of the tiniest atoms or electrons as much as the whirlings of the vastest Cosmic nebulae are expressions of the one great Rhythm. It is the power which draws them forth, supports them in their movements and into which again they are dissolved. In truth, it is not within them any more than the sun actually rises and sets. They are in It, not It in them, but such is the force of habit that we can but talk of it as being within them. Indeed, it is their very core, the heart of their being. It is the Light itself, they are its waves. Neither microscope nor telescope can compass its being. Cleave the minutest atom, it is there: Mount to the outer space beyond all stars; still we are within its all-enfolding arms. It is the Wondrous Being, the Dragon of Life and Wisdom. It soars majestic in the heavens and the starry worlds play like fireflies beneath the shadow of its outspread wings, and yet, at the same time, it dwells in the subtle central Well that is in the midst of the Caverns of the heart, the Well that is subtler than "the hundredth part of a hair." He is the "Breath" that blows the bubbles of the worlds.[23]
>
> —Sri Krishna Prem, *The Yoga of the Katha Upanishad*

THE SUPRAMENTAL TRANSFORMATION

According to Sri Aurobindo, a complete transformation of the physical, vital, and mental nature becomes possible with the awakening of the supramental consciousness. As the transformation proceeds, the characteristic dullness and inertia of the ordinary physical consciousness is replaced by an imperturbable Peace. The restless striving of the egoistic vital consciousness for domination and possession is transmuted into a "self-possessed power and illimitable act of force"; its suffering into a spiritual bliss. And the limited plodding intelligence of the ordinary mind becomes the swift illumination of an integral knowledge and understanding.

The individual whose mental, vital, and physical consciousness is thus transformed by the supramental Force would be

> aware of the transcendent reality, possess in the self-experience the supreme existence, consciousness, bliss, be one with *Sachchidananda*.[a] He will become one with cosmic being and universal Nature: he will contain the world in himself, in his own cosmic consciousness and feel himself one with all beings; he will see himself in all and all in himself, become united and identified with the Self which has become all existences. He will perceive the beauty of the All-Beautiful and the miracle of the All-Wonderful; he will enter in the end into the bliss of the *Brahman* and live abidingly in it and for all this he will not need to shun existence or plunge into the annihilation of the spiritual Person in some self-extinguishing *Nirvana*. As in the Self, so in Nature, he can realise the Divine. The nature of the Divine is Light and Power and Bliss; he can feel the divine Light and Power and Bliss above him and descending into him, filling every strand of his nature, every cell and atom of his being, flooding his soul and mind and life and body, surrounding him like an illimitable sea and filling the world,

---

a. *Sachchidananda* (often written as *Sat-Chit-Ananda*) is Sanskrit for "existence-consciousness-bliss."

suffusing all his feeling and sense and experience, making all his life truly and utterly divine. This and all else that the spiritual consciousness can bring to him the divine life will give him when it reaches its utmost completeness and perfection and the supramental truth-consciousness is fulfilled in all himself... All the infinite ranges of experience of the Infinite will be his and all the joy of the finite in the embrace of the Infinite.[24]

TOWARD THE FUTURE, NOW

In the introduction to this book we spoke of the current era as a time of unprecedented change. Some suggest we may be in the midst of a global renaissance resulting from the infusion of Asian spiritual wisdom into the world culture. Others say we may be seeing the end of a five-thousand-year age of empire leading to a new age of global collaboration. A further, and even more momentous possibility is that we are in the beginning stages of the emergence of a new consciousness altogether beyond the mind.

We close with some suggestions as to what might be happening.

> One thing seems obvious, humanity has reached a certain state of general tension—tension in effort, in action, even in daily life—with such an excessive hyperactivity, so widespread a trepidation, that mankind as a whole seems to have come to a point where it must either break through the resistance and emerge into a new consciousness or else fall back into an abyss of darkness and inertia.

> This tension is so complete and so widespread that something obviously has to break. It cannot go on this way... [But there is a hopeful sign which] we find traces of...in all countries, all over the world: the will to find a new, higher, progressive solution, an effort to rise towards a vaster, more comprehensive perfection.[25]

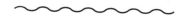

We are in a very special situation, extremely special, without precedent. We are now witnessing the birth of a new world; it is very young, very weak—not in its essence but in its outer manifestation—not yet recognized, not even felt, denied by the majority. But it is here. It is here, making an effort to grow, absolutely sure of the result. But the road to it is a completely new road which has never before been traced out—nobody has gone there, nobody has done that! It is a beginning, a universal beginning. So, it is an absolutely unexpected, an unpredictable adventure...

It is not a question of repeating spiritually what others have done before us, for our adventure begins beyond that. It is a question of a new creation, entirely new, with all the unforeseen events, the risks, the hazards it entails—a real adventure, whose goal is certain victory, but the road to which is unknown and must be traced out step by step, in the unexplored. Something that has never been in this present universe and that will never be again in the same way...

One must put aside all that has been foreseen, all that has been devised, all that has been constructed and then... set off walking into the unknown.[26]

APPENDIX A

SCIENCE AND YOGA

Science taken in its essence should stand only for a method and not for any special beliefs, yet as habitually taken by its votaries, science has come to be identified with a certain fixed general belief, the belief that the deeper order of nature is mechanical exclusively, and that nonmechanical categories are irrational ways of conceiving and explaining even such a thing as human life.[1]

—William James

How might we go about reconciling the yogic view of consciousness with that of science? In the Renaissance and post-Renaissance periods, scientists chose to focus their studies on the physical world in order to avoid conflict with religious authorities. Enlarging their sphere of study over the centuries, scientists in the past one hundred years have entered territory previously considered to be the province of religion. Having chosen to explore the nature of the subject—referred to variously as mind, consciousness, soul, or spirit—it is no longer possible to avoid conflict between science and religion by claiming, as did paleontologist Stephen J. Gould, that they investigate separate, non-overlapping fields of study.

From the yogic perspective, most modern versions of science, philosophy, and theology have something essential in common: They all make use of the reasoning capacity of the surface thinking mind as their primary tool of investigation. Scientific investigation adds one essential factor—careful use of the physical senses, augmented by various physical instruments and supported by complex mathematical analysis.

Sri Aurobindo describes the way of knowing common to the surface thinking mind as "separative knowledge." Our knowledge of people and the things of the world is limited because we take them to be essentially separate from ourselves. Because of the limitations of this way of knowing, scientists have had to develop compensatory means of gaining information and understanding, such as complex measuring instruments, statistical analyses, and painstaking peer review.

There is another kind of knowing, native to the inner or subliminal consciousness, which Sri Aurobindo refers to as "knowledge by direct contact." By means of this way of knowing it is possible to gain intimate knowledge of people and things that are physically external to ourselves. Once we awaken to the inner consciousness, we discover we have the capacity to know things apparently separate from us in time and space. Paranormal abilities, which are manifest in an extremely limited and unpredictable fashion as long as we are confined to the surface consciousness, become normal, fully utilizable capacities.

There is a still deeper way of knowing, which yogis say is the source of all other knowledge. According to Sri Aurobindo, this ultimate form of knowledge is altogether beyond the mind—"supramental"— though we can develop a reflection of it in the mind by cultivating our intuitive abilities. Sri Aurobindo describes this way of knowing as "knowledge by identity"; that is, we know something by becoming one in consciousness with that which we seek to know.

If we examine some of the latest scientific developments in the field of consciousness studies with regard to how they make use of these different ways of knowing, we may get a sense of what would be involved in developing a truly yogic science.

SEPARATIVE KNOWLEDGE: USING THE OUTER SENSES AND THE SURFACE THINKING MIND

Speculations Based on Preexisting Research

Several scientists have offered interesting speculations [a] regarding the relationship between consciousness and matter. For example, physicist

---

a. The limitations of such speculations in regard to the working of consciousness in matter were discussed earlier in chapter 5, "Second Challenge To the View."

Freeman Dyson, describing what he considers to be evidence of the operations of mind in matter, writes, "Atoms in the laboratory are weird stuff, behaving like active agents rather than inert substances. They make unpredictable choices between alternative possibilities according to the laws of quantum mechanics. It appears that mind, as manifested by the capacity to make choices, is to some extent inherent in every atom."[2] Dyson goes on to say that atoms and humans "may have minds that differ in degree but not in kind."[3]

Other scientists, reflecting on existing research, have offered more specific suggestions for possible ways that consciousness may relate to matter. Physicist Amit Goswami suggests that consciousness may make use of quantum processes to bring about the kind of creative mutations that lead to the appearance of new species. When it comes to helping a species become more stable within its environment, Goswami maintains that Darwinian natural selection plays an important role. However, he suggests that at the same time this process of stabilization is going on, potential mutations are accumulating in the form of quantum possibilities. These are passed down, in their potential form, to subsequent generations. When a change in the environment calls for it, a number of the potential mutations are then "chosen" to manifest simultaneously, resulting in a new species that will be suited to the new environment.

Aware that this makes no sense in the context of a purely materialistic perspective, Goswami proposes that the quantum possibilities for potential mutations are held in a nonphysical field. Both Ervin Laszlo and Daniel Benor propose kindred theories suggesting that nonmaterial fields of subtle energy are in part responsible for adaptive mutations. All three agree that consciousness appears to play a fundamental role in the evolutionary process.

Psychologist Alan Combs and neuroscientist Francisco Varela have developed intricate and compelling theories combining chaos and complexity theory as well as ideas about self-organization, which they suggest may contribute to understanding the role of consciousness in the material universe.

In each of these instances, scientists have analyzed existing data using their surface thinking minds in an attempt to discern meaningful patterns. They have then, without benefit of direct, intuitive knowledge, simply asserted a causal role for consciousness in bringing about or shaping these patterns. Let's see if there is anything more to be gained by conducting original research on the relationship of consciousness and matter while still using the surface mind as one's primary tool for understanding.

Conducting Research Using Conventional Scientific Methods

Biologist Rupert Sheldrake has conducted research suggesting that the experience of animals is somehow recorded in nonphysical "morphogenetic" (i.e., form-building) fields, making it easier for future generations to acquire certain behaviors. His research builds on the observations of others, including psychologist William McDougal, "who discovered quite by chance that untrained rats were quick to learn a task (escaping from a water maze) previously acquired by many earlier generations of rats of the same strain." Researchers in Scotland and Australia similarly found several years later that rats that had no training picked up the task almost immediately. Physiologist Ivan Pavlov also "observed a similar effect when he trained several generations of white mice to run to a feeding station at the sound of a bell. While the first generation required an average of about three hundred trials to learn the task, the second generation required only about one hundred trials. The third and fourth generations learned in thirty and ten trials respectively."[4]

After conducting numerous experiments on morphogenetic fields in relation to animals, Sheldrake has since conducted research on the relationship of these fields to human beings. Sheldrake theorizes that, when we focus our attention on something, our mind extends outward to connect us with the object of our attention. Thus, when a person is staring at someone, his field of vision "extends out to touch the person he is staring at." In addition, the person being looked at has a field around him as well, and the two fields interact—though this interaction may not be experienced consciously. Sheldrake suggests that these interacting fields may be the same as what yogis have referred to for centuries as *pranic* or vital energy fields.

Sheldrake has developed a simple experiment to test this theory. He has two people sit together, one designated as the starer, the other the person to be stared at. In each round of the experiment, the starer tosses a coin to decide whether he will look at the other person or not. He then signals the initiation of a ten-second period, during which the other person has to guess whether or not he is being stared at. Among the many trials Sheldrake has conducted, by far the largest number were carried out in Amsterdam, Holland, involving more than 18,700 pairs of subjects. He reports that "the statistical significance of the positive results is astronomical: The odds against chance are 10^{376} to 1."[5]

The work of psychiatrist Ian Stevenson, while also relying primarily on the use of the ordinary thinking mind, presents a strong challenge to conventional notions of the relationship between consciousness and matter. Over the course of several decades, Stevenson has conducted several thousand case studies of individuals (usually children) claiming to have recollections of a previous life. The prestigious *Journal of the American Medical Association* has written of his "meticulous and extended investigations," in which he has "painstakingly and unemotionally collected a detailed series of cases in which the evidence for reincarnation is difficult to understand on any other grounds... He has placed on record a large amount of data that cannot be ignored."[6]

As a young psychiatrist, prior to beginning this research, one of Stevenson's major interests had been psychosomatic medicine, the study of the relationship between mind and body. Later, in the course of conducting reincarnation research, he became intrigued by the many cases in which birthmarks in a current life could be correlated with wounds reportedly received in a previous life, suggesting the "mind's influence on the body across the gap of death."[7] In many cases, medical records, including autopsy reports, were found describing the precise location of a wound incurred by the person the child claims to have been in a previous life, and which matched the precise location of a birthmark in the current life. Sometimes a child in his current life was found to have a specific disease identical to that of the former personality, and which was entirely absent in the child's current genetic heritage.

In a particularly dramatic example, "a child in Turkey recalled being a bandit in his former life. He had committed suicide when about to be captured by the French police, [by wedging] the muzzle of his long rifle under the right side of his chin, resting the handle on the ground, and then [pulling] the trigger. In his new life, the boy was born with a huge gash mark under his chin. While Stevenson was investigating the case, an old man turned up who had remembered the bandit's death and seen the condition of his dead body."[8]

Stevenson conjectured, "If the bullet had gone through the brain in the manner described, there must be another scar where the bullet exited."[9] During his investigation, he asked the child if there was another scar, and one was found just to the left of the crown of his head, hidden under a thick crop of hair. In a presentation at the United Engineering Center in New York, Stevenson showed a slide tracing "the line of trajectory the bullet should have taken in its passage [from the gash under the jaw] through the brain…[which] was in perfect alignment with the scar mark on top of the head."[10]

Interesting though these observations and experiments may be, none of them involve the direct perception of the workings of consciousness. As physicist Arthur Zajonc notes:

> Physics, chemistry, and neuroscience provide accounts for the mechanism of consciousness but say nothing about the experience of consciousness itself[11]… Every science, if it would move beyond purely formal mathematical relationships, must incorporate qualities [i.e., subjective experience] into itself. All meaning inheres in qualities. The qualitative connects the formal treatment with experience… If our interest ultimately is consciousness, then we will require a means of investigation that is able to include the full range of conscious experience, and not merely a reduced set of variables easily amenable to quantification.[12]

As long as researchers continue to rely on the outer thinking mind and outer senses as the primary means of gathering and analyzing data, they will not gain an understanding of the nature of consciousness that is substantially different from that of mainstream science. Limited to the surface consciousness, which takes things to be essentially separate from each other, we have no direct awareness of the relationship between consciousness and the object of study. Even more fundamental, we cannot, using only the surface mind, develop a truly comprehensive understanding, because

> [m]ind in its essence is a consciousness which measures, limits, cuts out forms of things from the indivisible whole and contains them as if each were a separate integer. Even with what exists only as obvious parts and fractions, [m]ind establishes this fiction of its ordinary commerce that they are things with which it can deal separately and not merely as aspects of a whole.[13]

KNOWLEDGE BY DIRECT CONTACT: USING THE INNER MIND AND INNER SENSES

Recognizing the limits of conventional approaches, some scientists suggest that introspection would provide a more direct approach to the study of consciousness.[14] In an interesting instance of the interaction between theory and practice, psychiatrist Jeffrey Schwartz gained new insight into the mind-brain relationship as a result of teaching his patients to incorporate introspection as part of their treatment. He has developed a comprehensive program using mindfulness meditation—a form of introspection—for the treatment of obsessive-compulsive disorder. His treatment involves teaching patients to maintain a calm, nonjudgmental stance while passively observing arising thoughts and impulses. In his research Schwartz found that the simple act of focusing attention brings about specific and substantial changes in brain functioning that correlate with a substantial reduction of symptoms in his patients.

This use of introspection involves a more direct approach to the study of consciousness than other methods used by cognitive scientists. However, it differs from a yogic approach in three fundamental ways:

1) the focus of the subject's (or patient's) attention does not penetrate beyond the ordinary waking consciousness; 2) the researcher, in his analysis of results, relies on the limited, separative knowledge of the outer thinking mind; and 3) in a yogic approach to the study of consciousness, researcher and subject would be coparticipants, both making use of the inner consciousness, through which they could gain direct, unmediated knowledge of whatever "object" they seek to understand.

How might a researcher use his inner consciousness to conduct one of the experiments described earlier? With the inner consciousness it is possible to become directly aware of the interaction of the physical, vital, and mental consciousness in things. Consider, for example, research being conducted on mutations in bacteria. Currently, even with the compelling evidence amassed by such individuals as John Cairns, Barry Hall, and Eshel Ben-Jacob, the assumption that intelligence is involved in the process of mutation is not based on direct inner awareness, but rather indirect speculation. An individual who had sufficiently developed his inner consciousness could carry out similar experiments and perceive directly the role of the physical, vital, and mental consciousness in the process of mutation. Furthermore, given the greater intuitive capacity of the inner mind, he could understand the meaning and purpose of each step of the process in the context of the larger ecosystem and the entire cosmos, perceiving all as one interconnected physical-vital-mental whole. Such perceptions could be verified by having a number of yogic researchers observe the same phenomena and check for commonalities in their perceptions.

Developing the capacity for knowledge by direct contact which is native to the inner consciousness is only an intermediate step between the separative knowledge of the surface consciousness and the true knowledge by identity that characterizes the supramental consciousness. However, it is still such an immense change from our ordinary way of knowing, and still so subject to egoic distortion, that many safeguards would be needed to assure the validity of knowledge so acquired. Safeguards currently employed would continue to be useful: complex physical instruments to check for physical correlates of nonphysical perceptions, rigorous and refined experimental designs, statistical analyses, submission of results to the community of fellow scientists, and so on. However, another critical factor arises when the primary instrument of research is one's own consciousness.

Imagine if each time you looked through a microscope or telescope, the lens changed in wildly unpredictable ways. This is analogous to the way our minds function most of the time. There is, however, an important difference. Repairing a faulty physical instrument may require a great deal of work, but it does not call for a fundamental change in the person using it. On the other hand, when the instrument for looking is the mind of the researcher, the "repair" of the instrument calls for the involvement of the whole person. In other words, ethical considerations become paramount. With current methodologies, an individual scientist may very well be a highly ethical person, but that is not a requirement of the particular method he uses. By contrast, a scientist who employs inner or intuitive ways of knowing must live his life in a such a way that anger, craving, anxiety, and hatred do not prevent the mind from attaining an exquisitely refined and balanced level of attention. This has significant implications for the education of such scientists as it will require that they become highly trained, well-practiced contemplatives.

The research methodology suggested here may sound similar to psychologist Charles Tart's proposal for the development of "state-specific sciences."[15] Tart has observed that the "data" obtained in altered states of consciousness (e.g., the dream state) is often not only different from that obtained in the ordinary waking state, but difficult or even impossible to comprehend when not in the same altered state oneself. He therefore proposed that a complete science would require investigators to enter "altered states" in order to obtain the fullest understanding of data obtained in an altered state.

What is being described here is distinct from Tart's proposal in that it does not directly relate to a particular "state" of consciousness (i.e., waking or dream state). It may seem to do so because yogis have used the same terms ("waking state" and "dream state") to describe particular *ways of knowing*. In yogic terminology, the dream "state" (*swapna* in Sanskrit) refers to the *way of knowing* native to the inner consciousness, one in which we are in direct contact with that which we seek to understand. By contrast, the waking "state" (*jagrat*) refers primarily to the *way of knowing* characteristic of the surface or outer awareness, one in which we take ourselves to be separate from what we know. It is possible to employ knowledge by direct contact not only in what is commonly called the dream state, but in the waking state as well. Similarly, it is possible to employ separative knowledge both in the dream and waking states.

KNOWLEDGE BY IDENTITY: USING INTUITION

Though knowledge by direct contact is a more intimate way of knowing than the separative knowledge characteristic of the surface consciousness, knowledge by identity (what we've been referring to as "intuitive knowledge")[a] is a still more powerful and comprehensive way of knowing.[b] Physicist and philosopher of science Henri Bortoft in his book *The Wholeness of Nature*, writes of an intuitive approach to research based on the work of German writer Johannes Wolfgang von Goethe and Austrian philosopher Rudolf Steiner. Bortoft describes this research as involving a different kind of seeing, one that sees the whole reflected in the parts. This intuitive way of knowing can take in both the quantitative and qualitative in one integral glance.[16]

For example, studying a rose, the researcher would employ an intensely focused, highly disciplined awareness, making possible the discovery of a whole world of qualities not discernable by conventional quantitative methodology. To the extent he is able to identify his consciousness with the consciousness of the rose, he may actually experience it "coming-into-being." According to Bortoft, this method

---

a. We are using the term "intuition" broadly to refer both to the pure knowledge by identity characteristic of the supramental consciousness and the increasingly limited forms of intuition that are characteristic of the various mental planes, from the overmind down to the physical mind. See the section on intuition in chapter 18, "The Supramental Consciousness," for more details.

b. The brief descriptions offered in this section regarding intuitive yogic research methods are intended to provide no more than a hint of what is possible. Any description intended for practical use would require a great deal more written exposition. In order to make use of such a description, researchers would need extended contemplative training.

In addition to using intuition as a primary tool of research, the advanced yogic researcher, by virtue of having awakened the inner consciousness, would have a greatly expanded range of sensory data to work with. This would include the universal fields of physical, vital, and mental conscious-energy.

It would be interesting to see the extent to which a yogic methodology—utilizing both intuition and this expanded sensory capacity—could be applied to both the natural and social sciences. The use of intuition—which can "see" the whole in the part—may, in coming centuries, lead to a comprehension of large-scale sociocultural phenomena with a specificity beyond what even the most rigorous statistical analysis can provide. Similarly, with regard to physical phenomena, yogic research may yield a new understanding—perhaps in conjunction with further developments in external technology—of the movements of the galaxies and the course of biological evolution.

can lead to an understanding of the evolution of plant and animal forms that has so far eluded conventional methods of research.

However, Bortoft's descriptions still fall short of what one would expect at the highest levels of intuitive knowledge, as they lack an awareness of the inseparable relationship between the infinite and the finite.

What might a researcher with a highly developed capacity for knowledge by identity find, were she to examine the question of mutations in bacteria? Rather than focusing on the outer form of the bacteria, or even their inner qualities, she would enter into communion with the "Self" of the bacteria, which is the same as her own True Self. Knowing the bacteria as an appearance of the Divine, she would see the mutation as a purposeful unfolding of the Divine Consciousness and would know in the most intimate fashion the aspiration of that Consciousness to manifest more fully. In a single, unified act of knowing, she would comprehend the relationship between the Will of the Supreme Knower, the group-soul of the bacteria, the appearance of their evolving form, and the timing of the whole process.

The Indo-Tibetan tradition contains many sublime descriptions of knowledge by identity—particularly in the writings of Tibetan Buddhists and the great eleventh-century Tantric philosopher Abhinavagupta. Building upon this tradition, Sri Aurobindo gives some hints as to how intuitive knowledge may contribute to a radically new understanding of matter.

Sri Aurobindo's comments are offered here as scientific hypotheses to be tested. However, testing of these hypotheses, unlike those associated with conventional research, would require the use of a highly developed intuitive capacity. The level of requisite intuitive refinement is not one that could be easily achieved in a matter of weeks or even months. Rather, it would likely require an intensive, years-long training program along the lines of Alan Wallace's Samatha project. A number of researchers so trained might then be able to work collaboratively to reach an intimate knowledge of the relationship between matter and consciousness.

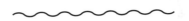

When science, instead of following the course of Nature upstream by analysis... shall begin to follow it downstream... and especially studying and utilizing critical stages of transition, then the secret of material creation will be solved, and Science will be able to create material life and not as now merely destroy it.[17]

—Sri Aurobindo, *Commentary on the Isha Upanishad*

A diamond is a diamond and a pearl a pearl, each thing of its own class, existing by its distinction from all others, each distinguished by its own form and properties. But each has also properties and elements which are common to both and others which are common to material things in general. And in reality each does not exist only by its distinctions, but much more essentially by that which is common to both; and we get back to the very basis and enduring truth of all material things only when we find that all are the same thing, one energy, one substance or, if you like, one universal motion which throws up, brings out, combines, realises these different forms, these various properties, these fixed and harmonised potentialities of its own being. If we stop short at the knowledge of distinctions, we can deal only with diamond and pearl as they are, fix their values, uses, varieties, make the best ordinary use and profit of them; but if we can get to the knowledge and control of their elements and the common properties of the class to which they belong, we may arrive at the power of making either a diamond or pearl at our pleasure: go farther still and master that which all material things are in their essence and we may arrive even at the power of transmutation which would give the greatest possible control of material Nature. Thus the knowledge of distinctions arrives at its greatest truth and effective use when we arrive at the deeper knowledge of that which reconciles distinctions in the unity behind all variations. That deeper knowledge does not deprive the other and more superficial of effectivity nor convict it of vanity. We cannot conclude from our ultimate material discovery that there is no original substance or Matter, only energy manifesting substance or manifesting as substance,—that diamond and pearl are non-existent, unreal, only true to the illusion of our senses of perception and action, that the one substance, energy or motion is the sole eternal truth and that therefore the best or only rational use of our science would be to dissolve diamond and pearl and everything else that we can dissolve into this one eternal and original reality and get done with their forms and properties for ever. There is an essentiality of things [the transcendent, infinite Spirit], a commonalty of things [the universal Spirit], an individuality of things [the individual Spirit]; the commonalty and individuality are true and eternal powers of the essentiality: that transcends them both, but the three together and not one by itself are the eternal terms of existence.

This truth which we can see, though with difficulty and under considerable restrictions, even in the material world where the subtler and higher powers of being have to be excluded from our intellectual operations, becomes clearer and more powerful when we ascend in the scale. We see the truth of our classifications and distinctions, but also their limits. All things, even while different, are yet one. For practical purposes plant, animal, man are different existences; yet when we look deeper we see that the plant is only an animal with an insufficient evolution of self-consciousness and dynamic force; the animal is man in the making; man himself is that animal and yet the something more of self-consciousness and dynamic power of consciousness that make him man; and yet again he is the something more which is contained and repressed in his being as the potentiality of the divine—he is a god in the making. In each of these, plant, animal, man, god, the Eternal is there containing and repressing himself as it were in order to make a certain statement of his being. Each is the whole Eternal concealed.[18]

—Sri Aurobindo, *The Life Divine*

APPENDIX B

AN OUTLINE OF YOGA PSYCHOLOGY

This summary is best approached as a kind of map—that is, a description of various terrains of consciousness as explored experientially by yogis (in the East and West) over the last several thousand years. The aim of the map is primarily to facilitate intuitive rather than intellectual understanding. However, there is a place for intellectual study; to the extent the mind is calm and can open to intimations of something deeper or higher, it can be an aid in clarifying experience.

Although some of the terms we use were coined by Sri Aurobindo (e.g., "physical mind," "vital mind," "supramental," etc.), we have tried to present what we understand to be—in spirit, though not in specifics—a "view" of the workings of consciousness common to contemplatives the world over.

PRELUDE: THE DANCE OF CONSCIOUSNESS

Consciousness is… the fundamental thing in existence—it is the energy, the motion, the movement of consciousness that creates the universe and all that is in it.[1]

—Sri Aurobindo, *Letters on Yoga*

The Divine is a radiant and joyful Reality, ecstatically bringing forth the universe from its own Being, within its own Consciousness, at every moment; playing out the infinite possibilities of its infinite Being, simultaneously in the eternal Now. It is the shift of Its attention that creates the sense of sequence in time, and the shift of its attention that creates the sense of movement through space. As the One Infinite Consciousness gazes in one way, the universe is birthed. As that gaze shifts, the stars are "born," planets and solar systems take shape, the adventure of evolution unfolds. Beyond time and space altogether, the supreme, infinite Conscious-Being sees within Itself its myriad, infinite possibilities, and in that very seeing joyfully, blissfully, manifests the all that we see around us.

All is the play of Conscious-Being and Conscious-Energy, *Shiva* and *Shakti*, Soul and Nature. In any act of "conscious-ing,"[a] that which is known (the "object") is a movement of Conscious-Energy. The movement is itself an act of will—a shift of attention of the Divine Conscious-Being (the "subject"). This movement (the "object" created by the shift of attention) is known as it is willed into being. Thus, the object is inseparable from the act of knowing it. The myriad objects of our universe—apparently separate but always one with the Infinite—are nothing more than infinite acts of shifting attention of the One Divine Being. These acts of knowing-and-willing—which manifest as the universe—exist inseparably within the Delight of the Divine Being. It is the movement of apparent separation and reunion that is experienced by different creatures as attraction and repulsion, pleasure and pain, love and hate, and ultimately as unbroken Delight by the fully awakened seer.

All is the One Conscious-Being knowing and feeling itself in infinite ways, in infinite forms. The individual Soul is a particular focus of consciousness, the various planes of consciousness each a particular kind of interaction between Conscious-Being and Its Conscious-Force, between Soul and Nature. When Consciousness is absorbed in the play of forms, identifying with a particular part of the Field, the result is Ignorance. Over the course of evolution there is a progressive freeing of the embodied consciousness from its exclusive identification with a small part of the Field. The essential Nature of this whole interaction between Soul and Nature, *Shiva* and *Shakti*, is infinite Joy, *Ananda*, Bliss.

---

a. Sri Krishna Prem (1988) notes that the word consciousness "suffers from the great drawback that it has no active verbal form. One can say 'to be conscious of' but not 'to conscious' such-and-such an object" (p. 195). To compensate for this, we've coined the awkward term "conscious-ing."

Involution: "Before" the "Big Bang"

Silence, utter stillness. In the "Beginning,"[a] the Knower is absorbed in silent, motionless contemplation of His own Being. The first distinction arises, between the Conscious-Being and His Conscious-Force, between the Knower and the Field, Soul and Nature, *Purusha* and *Prakriti*. There is a stirring, an infinitesimal vibration between the Two—He and She[b] —and the process of manifestation begins.

The Divine Shakespeare, imagining, dreaming of infinite possibilities, progressively limits His Consciousness, manifesting the various planes (grades) of consciousness in preparation for the great adventure of evolution. Various subtle, nonphysical worlds come into existence, worlds of conscious-energy that will be the immediate source for all that happens in the physical universe. Everything that is manifest in these worlds is a limited expression, a reflection of the infinite power of knowing, willing, and feeling of the Infinite Divine Being: matter, a reflection of *Sat*, Infinite Being; life, a reflection of *Shakti*, the Divine Conscious-Energy; the psychic being a reflection of *Ananda*, Infinite Bliss; and mind a reflection of *Vijñana*, the supramental Truth-Consciousness.

As these various planes of consciousness come into existence, the unlimited consciousness of the Knower becomes progressively more limited, more involved in the play of creation, until His Consciousness is completely absorbed in the workings of His Force. Of course, it is only the consciousness associated with the play of involution and evolution that is completely absorbed. The infinite, immeasurable Consciousness of the Knower[c] beyond all space and time remains completely free and untouched by the entire play. It is only an infinitesimal portion of the infinite Conscious-Being of the Knower that manifests as the various planes of consciousness.

---

a. The "Beginning," being outside of time, is Now, eternally.

b. The Divine is beyond all gender, but for the sake of our limited consciousness, "He" and "She" are more evocative than "It."

c. Strictly speaking, the *Purushottoma*—the Supreme Person—is as much "beyond" the Knower as it is beyond the Field. We take the perhaps inappropriate liberty here of conflating the two—Knower and the One or All "beyond" the Knower—in the interest of what may be a foolish, mental consistency (i.e., consistent with descriptions of the Infinite Knower earlier in the book).

It is what Sri Aurobindo calls the supramental consciousness, the Divine Intelligence, which guides the entire process of manifestation. Whatever that Supreme Consciousness sees in Its own Being is what comes into existence. As that Consciousness gazes, worlds arise; the universe is literally being "gazed" into existence. It is this Intelligence that manifests in the universe as what we refer to as the "laws" of nature as well as all the other meaningful patterns we may identify.

EVOLUTION: THE EMERGENCE OF CONSCIOUSNESS IN THE UNIVERSE

Again, Silence, utter stillness. At the nadir of involution, the Knower is completely absorbed—"exclusively concentrated," as Sri Aurobindo describes it—in His Conscious-Energy, seemingly forgetful of His True Self. It is because of this exclusive concentration that suffering exists in a universe that is contained within the Being of the All-Blissful Knower; that death can occur in a universe pervaded by Infinite Life; that unconscious matter seems to exist in a universe made of Conscious-Energy. There appears to be an essential separation between the Field and its Knower. It is this misperception, this ignorance of the essential Oneness of Knower and Field, that is responsible for all the suffering and travail that occur in the course of evolution.

Before the journey of evolution begins, there is no movement of Conscious-Energy—all is potential. Again, a stirring occurs—a vibration, an interaction between the hidden Being of the Knower (Soul) and His Field (Nature, the potential Conscious-Energy). This vibratory interaction is occurring at every moment—an inflowing or "return" of the cosmic energies to the Silence, and the outflowing or reemergence of these energies once again from the Silence into manifestation. This vibration—the dance between Soul and Nature—is manifest in our world in all the rhythms and polarities of nature: the negative and positive polarity of the atom, the alternation of day and night, the inbreath and outbreath of every living organism.

Over the course of evolution there will be a slow reversal of the absorption of the Knower in the Field, an undoing of the exclusive concentration. As the Knower's gaze shifts, his attention is gradually freed from absorption in the Field, and the various grades of consciousness that are yet hidden begin to emerge: from Matter to Life, Mind, and beyond. The same essential process, the freeing of attention, occurs on all scales of development: over the course of billions of years of evolution, in the lifetime of an individual human being, and in every moment of our lives.

The Knower is hidden in the Field as the infinitesimal spark, the Soul, what Sri Aurobindo calls the psychic entity. This Soul-essence remains and puts forth a growing soul-personality, the psychic being. The consciousness of the evolving Soul is diffuse in matter, and becomes slowly more organized over the course of evolution. In animals, a further organization of the consciousness of the Soul takes place and there emerges a kind of "group-soul," which coordinates the consciousness of each animal of a particular species. With the emergence of the human being, a further organization of this consciousness takes place, and there emerges the individual psychic being.

Karma and the Process of Evolution

How does the growing psychic being awaken? There is a constant interaction throughout the course of evolution between the hidden Knower, the growing Soul, and the Field which is its environment. With every impact of the environment, there is a disturbance of the surface consciousness which, like the "rubbing of tinders,"[2] impacts the slumbering Soul, leading to further awakening.

But this process of awakening is not so simple. When the energies of the Field come knocking at the door of the psychic being, it does not automatically awaken in response. Because the Divine intends this to be an adventure, a game of hide-and-seek, there is a challenge built in—the challenge of apparent separation. The awakening consciousness of the Knower mistakenly identifies itself with a finite, limited formation of the Field. Remaining subconscious in matter, plants, and animals, the process becomes conscious in human beings.[a]

---

a. This does not mean that every human being is conscious of the whole process of mistaken egoic identification; rather it means that the human being, unlike other creatures, consciously experiences himself as an individual separate from others and the world.

Every action, every disturbance or reaction of the surface consciousness that arises out of apparent separation, because it is out of harmony with the Oneness of things, leaves behind a karmic trace, a physical/vital/mental impression. This subconscient impression intensifies the sense of separation, thus increasing the aspiration of the psychic being to awaken and recover its essential Oneness. It is the momentum of karma, in tandem with the aspiration of the Soul to awaken—guided by the Will of the Divine Intelligence—that drives the entire process of evolution.

The whole process of karmic action and reaction involves the registration of a stimulus (knowing), an inner modification (feeling), and an active response (willing). Knowing, willing, and feeling, while present in matter, are negligible. As evolution proceeds, each becomes more complex, leading to a quickening in the pace of evolution. Underlying the momentum of the evolutionary force is the energy of the Soul's aspiration and the energy of the Divine Will moving the whole process forward.

As the consciousness grows at any given level of development, the capacities of knowing, willing, and feeling grow richer, more varied, and more integrated. In terms of form, for example, the brain develops a new more complex structure that allows for more differentiation in its functioning. At the same time, more neural connections develop so that the different functions are more integrated. Regarding consciousness, at any given level, abilities become richer, with greater integration among them as well. For example, during the stage where the child is influenced primarily by the inner vital being, there may be an increase in her emotional sensitivity, an increase in her capacity for selective attention, and along with this widening of ability, a greater capacity to integrate her thoughts, feelings, and actions.

As this process of growth continues over millions and even billions of years, widening the capacity for knowing, feeling, and willing, it reaches the point where a leap occurs, and a new, more complex grade of consciousness emerges. The attention, freed from its prior absorption, its exclusive concentration in a particular portion of the Field, shifts or expands into the new level of consciousness. Out of Matter, Life and Mind evolve. Along with this ascent or emancipation of consciousness, an integration occurs between the new, more complex layers of consciousness and those that preceded it. The physical matter that makes up the body of a plant or animal is transformed by the emergence of Life and Mind; the vital and mental consciousness of the human being will be transformed by the emergence of the supramental consciousness.

At the time the universe is born, only the physical consciousness is manifest. It is dull, mechanical, and inert because the Consciousness of the Knower is most hidden at that point in the evolutionary process. The vital consciousness—a reflection of the Divine Conscious-Energy—has to struggle to emerge from the dull, unconsciousness of matter. Because of this, the vital desire for mastery and enjoyment takes the form of a struggle against the inconscience of matter. When the mental consciousness first evolves, there is no integrating principle on the surface that can harmonize it with the vital and physical consciousness. Because of this, there tends to be frequent conflict between the different grades of consciousness. This conflict is less intense early on in evolution when only the first functions of mind—sensing and perceiving—have emerged. Associated with these two functions, only the physical mind (responsible for organizing sensations) and the vital mind (responsible for organizing the various levels of vital consciousness) have emerged. When the more complex functions of the thinking mind, along with more complex volition, emerge, there is both a greater potential for integration and at the same time a greater potential for conflict.

HUMAN EVOLUTION: COLLECTIVE

With the emergence of the thinking mind in human beings, there arises the possibility—which for a long time remains merely a potential—of conscious cooperation with the process of evolution.[a] The thinking mind brings an enormous range of new abilities—new, richer capacities of feeling, memory, attention, imagination, creativity, and reasoning as well as a

---

a. This new possibility for conscious cooperation with the Divine Will is symbolized in the biblical tale of Adam (*Purusha* or Conscious-Being) and Eve (*Prakriti* or Conscious-Energy) in the Garden of Eden.

more refined physical consciousness. But it also strengthens the ego, the sense of separation, further intensifying desire by distorting the Soul's aspiration. The strengthening of the physical, vital, and mental ego has resulted in a profound distortion of the human consciousness. It is the play of increased capacities along with the falsifying action of the ego that are responsible for the unfathomable complexity of human history.

All human history can be understood as reflecting the unfolding of the mental consciousness of the Divine. In early humanity the thinking mind was largely under the influence of the physical consciousness. Over millennia, as the cosmic energy manifesting in humanity ascended the scale of consciousness, there was a successive influence of various levels of the vital consciousness, until the thinking mind became free, to some degree, from the domination of the vital and physical. However, one might say it overshot the mark, dominating them in turn, in the process becoming alienated from the larger, inner consciousness, and to some extent limiting its own activity to a small portion of the analytic reasoning mind.

While this description may be an accurate depiction of general trends, the actual evolution of humanity has occurred (and continues to occur) along many different and overlapping lines of physical, vital, and mental karma. Different cultures, for example, have reflected different predominant aspects of consciousness: nineteenth-century England, the physical mind; eighteenth and nineteenth-century Russia, the vital mind; Italy during the Renaissance, and Athens in the early centuries B.C.E., embodied what Sri Aurobindo refers to as the aesthetic mind; Spartan Rome and early Puritan America, the ethical mind; eighteenth and nineteenth-century Germany, the thinking mind proper; India during the time of the Upanishads, and Tibet during the Middle Ages, the intuitive mind. [a] There is also a collective ego of a people—of a tribe, a community, a nation; and underlying that, the soul of the culture, a group-soul seeking to express its true nature. The karmic process of action and reaction takes place on the collective scale as well, and, combined with the aspiration of the group-soul, drives the evolution of human consciousness.

---

a. These correlations of aspects of consciousness with various cultures are drawn largely from Sri Aurobindo's work, *The Human Cycle;* in particular, chapters 2, 4, and 10.

Human Evolution: Individual

The surface layer of the evolving Field is made up of various layers of physical, vital, and mental consciousness. These can be subdivided in various ways, though actually they make up a continuum. Using Sri Aurobindo's terminology (based on the original prephilosophic Vedanta of the Upanishads), the outer or surface nature, ascending vertically, consists of the following grades of consciousness: physical (material physical, physical, vital physical, mental physical); vital (physical vital, lower vital, central vital, higher vital, mental vital); and mental (physical mind, vital mind, and the various subdivisions of the thinking mind).[a]

There is another layer of the evolving Field "behind" or deeper than the surface nature—the inner or subliminal consciousness. There is an inner mind, inner vital, and inner subtle physical consciousness, each of which includes all the subdivisions of the outer nature mentioned above (inner higher vital, inner central vital, etc.). This wider, vaster consciousness is in direct connection with the universal fields of physical, vital, and mental consciousness and is the immediate source of much of the content of the outer nature. Most of our thoughts and feelings come either from this inner consciousness or from the layers of the personal or universal subconscient.[b]

Still deeper within than either the outer or inner Field is the individual Knower—the psychic being (*Chaitya Purusha*; the Being in the Heart) which is the basis of everything that occurs in the inner and

---

a. The second of the double terms is the layer of consciousness that is influenced by the first. For example, the term "mental vital" refers to that grade of the vital consciousness which is most strongly influenced by the mind. Sri Aurobindo uses a variety of terms describing layers or dimensions of the thinking mind, such as aesthetic mind, ethical mind, reasoning mind, externalizing mind (distantly related to what psychologists refer to as the capacity for expressive and receptive language), and dynamic mind (the volitional aspect of the thinking mind). All verbal terms should be taken as provisional; the purpose of the terminology is primarily to provide clarification of experience, and intellectual understanding only secondarily.

b. Rarely, something may come through from the Soul or superconscient, but usually this will be in a highly distorted form once it reaches the surface consciousness.

outer nature.[a] In each moment, behind every thought, every feeling, every sensation, is the consciousness of the psychic being, directing and ultimately giving its consent to all movements of the inner and outer nature. Its attention, when focused at the higher chakras, brings the mind into play. Shifting attention to the lower chakras, the Soul brings into play the vital or physical consciousness.

Behind the evolving psychic being is the individual Soul, what Sri Aurobindo calls the "psychic entity." This is a reflection in the Field of the individual Spirit (*Jivatman*; Conscious-Being) which exists forever beyond time and space.[b] This individual Spirit is a particular "focus" (though not separate as with egoic consciousness) of the Infinite, transcendent Knower (*Purushottoma*; Supreme Conscious-Being), a particular window or (nonmental) perspective through which He can experience his Infinitudes.

At each level of the Field there is a reflection of the Spirit. In the ancient Vedanta these are referred to as the physical being (*annamaya purusha*, literally, the being made of food); vital being (*pranamaya purusha*, the being of *prana* or life), and the mental being (*manomaya purusha*, the being of mind). These three "beings" can be experienced deep within as the inner witness, behind the various layers of the inner consciousness.[c]

---

a. Sri Aurobindo sometimes speaks of the "true mental," the "true vital," and the "true physical" consciousness as being "between" the inner and psychic consciousness. At this level of subtlety, spatial dimensions can be misleading. For those with sufficient experience, extensive comments regarding this domain may be helpful and can be found in the section "Planes and Parts of the Being" in Sri Aurobindo's book *Letters on Yoga*, Volume 1.

b. The Soul is also beyond time and space but has a more direct relation to the evolving Field than the individual Spirit. Here, more even than with the terms that describe the layers of the Field, words like "Soul" and "Spirit" are difficult to understand without some experience of that to which they refer. If taken as labels or definitions, they will seem contradictory or even paradoxical. For example, how can Being, which is one, be divided up into psychic being, Soul, Spirit, and so on? It can't be divided, but different aspects can be distinguished—though not by the mind unless supported by spiritual discernment.

c. This experience of the inner witness is often confused with full enlightenment. This theoretical distinction—between the inner witness and, deeper within, the

The Process of Development

To the outer mind, human development appears to involve the maturation of the mind, emotions, and body. From the inner perspective, it is ultimately the psychic being that is developing, even when the outer consciousness is entirely unaware of it. Both dimensions of growth—the development of the Field (the mental, vital, and physical consciousness), and of the individual Knower (the growing Soul)—occur simultaneously. However, the development of the Field is purely for the sake of the Knower—to provide a more complex and versatile instrument through which the Knower can express Himself. One might speak of the evolving Field in terms of a vertical axis of development. This would include, in ascending order, the following levels: inconscient,[a] subconscient, physical, vital, mental; the planes of spiritual mind[3] (higher mind,[b] illumined mind, intuitive mind, overmind); and the planes of the "higher hemisphere": the *Vijñana* (supramental), *Ananda* (bliss), *Chit* (Conscious-Force), and *Sat* (Being).

The development of the individual, as was the case collectively over the course of human history, involves the gradual freeing of the thinking mind from domination by the physical and vital consciousness. Looking solely at the outer nature, one may be led to believe that a person with the highest level of development would be the one who has access to the most complex levels of the thinking mind. But from the yogic perspective, an individual may have developed an extremely complex thinking mind but still be ruled from within by the physical being or vital being. The inner beings—physical, vital, and mental—play an important role in the development of the outer nature, though not the central role, which belongs to the psychic being. This distinction is important, because often we wrongly take the experience of the

---

Infinite Knower—has been made by various writers. However, in practice, the overwhelming perception of the inseparability of the Knower and the Field that accompanies the witnessing experience may lead the individual to confuse it with the pure, non-dual awareness of the Knower.

a. See Figure 3 in chapter 18, "Supramental Consciousness."

b. See Figure 3 in chapter 18, "Supramental Consciousness."

inner being to be a soul-experience.[a]

Ultimately the degree of "awakeness" of the psychic being is the true measure of an individual's level of development. A person who is profoundly retarded, whose thinking mind will never progress beyond that of a one or two-year-old child, may be a highly evolved Soul. In fact, the psychic being may have chosen to be born in a body with a defective brain in order to more fully develop certain emotional capacities or still deeper soul qualities.

The Role of Ego in the Developmental Process

The physical, vital, and mental consciousness do not function as pure instruments because of the original (apparent, though not actual) separation of the Knower and the Field. For example, the true role of the lower vital consciousness is simply enjoyment of the world. However, because of ego, this enjoyment is distorted into craving and attachment. The same thing occurs with respect to all the instruments—the will to mastery of the central vital becomes an urge toward domination; the pure love of the Soul become in the surface vital a constant war of like and dislike, love and hate. The pure aspiration of the Soul is hijacked by the ego-dominated nature and turned into the energy of desire. The mind, intended to be the pure seeker of Truth, becomes instead a justifier of vital desires. When working as a pure instrument of the supramental consciousness above, the sole function of the mind would be to express that infinite Intelligence in finite forms. Distorted by ego, the mind sees the world as made up of separate and distinct entities, and is unable to perceive the underlying Oneness.

Because the surface (and to a large extent, the inner) consciousness

---

a. Regarding the importance of the inner beings in psychological development, it is possible, for example, for someone to have a very-well-developed intellect but be ruled by the physical consciousness. In this case, regardless of their mental capacity, their mental activity would likely be rigid and dominated by prejudice and dogmatism. Conversely, it is possible for someone to have a poorly developed intellect and be ruled by the mental being. This is sometimes seen in retarded individuals who have a high degree of self-awareness.

is shaped by ego, all its actions create further karma, strengthening the web of attachments that bind the Soul in countless ways. Not only are all the workings of each individual instrument distorted, but because the Soul is not yet sufficiently awake to function as an integrating factor, each instrument is in conflict with the other. The desires and cravings of the vital lead to physical illness and mental confusion; the separative will of the mind overrides the needs of the body and the pure expression of the vital. The inertia and dullness of the physical consciousness impede the free flow of emotion and the clear, unbiased working of the mind.

Complicating this process still further, various enduring patterns of physical, vital, and mental consciousness come together to form a multitude of personalities. Accumulated over many lifetimes, we have hundreds, even thousands of these subpersonalities influencing us from the various subconscient levels of our being.

PREPARATION FOR AWAKENING AND TRANSFORMATION

The Soul accepts this web of ego and karma as part of the adventure of evolution. In fact, when the individual begins to awaken, it is possible to see the sanction of the psychic being behind virtually every vibration of the inner and outer nature. It can be seen that, in a way, the intention of the psychic being is ultimately required for any movement of the physical, vital, or mental consciousness.

The psychic being is always seeking in some way to express—in whatever limited fashion available to it in the nature—its innate soul qualities of love, wisdom, strength, and the like. At some point in development—in one lifetime or another—the psychic being is no longer content to have only an indirect influence on the surface consciousness. It is only by fully awakening that the psychic being can fully express its native qualities.

The awakening of the psychic being may seem to come about suddenly, brought on perhaps by some kind of traumatic shock. However, it usually involves many lifetimes in which the Soul has gradually purified and harmonized the instruments of the nature. The mind, through calm, nonjudgmental attention, can work to align the vital and physical consciousness with the Soul. It can do this to the extent it is guided by true faith—*shraddha*—always listening intently for intimations of the voice of the true Conscience, the influence of the psychic being in the outer nature.

Through such mindful (and heartful) attention, the mind can minimize the constant conflict between the various grades of physical, vital, and mental consciousness, enabling them to perform their appropriate functions. The ego will still be active, distorting the working of the nature, but through calm, mindful attention to the promptings of the psychic being, its influence can be minimized.

Though this process of attention can be fruitful, as long as the consciousness is confined to the surface, its capacity is extremely limited. The surface consciousness knows things only as separate from itself. The mind, for example, cannot understand the vital, because it cannot enter into direct communion with it. When we enter within, however, we know things by direct contact. Not only are we in intimate contact with the various parts of our own nature, we can directly touch the consciousness of other people (and even of physical objects) in a way impossible for the surface consciousness. The inner consciousness, unlike the outer consciousness, is also open to the powerful energy of the universal physical, vital, and mental fields, thus giving it potentially greater power to change the nature. Most important, the inner consciousness, being closer to the Soul, is more open to its influence than is the outer consciousness.

AWAKENING AND TRANSFORMATION: INDIVIDUAL

Once the psychic being has awakened, it is possible to bring its influence directly to bear on the outer nature, allowing for the fuller manifestation of the *swabhava*—the true nature of the Soul. The whole process—the initial purification of the nature, the opening to the inner consciousness, and the awakening of the Soul—is hastened to the extent the individual is open to the direct influence of the Force, the Conscious-Energy *(Chit-Shakti)* of the Divine. Aligning one's will with that of the Divine, the outer instruments gradually become trans-formed, guided now at every step by the awakened psychic being.

The person, when awakened, discovers a method of "control" that is entirely different from that of the unawakened outer nature. He realizes that the Soul's consent is needed for every movement of con-sciousness. Rather than willfully dominating or controlling one part or another of his consciousness, he comes to see that merely removing that consent is sufficient to reject the distorted, egoic movements. He can also develop penetrating insight, by means of which he can learn to see every layer and every detail of the complex karmic web woven by ego. By this spiritual insight, and by remaining open to the working of the Divine Force, the egoic distortions can not only be rejected, they can be transformed, restoring the proper function of each instrument.

But the capacity of the Soul to fully express its true nature will be limited as long as the instruments of the nature are confined to the physical, vital, and ordinary mental consciousness. It is possible to awaken levels of consciousness beyond the thinking mind, which in turn allows a greater power of Divine Force to descend, further transforming the nature. Ultimately the individual consciousness can ascend beyond the mind altogether, awakening the supramental con-sciousness, which will allow for the descent of a Force so powerful, it will be possible to utterly transform not only the mind and vital but the physical body itself.

AWAKENING AND TRANSFORMATION: COLLECTIVE

The same evolutionary processes are at work on the collective as on the individual level. At the collective level there is both a group ego and group-soul. The actions of the family, community, and nation accumu-late karmic impressions, which are collected in the group-subconscient. As in the individual, the weight of these karmic traces intensifies the aspiration of the group-soul to awaken and manifest its true nature. As each individual member of the family or community awakens and transforms his individual consciousness, it becomes more possible for this to happen on the collective level.

Just as with the individual, a collaborative effort toward purification and harmonization of the workings of the collective physical, vital, and mental consciousness can prepare the ground for this awakening and transformation. Even now, the world may be going through a collective process leading to the next and potentially dangerous step, an opening to the influence of the vaster inner realms of consciousness. In the inner realm, the forces of ego and distortion are far more powerful and potentially destructive. Thus, it is imperative that we learn to open ourselves to the influence of the Divine Soul at the heart of things as we take this step.

Someday we will all awaken. Guided by the Divine, we will be able to manifest the Divine Nature, creating together a world in which we consciously recognize all matter as the body of the Spirit, life as the movement and play of Spirit, and mind as a subordinate working of the Truth-consciousness beyond mind. We will see the "one Divine in all"; we will live in the awareness that "all are in the Divine, all are the Divine and there is nothing else in the Universe."[4]

> Lift your eyes towards the Sun; He is there in that wonderful heart of life and light and splendor. Watch at night the innumerable constellations glittering like so many solemn watchfires of the Eternal in the limitless silence which is no void but throbs with the presence of a single calm and tremendous existence; see there Orion with his sword and belt shining...Sirius in his splendor, Lyra sailing billions of miles away in the ocean of space. Remember that these innumerable worlds, most of them mightier than our own, are whirling with indescribable speed at the beck of that Ancient of Days whither none but He knoweth, and yet that they are a million times more ancient than your Himalaya, more steady than the roots of your hills and shall so remain until He at his will shakes them off like withered leaves from the eternal tree of the Universe. Imagine the endlessness of Time, realize the boundlessness of Space; and then remember that when these worlds were not, He was, the Same as now, and when these are not, He shall be, still

the Same; perceive that beyond Lyra He is and far away in Space where the stars of the Southern Cross cannot be seen, still He is there.

And then come back to the Earth and realize who this He is. He is quite near to you. See yonder old man who passes near you crouching and bent, with his stick. Do you realize that it is God who is passing? There a child runs laughing in the sunlight. Can you hear Him in that laughter? Nay, He is nearer still to you. He is in you, He is you. It is yourself that burns yonder millions of miles away in the infinite reaches of Space, that walks with confident steps on the tumbling billows of the ethereal sea; it is you who have set the stars in their places and woven the necklace of the suns not with hands but by that Yoga, that silent actionless impersonal Will which has set you here today listening to yourself in me. Look up, O child of the ancient Yoga, and be no longer a trembler and a doubter; fear not, doubt not, grieve not; for in your apparent body is One who can create and destroy worlds with a breath."[5]

—Sri Aurobindo, *Commentary on the Isha Upanishad*

APPENDIX C

BIOGRAPHICAL SKETCHES OF SRI AUROBINDO AND MIRRA ALFASSA

There should be somewhere upon earth a place that no nation could claim as its sole property, a place where all human beings of good will, sincere in their aspiration, could live freely as citizens of the world, obeying one single authority, that of the supreme Truth, a place of peace, concord, harmony...[1]

—*Mirra Alfassa*

In 1872, the year Aurobindo Ghose (later known as "Sri Aurobindo") was born in Calcutta, India, the idea of Yoga as a means of escape from the world was prevalent not only in Europe but in India as well. Aurobindo's father, a thoroughly anglicized Indian, was concerned that his children not be infected with the religious outlook he felt to be the cause of the poverty and backwardness so pervasive in his country. For this reason, when Aurobindo was seven years old, he sent him to England to be educated, with the strict mandate that he not be given any instruction regarding the history or culture of his native land. After attending the best schools in London, Aurobindo matriculated at Cambridge University, where he studied Greek and Latin classics. In 1893 he returned to India with a strong interest in its liberation.

Some years later, Aurobindo began writing and giving speeches, and by 1906 had become a leader in the freedom movement for Indian independence. His work in developing the principles for the non-cooperation movement helped lay the foundation for the satyagraha campaign of Mahatma Gandhi. In 1908, after being falsely accused of involvement in a bombing incident that resulted in the death of several women, Aurobindo was detained for one year as a prisoner in the Alipore jail. During that year of forced isolation, he had a series of powerful spiritual experiences that played a pivotal role in changing his life from its outward orientation to an intensely inward one.

When acquitted of the charges, Sri Aurobindo realized he could not continue his work under the eye of the British police, and in 1910 moved to the French colony of Pondicherry in South India, where he remained for the rest of his life. His spiritual awakening while in prison had led him to the conviction that "it is not just a revolt against the British empire that we must wage, but a revolt against the whole universal Nature!"[2] Soon after, he retired from political work to dedicate himself more fully to the practice of yoga.

Mirra Alfassa was born in Paris in 1879 to Sephardic Jews who had previously lived in Turkey and Egypt. She began having spiritual experiences at a very young age and by early adolescence, a vision of her work in the world slowly became clear to her:

> Between the ages of 11 and 13 a series of… spiritual experiences revealed to me not only the existence of God, but man's possibility of uniting with Him, of realizing Him integrally in consciousness and action, of manifesting Him upon earth in a life divine.[3]

Mirra studied music and art throughout her childhood, and as a young adult became part of the circle of French painters in turn-of-the century Paris. Around the same time, she began leading a group of spiritual seekers, giving talks and establishing a vision of a "progressing universal harmony."[4]

In 1910 her husband, Paul Richard, became involved in French politics in Pondicherry and, while there, met Sri Aurobindo. They maintained a correspondence after Paul's return to France. In 1914, Paul and Mirra returned to India together, and along with Sri Aurobindo, the three began publishing a monthly journal, *The Arya*.

Its purpose was to be "a systematic study of the highest problems of existence," and to arrive at "the formation of a vast synthesis of knowledge, harmonizing the diverse religious traditions of humanity, occidental as well as oriental."[5] Sri Aurobindo's major writings, including *The Life Divine, The Synthesis of Yoga, Essays on the Gita* and

The Secret of the Vedas, were originally published in serial form during the six-year publication cycle of *The Arya*, laying the foundation for his integral vision of yoga psychology. This vision was further refined over the next thirty years, as reflected in three volumes of letters to his disciples and his epic poem *Savitri*. Paul Richard eventually left Pondicherry, while Mirra remained in India to devote herself to the spiritual work of Sri Aurobindo.

Both Mirra and Sri Aurobindo had studied the philosophies and spiritual practices of Asia, Europe, and Africa, and they brought this broad body of knowledge to their work. Their yogic practice was a comprehensive one that integrated action, contemplation, and devotion. It unified nontheistic and theistic approaches to spirituality, recognizing a Reality greater than either the exclusively personal or exclusively impersonal Divine spoken of in many of the spiritual philosophies they had studied.

In 1926, Mirra took responsibility for administering the affairs of the ashram, which had begun with a dozen students and grew during the next several decades to a community of over a thousand. Following Sri Aurobindo's death in 1950, she became both administrator and spiritual head of the ashram. In 1952 she established the Sri Aurobindo International Centre of Education, which remains a first-rate center for experiments in integral education, encompassing physical, emotional, intellectual, and spiritual growth and development. Fulfilling her earlier vision for the establishment of an ideal society, in 1968, Mirra arranged for children from over 120 nations to bring a handful of earth from their native lands in order to pour it into a common urn at the center of the land she called "Auroville," the city of dawn.

Echoing words she had written in Paris more than a half century earlier, she declared, "Auroville wants to be a universal town where men and women of all countries are able to live in peace and progressive harmony, above all creeds, all politics and all nationalities. The purpose of Auroville is to realize human unity."[6]

APPENDIX D

A TRIBUTE TO INDRA SEN

The first person to diligently cull the psychological elements from Sri Aurobindo's writings was Dr. Indra Sen. Dr. Sen had been a professor of philosophy and psychology at the University of Delhi and later went on to become president of the psychology section of the Indian Science Congress. He was also the recipient of the Eastern-Western psychology lecture award of the Swami Pranavananda Psychology Trust.

In the mid-1930s he wrote an essay using the term "Integral Psychology" to refer to the psychological understanding contained within Sri Aurobindo's writings. Over the course of the next forty years, Dr. Sen wrote a number of journal articles which, in 1986, were published collectively in a book entitled *Integral Psychology: The Psychological System of Sri Aurobindo*. His daughter, Aster Patel, is currently working on bringing out a third edition of that book as well as collections of his other writings.

ENDNOTES

Cover Page

1. Sri Aurobindo, *Essays on the Gita,* p. 360.

Preface

1. Both Geraldine Costner and Alan Weinstock have published books with the title *Yoga Psychology.*

2. Sri Aurobindo, *Essays Divine and Human,* p. 322.

Introduction

1. T. Hartmann, *The Last Hours of Ancient Sunlight,* p. 1.

2. See http://www.photonics.cusat.edu/article2.html; Dr. D. P. Girijavallabhan, *Indian Influence on the Development of Quantum Mechanics.*

3. See J. Niimi, "Buddhism and the Cognitive Scientist," at http://home.uchicago.edu~jniimi/buddcogsci/paper.html. According to Niimi, "When the Buddhist spokesman Dharmapala attended one of James' lectures at Harvard, James was quoted as having said to him, 'Take my chair. You are better equipped to lecture on psychology than I,' and after one of Dharmapala's own lectures, James declared, 'This is the psychology everybody will be studying twenty-five years from now.'"

4. D. Goleman, *The Meditative Mind,* p. 174.

5. A comprehensive review of the effects of meditation—including improvements in perceptual and cognitive abilities, changes in the nervous, metabolic, respiratory, and other systems of the body, and a variety of other effects—can be found in M. Murphy, *The Physical and Psychological Effects of Meditation.*

6. H. Benson, *Timeless Healing,* p. 155.

7. In answer to a question as to whether parapsychology violates physical laws, Josephson said, "My feeling is that to some extent [parapsychology lies within the bounds of physical law], but physical law itself may have to be redefined. It may be that some effects in parapsychology are ordered-state effects of a kind not yet encompassed by physical theory." In Radin, *The Conscious Universe,* p. 281.

8. In 2001, Robert Thurman and Rajiv Malhotra (founder/director of the

Infinity Foundation) settled upon the phrase "yoga psychology" as the name of an online discussion group that was inclusive of both Buddhist and Hindu traditions. Personal communication.

9. Cognitive-behavioral therapy has demonstrated great success in helping people relieve psychological problems by changing their views, and is based on several decades of both clinical and laboratory research. Leading theorists and researchers include Beck, Bandura, Ellis, Meichenbaum, and Barlow.

10. See B. Swimme and T. Berry, *The Universe Story.*

11. See P. Ray, and S. Anderson, *The Cultural Creatives.* Ray distinguishes between a larger group that has some interest in spirituality from a smaller, core group that seeks to fully integrate their lives around a spiritual vision.

12. See R.Forman, *Grassroots Spirituality.*

13. H. Benson, *The Healing Power of Faith.*

14. L. Dossey, *Healing Beyond the Body,* pp. 319–20.

15. See more about the idea of the "Second Renaissance" at www.bobthurman.com.

16. Riane Eisler is a cultural historian and David Loye is a social psychologist. For more on their evolutionary vision, see their website, www.partnershipway.org.

17. Tolle writes about what he sees as a great potential for a widespread change of consciousness in *A New Earth.* The core theme of Sri Aurobindo's writings is the imminent emergence of a profoundly new grade of consciousness, what he calls the "supramental" consciousness.

Book I, Chapter 2: The Story of the Evolution of Consciousness

1. F. Dyson, Gifford Lectures, at http://en.wikiquote.org/wiki/Freeman_Dyson.

2. J. Darby, *Intelligence in Nature,* pp. 83–84.

3. Ibid., p. 96.

4. Ibid.

5. M. Donald, *A Mind So Rare,* p. 114.

6. I. Barbour, *When Religion Meets Science,* p. 111.

7. A. Hobson, *Consciousness,* p. 223.

8. In the eighteenth century, philosopher Immanuel Kant declared "knowing,

willing and feeling" to be the fundamental components of the mind. Philosopher Charles Pierce, following Kant, described the "triad" of knowing, willing and feeling in psychology. After several decades of narrowly focusing on cognition, neuroscientists have come to see that, in addition to cognitive science, there is a need for a "volitional" and "affective" neuroscience—in other words, knowing, willing, and feeling.

9. H. Bloom, *Global Brain*, p. 36.

10. J. Darby, *Intelligence in Nature*, p. 60.

11. S. Blakeslee, *Minds of Their Own*.

12. J. Darby, *Intelligence in Nature*, p. 159.

13. D. Glenn, "Sharing the World with Thinking Animals," at http://www.animalsvoice.com/PAGES/writes/intros/sentience.html.

14. Information on Koko is available at www.koko.org.

15. Some biologists speak of "culture" as beginning with birds and mammals, who, like primates, are capable of passing along acquired knowledge to their young.

16. Or as Piaget would say, it has become decentered. Piaget did not explicitly describe decentering as involving a shift of attention. We have based our interpretation of Piaget's work on the writings of psychologist Robert Kegan. See chapter 1, *"The Unrecognized Genius of Jean Piaget,"* in *The Evolving Self*.

17. R. Kegan, *The Evolving Self*, p. 30.

18. Ibid., p. 79.

19. Ibid.

20. Ibid., p. 80.

21. Ibid.

22. Ibid., p. 81.

23. Ibid., pp. 88–89.

24. Ibid., p. 89.

25. The material in this section is based on J. Hayward, *A Rdzogs-chen Buddhist Interpretation of the Sense of Self*.

26. W. James, in B. Mangan, "Sensation's Ghost," at http://psyche.consciousness.monash.edu.au/v7/psyche-7-18-mangan.html.

27. See Allan Combs' *The Radiance of Being* for an extensive discussion of the application of complexity and chaos theory to the evolution of consciousness and the possibility of inner freedom.

Book II, Chapter 3: The View from Nowhere

1. A. Eddington, in J. Randall, *Parapsychology and the Nature of Life*, pp. 217–18.

Book II, Chapter 4: The First Challenge

1. This is a paraphrase of a passage from Samuel Coleridge's *Anima Poetae*. Here is the original: "If a man could pass thro' Paradise in a Dream, & have a flower presented to him as a pledge that his Soul had really been there, & found that flower in his hand when he awoke — Aye ! and what then?"

2. This sequence of dreams and false awakenings is based on the experience of someone we know. The name in the text is a pseudonym.

3. Jonathan Bricklin, in "Sciousness and Con-Sciousness," points out that for William James, "consciousness is not *of* something (internalized) but *as* something (neither internalized nor externalized.") Bricklin further offers this sentence from James as a kind of Zen Koan: "How, if 'subject' and 'object' were separated 'by the whole diameter of being,' and had no attributes in common, could it be so hard to tell, in a presented and recognized material object, what part comes in through the sense-organs and what part comes 'out of one's own head'?" See J. Bricklin, "Sciousness and Con-Sciousness," at http://primereality.org/sciousness.pdf. Sri Krishna Prem (1988), along similar lines, notes that the word consciousness "suffers from the great drawback that it has no active verbal form. One can say 'to be conscious of' but not 'to conscious' such-and-such an object" (p. 195).

4. S. K. Prem, *The Yoga of the Bhagavad Gita*, pp. 123–24.

5. C. Tart, *Open Mind, Discriminating Mind*, p. 167.

6. D. Chalmers, *The Puzzle of Conscious Experience*, pp. 62–68.

7. We are not saying we agree with those who use this example from physics to claim that what is "really" "out there" are quality-less abstract waves and particles. This and other examples in this section are meant to be what the Buddhists refer to as "skillful means." Rather than philosophic statements, they are meant to be pointers, challenging our conventional assumptions.

8. C. Tart, *Open Mind, Discriminating Mind*, pp. 159–60.

9. Neither we nor Tart endorse the naïve, Cartesian view of a homonculous "sitting" in the brain. Tart's novice pilot example is only meant as a loose metaphor.

10. L. Govinda, *Buddhist Reflections*, p. 4.

11. B. A. Wallace, *Choosing Reality*, p. 115.

12. W. James, *Varieties of Religious Experience*, at www.csp.org/experience/

james-varieties/james-varieties16.html.

13. E. Hartmann, *The Philosophy of the Unconscious*, cited at www.ccel.org/ccel/orr/view.ix.html

14. See B. F. Skinner, *Beyond Freedom and Dignity*.

15. J. Kilhstrom, in M. Velmans, *The Science of Consciousness*, p. 38.

16. Bernard Baars (1996) uses the metaphor of consciousness as a spotlight.

17. However hard we try, that is, without extensive contemplative training. Some experiments have been done with tachistoscopes—machines that present images in increments of a few milliseconds—showing that advanced meditators may actually be able to distinguish images flashing at the rate of twenty-four per second.

18. G. Rawlinson, "The Significance of Letter Position in Word Recognition," at http://www.mrc-cbu.cam.ac.uk/~matt.davis/Cmabrigde/rawlinson.html.

19. Klein, in B. Mangan, "Sensation's Ghost," at http://psyche.consciousness.monash.edu.au/v7/psyche-7-18-mangan.html.

20. E. Hilgard in B. Lancaster, *Mind, Brain, and Human Potential*, p. 161.

21. Ibid., p. 163.

22. Ibid.

23. Ibid., p. 164.

24. C. Tart, *Open Mind, Discriminating Mind*, p. 343.

Book II, Chapter 5: The Second Challenge

1. J. Schwartz, *The Mind and the Brain*, p. 364.

2. D. Hoffman, *Visual Intelligence*, p. 196. Though Hoffman did not mention it, one might add that scientific data are equally compatible with other philosophic views such as panpsychism, dual-aspect monism, and panexperientialism.

3. P. Chodron, *The Wisdom of No Escape*, p. 53.

4. This is not to say that all three-card monte players work this way. Some claim to be exceptionally fast shufflers. However, according to a number of New York City street players, the most common way of playing is to remove the card from the deck altogether. The analogy of three-card monte to the removal of God as an explanation for the laws of nature comes from R. Dixey, p. 138.

5. B. Russell, *Mysticism and Logic*, p. 46.

6. L. Wittgenstein, *Tractatus Logico-Philosophicus*, 6.37ff.

7. R. A. Varghese, *The Wonder of the World*, p. 322.

8. H. Stapp, *Mind, Matter and Quantum Mechanics*, p. 93.

9. D. Dennett, in I. Barbour, *When Science Meets Religion*, p. 95.

10. R. Dawkins, in ibid., p. 94.

11. S. Hawking, in R. Sheldrake, *The Rebirth of Nature*, p. 130.

12. Ibid., pp. 129–30.

13. R. Feynman, in B. A. Wallace, *Choosing Reality*, p. 53.

14. A. G. Cairns-Smith, *Evolving the Mind*, p. 49.

15. G. K. Chesterton, *The Ethics of Elfland*. See http://ccel.wheaton.edu/c/chesterton/orthodoxy/orthodoxy.html.

16. See W. Dembski, *The Design Inference*.

17. J. Campbell, in L. Smith, *Intelligence Came First*, p. 158.

18. B. Hall, in H. Bloom, *Global Brain*, p. 45.

19. Ibid, p. 46.

20. Ibid., pp. 45–46.

21. R. Thompson, *Mechanistic and Nonmechanistic Science*, p. 203.

22. S. J. Gould, in ibid.

23. See R. Sheldrake, "How Widely Is Blind Assessment Used in Scientific Research?" See http://sheldrake.org/articles/pdf/29/pdf.

24. H. L. F. von Helmholtz, in L. Leshan, and H. Margenau, *Einstein's Space and Van Gogh's Sky*, p. 206.

25. D. O. Hebb, in D. Radin, *The Conscious Universe*, p. 214.

26. W. Weaver, in L. Leshan, and H. Margenau, *Einstein's Space and Van Gogh's Sky*, p. 206.

27. In J. Hayward, *Perceiving Ordinary Magic*, p. 73.

28. In W. Harman, *Global Mind Change*, p. 61.

29. See J. A. Hobson, *Consciousness*.

30. R. Melzack, *Phantom Limbs*, pp. 1–2.

31. F. Crick, *Astonishing Hypothesis*, p. 3.

32. S. Pinker, in R. A. Varghese, *Wonder of the World*, p. 56.

33. J. Fodor, *The Big Idea*, p. 5.

34. See C. Tart, "Transpersonal Realities or Neurophysiological Illusions: Toward an Empirically Testable Dualism," at http://www.paradigm-sys.com/display/ctt_articles2.cfm?ID=55.

35. D. Radin, *The Conscious Universe*, p. 3.

36. Ibid., pp. 105–6.

37. H. Sidgwick, in J. Randall, *Parapsychology and the Nature of Life*, p. 114.

38. G. Price, in ibid., p. 113.

39. J. Utts, in R. Targ, and J. Katra, *Miracles of Mind*, p. 25.

40. R. Hyman, in D. Radin, *The Conscious Universe*, p. 103.

41. R. Hyman, in L. Dossey, *Healing Beyond the Body*, p. *237*. Hyman concluded with a neutral observation, writing, "Inexplicable statistical departures from chance, however, are a far cry from compelling evidence for anomalous cognition."

42. The INSCOM experiment is described in P. Pearsall, *The Heart's Code*, p. 43.

43. E. Laszlo, *Science and the Akashic Field*, p. 96.

44. D. Radin, personal communication.

45. E. Laszlo, *Science and the Akashic Field*, p. 99.

46. D. Radin, *The Conscious Universe*, p. 277.

47. L. Dossey, *Healing Beyond the Body*, pp. 252–53.

48. E. Laszlo, *Science and the Akashic Field*, p. 79.

49. For more on quantum coherence, see M. Wan-Ho, *The Rainbow and the Worm*.

50. F. Dyson, *Gifford Lectures*, at http://en.wikiquote.org/wiki/Freeman_Dyson.

51. F. Dyson, ibid.

52. A. Zajonc, "Toward an Adequate Epistemology and Methodology for Consciousness Studies," at http://www.infinityfoundation.com.

53. R. Jahn, http://www.princeton.edu/~pear/.

54. R. Jahn, in L. Dossey, *Healing and the Body*, p. 249.

55. Ibid, p. 250.

56. W. James, in E. Laszlo, *Science and the Akashic Field*, pp. 103–4.

Book III, The Journey

1. Sri Aurobindo, *Essays Human and Divine*, p. 423.

Third Challenge

1. Sri Aurobindo, *Letters on Yoga*, p. 236.

Book III, Part I, Chapter 6: The View from Infinity

1. Sri Aurobindo, *Letters on Yoga*, p. 236.

2. Regarding postmodernists' concerns about "totalizing" systems: The "view from infinity" is neither a system nor a view.

3. Acts, 17:26–28.

4. Exodus, 3:14.

5. A. Heschel, *God in Search of Man*.

6. Sri Aurobindo, *Savitri*, book I, canto II, verse 37.

7. The *Bhagavad Gita*, chapter 13, verse 2. For a translation, see Sri Aurobindo, *Essays on the Gita*.

8. *Kena Upanishad*, part I, verses 6 and 7.

9. E. Tolle, *The Power of Now*, p. 14.

10. Sri Aurobindo, *Essays on the Gita*, p. 416.

Book III, Part II, Overview

1. T. V. P. Sastry, *Collected Works*, p. 10.

Book III, Part II, Chapter 7: Matter

1. Sri Aurobindo, *Letters on Yoga*, pp. 236–37.

2. P. Russell, www.peterussell.com/WUIT/accel.html.

3. I Corinthians 13:12.

Book III, Part II, Chapter 8: Life

1. Sri Aurobindo, *Letters on Yoga*, pp. 236–37.

2. L. Thomas, *The Lives of a Cell*. p. 170.

3. Ibid., p. 170.

4. H. G. Wells, in O. Sacks, *A Neurologist's Notebook*. p. 60.

5. In a sense, one might say we are each a human being with a human (i.e., mental) consciousness, but we have also within us the consciousness of a stone (i.e., physical consciousness), a plant, and an animal (i.e., vital and vital-mental consciousness).

6. B. Heinrich, in Barber, T. X., "Scientific Evidence that Birds are Aware, Intelligent and Astonishingly Like Humans: Implications and Future Research Directions," at http://www.psyeta.org/hia/vol8/barber.html.

7. R. Carrington, "Theory of Mind and Insight in Chimpanzees, Elephants and other Animals?" At http://www.is.wayne.edu/mnissani/ElephantCorner/conscrev.htm.

8. L. Tangley, "Natural Passions," at http://www.nwf.org/internationalwildlife/2001/emotionso01.html.

9. J. Goodall, in ibid.

10. Bekoff, M., in ibid.

11. L. Howard, in T. Barber, *"Scientific Evidence that Birds are Aware."*

12. This phrase is known in Islam as a "Hadith qudsi," or "sacred tradition." Passed down through the ages, it is a particular favorite of the Sufis, an Islamic mystical sect.

Book III, Part II, Chapter 9: Animal Mind

1. Sri Aurobindo, *Letters on Yoga*, pp. 236–37.

2. In his commentary on the Kena Upanishad, Sri Aurobindo makes this assertion regarding the Upanishads, though he does not cite the source. He gives the following Sanskrit terms as the equivalent of these four mental functions: Sanjnana, Prajnana, Ajnana, Vijnana. He adds that the origin of these functions is in the Supramental consciousness. As they manifest in the mental consciousness, these functions are limited reflections of a far greater consciousness beyond the mind.

3. See Sri Aurobindo's book, *Letters on Yoga*, for a detailed explanation of the relationship between the terms *physical mind* and *manas*.

4. There is a strong correspondence between the qualities of the physical, vital, and mental consciousness and what in Sanskrit is referred to as the three *gunas* or qualities of nature: *tamas, rajas,* and *sattwa*. Sri Aurobindo describes how the *gunas* contribute to the shaping of personality in his books *Essays on the Gita* (first series, chapters 21 and 22; second series, chapters 14, 18, and 19), and *The Synthesis of Yoga* (part I, chapter X; part IV, chapter IX).

5. H. Bloom, *Global Brain*, p. 46.

6. M. Donald, *A Mind So Rare*, pp. 114-115.

7. Ibid., p. 115.

8. Ibid., p. 124.

9. Ibid.

10. Ibid.

11. Ibid., p. 125.

12. See K. E. Fichtelius, *Smarter Than Man?*

13. M. Donald, *A Mind So Rare*, p. 127.

14. See J. Poole, in "Not So Dumbo," at http://www.bbc.co.uk.nature/animals/features/302features1.shtml.

15. Ibid.

16. I. Pepperberg, "That Damn Bird: A Talk with Irene Pepperberg," at http://www.edge.org/3rd_culture/pepperberg03/pepperberg_index.html.

17. M. Tomasello, in I. Pepperberg, "That Damn Bird."

18. T. Barber, " Scientific Evidence That Birds Are Aware."

19. I. Pepperberg, "That Damn Bird."

20. F. Dewaal, in K. Wright, "The Tarzan Syndrome: Only Human Beings Can Conceive of Themselves and Others," in *Discover* 17, #11 (November 1996) at http://www.findarticles.com/p/articles/mi_m1511/is_n11_v17/ai_18762290.

21. R. Cooper, *The Evolving Mind*, p. 100.

22. K. Wright, *The Tarzan Syndrome.*

23. Ibid.

24. Ibid.

25. Sri Aurobindo, *Letters on Yoga*, p. 1429.

26. Ibid., p. 414.

27. O. Sacks, *A Neurologist's Notebook*, p. 68.

28. R. Sheldrake, *The Sense of Being Stared At*, p. 25.

29. Ibid.

30. Ibid., p. 28.

31. Ibid., p. 116. Most ornithologists believe that flock behavior can be explained without resorting to paranormal explanations. However, this does not mean that they are able to rule out the involvement of nonsensory communication. Occam's razor sometimes obscures more than it clarifies.

Book III, Part II, Chapter 10: Human Evolution I

1. Sri Aurobindo, *Letters on Yoga*, pp. 236–37.

2. H. Keller, *The World I Live In.*

3. O. Sacks, *An Anthropologist on Mars*, p. 126.

4. C. Turnbull, in T. G. Jordan-Bychkov, *Human Mosaic*, p. 305. Some have questioned Turnbull's interpretation of Kenge's reaction, suggesting that he in fact did have normal distance perception and was playacting. Whether or not Turnbull's account was accurate, psychologist Richard Gregory and other experts on perception have reported and verified similar stories.

5. O. Sacks, *An Anthropologist on Mars*, p. 108.

6. Ibid., p. 114.

7. Ibid., pp. 114–15.

8. Ibid., pp. 120–21.

9. Ibid., p. 120.

10. Ibid., p. 268.

11. Ibid., p. 259.

12. H. Bortoft, *The Wholeness of Nature*, pp. 312–13.

Book III, Part II, Chapter 11: Human Evolution II

1. Psychologist Clare Graves developed an interesting theory regarding stages of cultural development, though without an explicit spiritual foundation. For more on Graves's work, see www.claregraves.com.

2. D. Elgin, *Awakening Earth*, pp. 33–35.

3. Though anthropologists recognize the species *homo habilis* as being transitional between Australopithecus and *homo erectus*, from the yogic perspective the descriptions of both Australopithecus and *homo habilis* seem to us to reflect a similarly predominant influence of the physical consciousness on the thinking mind.

4. J. Gebser, *The Ever-Present Origin.* p. 75.

5. N. Mann, "Petrarch at the Crossroads," at http://petrarch.petersadlon.com/submissions/Mann.pdf.

6. See J. Gebser, *The Ever-Present Origin*, chapter 3.

7. D. Elgin, *Awakening Earth*, p. 51.

8. Sri Aurobindo, *The Human Cycle*, p. 7.

9. S. K. Prem, *Initiation Into Yoga*, pp. 55–56.

10. E. Podvoll, *The Seduction of Madness*, p. 86.

11. Ibid., p. 83.

12. Ibid., p. 76.

13. Ibid., p. 88.

14. J. Custance, in E. Podvoll, *The Seduction of Madness*, p. 84.

15. Ibid.

16. Sri Aurobindo, *The Life Divine*, p. 214.

17. C. Darwin, in Schumacher, *Small is Beautiful*, p. 98.

18. J. Gebser, *The Ever-Present Origin*. pp. 94–95.

19. Sri Aurobindo, *The Life Divine*, p. 163.

Book III, Part III: The Knower of the Field, Overview

1. T. V. P. Sastry, *Collected Works*, p. 10.

Book III, Part III, Chapter 12: The Soul and the Psychic Being

1. Sri Aurobindo, *Letters on Yoga*, pp. 236–37.

2. Sri Aurobindo, *The Life Divine*, p. 225.

3. S. K. Prem, *The Yoga of the Kathopanishad*, pp. 214–15.

4. Ibid., pp. 215–16.

5. L. Vaughan-Lee, *The Face before I Was Born*, p. 278.

6. Sri Aurobindo, *Essays Human and Divine*, p. 100.

7. Sri Aurobindo, *The Life Divine*, p. 225.

8. M. Alfassa, *Questions and Answers*, vol. 3, p. 72.

9. Sri Aurobindo, *The Synthesis of Yoga*, pp. 153–54.

10. Ibid., p. 351.

11. W. Wordsworth, *Intimations of Immortality*.

12. Sri Aurobindo, *Letters on Yoga*, p. 22.

13. B. A. Wallace, *The Taboo of Subjectivity*, p. 168.

14. Sri Aurobindo, *The Synthesis of Yoga*, p. 771.

15. Sri Aurobindo, *The Life Divine*, p. 226.

16. Ibid., p. 226.

17. S. K. Prem, *The Yoga of the Kathopanishad*, p. 214.

18. M. Alfassa, *Questions and Answers*, vol. 9, p. 309.

19. Benjamin Franklin, epitaph, composed at age twenty-two.

20. Sri Aurobindo, *The Life Divine*, p. 225.

21. L. A. Govinda, *The Way of the White Clouds*, pp.132-133

22. We realize some readers may protest our use of "soul" in conjunction with Buddhism. There are a number of excellent writers on Buddhism who present an understanding of rebirth that is compatible with Sri Aurobindo's description of the evolving psychic being. Some excellent sources include Lama Govinda's *Creative Meditation and Multi-Dimensional Consciousness;* Sri Krishna Prem's *Yoga of the Bhagavad Gita* (see especially his appendix on after-death states); Robert Thurman's *Tibetan Book of the Dead* and Philip Kapleau's *Three Pillars of Zen* (see especially the story of the Canadian housewife and Yaeko Iwasaki's enlightenment letters).

23. L. A. Govinda, *The Way of the White Clouds*, pp. 133–34.

24. Ibid., p. 134.

25. Ibid., p. 135.

26. Ibid., p. 136.

Book III, Part III, Chapter 13: Ego

1. Sri Aurobindo, *Letters on Yoga*, pp. 236–37.

2. Sri Aurobindo, *The Synthesis of Yoga*, pp. 59–60.

3. Ibid., p. 59.

4. S. K. Prem, *The Yoga of the Bhagavad Gita*, p. 35.

5. Sri Aurobindo, *The Synthesis of Yoga*, p. 72.

6. R. Cooper, *The Evolving Mind*, p. 61.

7. Sri Aurobindo, *The Synthesis of Yoga*, p. 112.

8. Sri Aurobindo, *The Life Divine*, p. 303.

9. R. Tagore, *The Religion of Man*, p. 25.

10. Sri Aurobindo, *Essays on the Gita*, p. 382.

11. Sri Aurobindo, *The Life Divine*, p. 109.

12. There are several references to this statement on the Internet; we could not find the original source. It may be in M.'s biographical work, *The Gospel of Ramakrishna.*

13. *Coriolanus*, act IV, scene V. This quote was drawn from Chris Hedges' book *War Is a Force That Gives Life Meaning*. We drew on Hedges' insightful observations about war as the basis for this section.

14. C. Hedges, *War Is a Force That Gives Life Meaning*, p. 6.

15. Ibid., p. 7.

16. Ibid.

17. Sri Aurobindo, *The Synthesis of Yoga*, p. 679.

Book III, Part IV, Overview

1. T. V. P. Sastry, *Collected Works*, p. 10.

Book III, Part IV, Chapter 14: The Play of Karma in the Individual

1. Sri Aurobindo, *Letters on Yoga*, pp. 236–37.

2. Sri Aurobindo, *The Problem of Rebirth*, p. 428.

3. Ibid., p. 331.

4. Sri Aurobindo, *Letters on Yoga*, p. 335.

5. The description in this section of the contribution of the karmic process to evolution is based in part on Swami Ramananda's unpublished manuscript *Evolutionary Spirituality*.

6. Sri Aurobindo, *The Synthesis of Yoga*, p. 656.

7. Sri Aurobindo, *The Upanishads*, p. 145.

8. Neuroscientist Walter Freeman, applying chaos theory to the study of the brain, has developed an extremely interesting theory regarding the way neural patterns are built that bears much resemblance to the process by which karmic impressions accumulate. These similarities could provide the basis for an extremely interesting collaboration between neuroscientists and expert contemplatives whose inner vision is sufficiently developed to "see" the working of the subtle (i.e., nonphysical) karmic patterns associated with brain activity.

9. Sri Aurobindo, *Letters on Yoga*, p. 313.

10. Ibid., p. 1258.

11. Sri Aurobindo, *The Life Divine*, p.538.

Book III, Part IV, Chapter 15: Collective Karma

1. Abraham Lincoln is reported to have said this in reply to the comment of a

visitor to the White House, who expressed his hope that "God is on our side."

2. E. Taylor, *Desperately Seeking Spirituality*, p. 54.

3. E. Taylor, *Shadow Culture*, p. 15.

4. Ibid., p. x.

5. Ibid., p. 21.

6. Ibid., p. 18.

7. Ibid., p. 18.

8. M. Boot, *The Case for American Empire*.

9. Sri Aurobindo, *Essays on the Gita*, pp. 472–73.

10. K. Armstrong, *The Battle For God*, p. 78.

11. Ibid., p. 78.

12. Ibid., p. 79.

13. Ibid.

14. Ibid., p. 80.

15. A. Schlesinger, *Forgetting Reinhold Niebuhr*.

16. Ibid.

17. Ibid.

18. R. Jewett, and S. Lawrence, *Captain America and the Crusade Against Evil*, p. 70.

19. Ibid., p. 72.

20. Ibid., p. 63.

21. Ibid., p. 70.

22. Ibid., p. 71. We may feel comfort in the thought that nobody today would express such sentiments as Beveridge did so unabashedly. However, it was only a few years ago that one of the leading proponents of the current "war on terror," on a trip to the Philippines, spoke of meeting a Filipino and observing that "his smiling, naïve eyes cried out for what we in the West call colonialism." From R. Kaplan, *Imperial Grunts*.

23. A. Schlesinger, Forgetting Reinhold Niebuhr.

24. Ibid.

25. A. Lincoln, "Second Inaugural Address," March 4, 1865.

26. A. Lincoln, "Letter To Thurlow Weed," at http://showcase.netins.net/web/creative/lincoln/mind/.

27. A. Lincoln, "Second Inaugural Address."

28. M. Alfassa, *Psychic Education and Spiritual Education*, p. 33.

Book III, Part IV, Chapter 16: Psychic Awakening and the Transformation of the Individual

1. Sri Aurobindo, *Letters on Yoga*, p. 236.

2. Sri Aurobindo, *The Life Divine*, p. 907.

3. Frank Oppenheimer, in "The Day after Trinity: J. Robert Oppenheimer and the Atomic Bomb," video documentary available at www.pyramiddirect.com.

4. Freeman Dyson, in "The Day after Trinity."

5. See G. E. Schwartz, *Psychobiology of Health*.

6. "Swami Rama: Researcher/Scientist," at www.kumbhamelatimes.org/swami/researcher.html.

7. M. Wan-Ho, "The Organic Revolution in Science and Implications for Science and Spirituality", at www.ratical.org/co-globalize/MaeWanHo/.

8. The Buddha, *The Dhammapada*, verses 1 and 2. (trans.) Max Muller.

9. Sri Aurobindo, *The Life Divine*, p. 533.

10. See L. S. Greenberg, L. N. Rice, and R. Elliot, *Facilitating Emotional Change*.

11. Sri Aurobindo, *The Synthesis of Yoga*, p. 112.

12. Ibid., p. 693.

13. Sri Aurobindo, *Letters on Yoga*, p. 638.

14. L. Dossey, *Space, Time and Medicine*, p. 170

15. Ibid., p. 171.

16. T. Palmo, *Cave in the Snow*, p. 118.

17. Ramana Maharshi, *The Teachings of Ramana Maharshi*, p. 207.

Book III, Part IV, Chapter 17: Psychic Awakening and the Transformation of Society

1. V. Havel, in W. Cappas, "Interpreting Vaclev Havel," at www.crosscurrents.org/capps.htm.

2. O. Arias, "Peace in Their Time?" At www.numag.neu.edu/9801/arias.html.

3. T. Hartmann, *The Last Hours of Ancient Sunlight*, p. 1.

4. United Nations 1998 Human Development Report, in D. Elgin, *Promise Ahead*, pp. 126–27.

5. O. Arias, speech at Hunter College, April 20, 1999. See www.ervk.org/oscararias.htm.

6. D. Korten, V, Shiva, and N. Perlas, "Global Civil Society: The Path Ahead," at www.pcdf.org/civilsociety/default.htm.

7. Ibid.

8. World Values Survey, 1990–91, in D. Elgin, *Promise Ahead*, p. 83.

9. Paul Ray makes this distinction in his reference to "Cultural Creatives" versus "Core Cultural Creatives." See P. Ray and S. Anderson, *The Cultural Creatives*.

10. Information on Ithaca Hours is from www.wikipedia.org/wiki/Ithaca_Hours.

11. Ibid.

12. Ibid.

13. P. Glover, "Grassroots Economics," at http://www.geocities.com/RainForest/7813/ccs-ithi.htm.

14. Ibid.

15. P. Lugari, in A. Weisman, "Oasis of the Imagination," at http://www.yesmagazine.org/article/asp?ID=842.

16. A. Weisman, *Gaviotas*, p. 7.

17. Ibid., p. 8.

18. Ibid., p. 164.

19. Ibid., p. 165.

20. P. Lugari, in ibid., p. 175.

21. P. Lugari, "Dialogue on Innovation and Perseverance," at http://www.planeta.com/planeta/02/0209gaviotas.html.

22. Sri Aurobindo, *The Human Cycle*, p. 256.

23. M. Wan-Ho, *The Organic Revolution in Science*.

24. G. Bond, *Buddhism at Work*, p. 7.

25. The Hunger Project Website, http://www.thp.org/sac/unit3/awake.htm.

26. G. Bond, *Buddhism at Work*, p. 2.

27. G. Bond, in D. Hoang, "A Buddhist Socioeconomic System," at http://www.buddhanetz.org/texte/sarvoday.htm.

28. Ibid.

29. A. T. Ariyaratne, at http://www.thp.org/sac/unit3/awake.htm.

30. See http://www.bread.org/learn/hunger-reports/hunger-report-pdfs/hunger-report-2006/Chap-5-Emergencies.pdf.

31. A. T. Ariyaratne, in G. Bond, *Buddhism at Work*, p. 29.

32. Ibid.

33. Ibid.

34. Description of the aims of CMS is at http://wwworiononline.org/pages/ogn/vieworg.cfm?action=one&ogn_org_ID=883&viewby=name.

35. M. Bush, "Interview with Mirabai Bush," http://www.contemplative-mind.org/programs/business/corpculture.html.

36. Description of the aims of CMS is at http://www.oriononline.org/pages/ogn/vieworg.cfm?action=one&ogn_org_ID=883&viewby=name.

37. M. Bush, "Interview with Mirabai Bush," http://www.contemplative-mind.org/programs/business/corpculture.html.

38. Ibid.

39. Ibid.

40. See the Santa Barbara Institute website at http://www.sbinstitute.com/news.

41. An interview of Alan Wallace, by Tom McFarlane, at www.centerforsacredsciences.org.

42. Ibid.

43. Ibid.

44. Ibid.

45. Opening page of Santa Barbara Institute, at http://www.sbinstitute.com/news.

46. Alan Wallace, in *Buddhadharma Journal*, (fall 2004); interview with Jeff Pardy.

47. An interview of Alan Wallace, by Tom McFarlane, at www.centerforsacredsciences.org.

48. Ibid.

49. Ibid.

50. Ibid.

51. See A. Ardagh, *The Translucent Revolution.*

52. Insight meditation teacher Greg Kramer has developed an excellent practice to help people learn to integrate meditative awareness with dialogue, which he calls "Insight Dialogue." For more information on this practice, see www.metta.org.

53. S. K. Prem, *Initiation into Yoga*, p. 107.

54. Sri Aurobindo, *Essays on Philosophy and Yoga*, pp. 77–78.

Book III, Part IV, Chapter 18: Spiritual and Supramental Awakening and Transformation

1. Sri Aurobindo, *Letters on Yoga*, pp. 236–37.

2. M. Alfassa, *On Education*, pp. 33–34.

3. E. Underhill *Practical Mysticism*, p. 138.

4. S. K. Prem, *The Yoga of the Bhagavad Gita*, p. 56.

5. E. Underhill *Practical Mysticism*, pp. 110–13.

6. J. Blofeld, *The Secret and Sublime*, p. 209–10.

7. Sri Aurobindo, *Letters on Yoga*, p. 1167.

8. E. Underhill *Practical Mysticism*, p. 137.

9. Sri Aurobindo, *The Life Divine*, pp. 913–14.

10. Sri Aurobindo, *The Upanishads*, p. 36.

11. Sri Aurobindo, *The Life Divine*, p. 62.

12. S. K. Prem, *Initiation Into Yoga*, p. 67.

13. Ibid.

14. Ibid.

15. The stories of "Luke" and "Laura" refer to actual events; only the names have been changed.

16. A. Reber, *The Dictionary of Psychology.*

17. This story is recounted in E. Wood, Mind and Memory Training, pp. 128–29. Olcott was known to embellish his accounts of what he witnessed in India, but Wood personally witnessed feats of memory greater than those told by Olcott, and describes one in his book that is more remarkable than the one described here.

18. L. Dossey, *Healing beyond the Body*, p. 265. Joseph Chilton Pearce, who has also made a study of savants, adds the interesting point that in at least

some cases, as far as can be observed, they have not acquired their extraordinary information by ordinary means. In fact, their cognitive limitations would make that impossible.

19. Ibid., p. 286.

20. P. Garfield, *Creative Dreaming*, p. 45.

21. Sri Aurobindo, *The Upanishads*, p. 189.

22. Plotinus, *Enneads* V, Tractate 8.

23. S. K. Prem, *The Yoga of the Kathopanishad*, p. 94.

24. Sri Aurobindo, *Essays in Philosophy and Yoga*, pp. 563–64.

25. M. Alfassa, *Questions and Answers*, vol. 9, pp. 296–97.

26. Ibid., p. 150.

Appendix A: Science and Yoga Psychology

1. W. James, in D. Lorimer, ed., "Manifesto for an Integral Science of Consciousness", at http://www.datadiwan.de/SciMedNet/manifesto.htm.

2. F. Dyson, "The Gifford Lectures," at http://en.wikiquote.org/wiki/Freeman_Dyson.

3. Ibid.

4. A. Combs, *The Radiance of Being*, p. 174.

5. R. Sheldrake, *The Sense of Being Stared At*, pp. 176–77.

6. L. King, Review of I. Stevenson, "Cases of the Reincarnation Type," in *Journal of the American Medical Association* 234 (December 1, 1975); 278.

7. Talk by Ian Stevenson, "My Journeys in Medicine," at www.childpastlives.org/stevensonarticle.htm.

8. S. Cranston and C. Williams, *Reincarnation*, p. 67.

9. Ibid.

10. Ibid.

11. This is not to say that it is not helpful to conduct research providing understanding of the mechanisms of consciousness. Psychiatrist Jeffrey Schwartz and physicist Henry Stapp have come up with an intriguing theory that attention serves to collapse two coexisting quantum possibilities in the brain—"release neurotransmitter" or "don't release neurotransmitter." Their fascinating description of the way in which this may work is in Schwartz's *The Mind and the Brain*. In this book and in an article for the *Journal of Consciousness Studies*, Schwartz

takes the step—quite bold within the current world of neuroscience—of asserting that the mind has causal efficacy in regard to the brain.

12. A. Zajonc, "Toward An Adequate Epistemology and Methodology for Consciousness Studies," at http://www.infinityfoundation.com.

13. Sri Aurobindo, *The Life Divine*, p. 162.

14. The introspective approach has recently been referred to as a "view from within." See F. Varela, and J. Shear, *The View From Within*.

15. For more on state-specific science, see C. Tart, *Open Mind, Discriminating Mind*.

16. For a masterful account of a new approach to scientific methodology inspired by this way of knowing, see H. Bortoft, *The Wholeness of Nature*.

17. Sri Aurobindo, *The Upanishads*, p. 128.

18. Sri Aurobindo, *The Life Divine*, p. 381.

Appendix B: An Outline of Yoga Psychology

1. Sri Aurobindo, *Letters on Yoga*, p. 236.

2. Sri Aurobindo, *The Life Divine*, p. 616.

3. Some writers—the psychologist Alan Combs for example—identify the term "Higher Mind" with the level of postformal operations of some developmental psychologists (Robert Kegan's fifth stage, for example). However, as used by Sri Aurobindo, the term "Higher Mind" refers to "a first plane of spiritual consciousness where one becomes constantly and closely aware of the Self, the One everywhere and knows and sees things habitually with that awareness." Developmental psychologists have proposed a number of cognitive levels beyond Piaget's formal operations; for example, the second tier levels proposed by Don Beck based on the work of psychologist Clare Graves. All these postformal levels can be understood, from the perspective of yoga psychology, as increasingly refined functioning of the thinking mind, representing a progressive freeing of the thinking mind from the influence of the egoic vital and physical consciousness. It may help to keep in mind that even the realization of nondual awareness does not require vertical development—a rising above concrete operations, much less any level of formal operations. Nondual awareness does not involve a change in the Field, but rather an awakening to the ever-present Knower "behind" (or rather, embracing and containing) the Field.

4. Sri Aurobindo, *The Synthesis of Yoga*, p. 112.

5. Sri Aurobindo, *The Upanishads*, pp. 475–76.

Appendix C: Biographical Sketches of Sri Aurobindo and Mirra Alfassa

1. The Mother, "A Dream," in *The Essential Aurobindo*, ed. R. McDermott, p. 236.

2. Sri Aurobindo, in *The Adventure of Consciousness*, p. 325.

3. The Mother, at www.sriaurobindosociety.org.in/mother/motherlf.htm

4. The Mother, Collected Works of the Mother, Vol. 2, p. 47.

5. Sri Aurobindo, in *Mahayogi: Life, Sadhana, and Teachings of Sri Aurobindo*, p. 77.

6. The Mother, at www.auroville.org.

BIBLIOGRAPHY

Abraham, F. D., and A.R. Gilgen, eds. (1995). *Chaos Theory in Psychology*. Westport, CT: Praeger Publishers.

Achterberg, J. (1985). *Imagery in Healing: Shamanism and Modern Medicine*. Boston: Shambhala Publications.

Alcock, J., J. Burns, A. Freeman, eds. (2003). *Psi Wars: Getting To Grips with the Paranormal*. Exeter, UK: Imprint Academic.

Alexander, C. N., and E. J. Langer (1990). *Higher Stages of Human Development*. New York: Oxford University Press.

Alfassa, M. (The Mother). (1978). *Questions and Answers, 1929–31*. Collected Works of The Mother. Vol. 3. Pondicherry, India: Sri Aurobindo Ashram.

———. (The Mother). (1978). *Questions and Answers, 1957—58*. Collected Works of The Mother. Vol. 9. Pondicherry, India: Sri Aurobindo Ashram.

———. (The Mother). (1978). *On Education*. Collected Works of The Mother. Vol. 12. Pondicherry, India: Sri Aurobindo Ashram.

Andresen, J. "Meditation Meets Behavioral Medicine: The Story of Experimental Research on Meditation." *Journal of Consciousness Studies* 7, No. 11-12, November/December 2000, pp. 17-73.

Ardagh, A. (2005). *The Translucent Revolution: How People Just Like You Are Waking Up and Changing the World*. Novato, CA: New World Library.

Armstrong, K. (2000). *The Battle for God*. New York: Ballantine Books.

Artigas, M. (2000). *The Mind of the Universe: Understanding Science and Religion*. Philadelphia: Templeton Foundation Press.

Augros, R., and G. Stanciu (1987). *The New Biology: Discovering the Wisdom in Nature*. Boston: New Science Library.

———. (1986). *The New Story of Science: How the New Cosmology Is Reshaping Our View of Mind, Art, God…and Ourselves*. New York: Bantam Books.

Aung San, S. K. (1997). *The Voice of Hope: Conversations with Alan Clements.* London: Penguin Books.

Aurobindo Ghose, Sri. (1972). *The Life Divine.* Sri Aurobindo Birth Centenary Library. Vols. 18–19. Pondicherry, India: Sri Aurobindo Ashram.

———. (1981). *The Upanishads: Texts, Translations, and Commentaries.* Pondicherry, India: Sri Aurobindo Ashram.

———. (1997). *Essays on the Gita.* Collected Works of Sri Aurobindo. Vol. 19. Pondicherry, India: Sri Aurobindo Ashram.

———. (1997). *Savitri.* Collected Works of Sri Aurobindo. Vols. 33–34. Pondicherry, India: Sri Aurobindo Ashram.

———.(1998). *Essays Divine and Human.* Collected Works of Sri Aurobindo. Vol 12. Pondicherry, India: Sri Aurobindo Ashram.

———. (1998). *Essays in Philosophy and Yoga.* Collected Works of Sri Aurobindo. Vol. 13. Pondicherry, India: Sri Aurobindo Ashram.

———. (1998). *The Human Cycle.* Collected Works of Sri Aurobindo. Vol. 25. Pondicherry, India: Sri Aurobindo Ashram.

———. (1999). *The Synthesis of Yoga.* Collected Works of Sri Aurobindo. Vols. 23–24. Pondicherry, India: Sri Aurobindo Ashram.

Baars, B. J. (1997). *In the Theatre of Consciousness.* Oxford, UK: Oxford University Press.

Ballentine, R. (1999). *Radical Healing: Integrating the World's Great Therapeutic Traditions to Create a New Transformative Medicine.* New York: Three Rivers Press.

Barber, B. R. (1995). *Jihad vs. McWorld: How Globalism and Tribalism are Reshaping the World.* New York: Ballantine Books.

Barbour, I. G. (1997). *Religion and Science: Historical and Contemporary Issues.* San Francisco: HarperSanFrancisco.

———. (2000). *When Science Meets Religion: Enemies, Strangers, or Partners?* San Francisco: HarperSanFrancisco.

Barfield, O. (1965). *Saving the Appearances: A Study in Idolatry.* Hanover, NH: Wesleyan University Press.

———. (1977). *The Rediscovery of Meaning and Other Essays.* Middletown, CT. Wesleyan University Press.

Barrell, J. (1990). *The Experiential Method: Exploring the Human Experience.* Acton, MA: Copley Publishing Group.

————. (1986). *A Science of Human Experience*. Acton, MA: Copley Publishing Group.

Barrows, P. (1998). *Beyond the Self: Consciousness, Mysticism and the New Physics*. London: Janus Publishing.

Basu, S. (1981). *Social and Political Evolution of Man as Visioned by Sri Aurobindo: A Brief Study*. Pondicherry, India: World Union International.

Beck, A. T. (1979). *Cognitive Therapy and the Emotional Disorders*. New York: Penguin Group.

Benor, D. J. (2002). *Spiritual Healing: Scientific Validation of a Healing Revolution*. Southfield, MI: Vision Publications.

H. Benson, (1997). *Timeless Healing: The Power of Biology and Belief*. New York: Fireside.

Berry, T. (1990). *The Dream of the Earth*. San Francisco: Sierra Club Books.

Blackmore, S. (2004). *Consciousness: An Introduction*. New York: Oxford University Press.

Blakeslee, S. "Minds of Their Own: Birds Gain Respect." *New York Times*, February 1, 2005.

Blofeld, J. (1973). *The Secret and Sublime: Taoist Mysteries and Magic*. New York: E. P. Dutton.

Bloom, H. (2000). *Global Brain: The Evolution of Mass Mind from the Big Bang to the 21st Century*. New York: John Wiley & Sons.

Bohm, D. (1980). *Wholeness and the Implicate Order*. London: Ark Paperbacks.

Bond, G. D. (2004). *Buddhism at Work: Community Development, Social Empowerment, and the Sarvodaya Movement*. Bloomfield, CT: Kumarian Press.

Boot, M. "The Case for American Empire." *Weekly Standard* 7, No. 5 (October 15, 2001).

Bortoft, H. (1996). *The Wholeness of Nature: Goethe's Way toward a Science of Conscious Participation in Nature*. Hudson, NY: Lindisfarne Books.

————. "Goethe's Organic Vision." *Network* 65 (December 1997) 3–7.

Bricklin, J. (1999). "A Variety of Religious Experience: William James and the Non-Reality of Free Will." In Libet et al., eds (1999). *The Volitional Brain: Towards a Neuroscience of Free Will*.

Brunton, P. (1941). *The Hidden Teaching beyond Yoga*. York Beach, ME: Samuel Weiser.

———. (1984). *The Wisdom of the Overself.* York Beach, ME: Samuel Weiser.

Burger, W. C. (2003). *How Unique Are We?: Perfect Planet, Clever Species.* Amherst, NY: Prometheus Books.

Cairns-Smith, A. G. (1996). *Evolving the Mind: On the Nature of Matter and the Origin of Consciousness.* Cambridge, UK: Cambridge University Press.

Capra, F. (1996). *The Web of Life: A New Scientific Understanding of Living Systems.* New York: Anchor Books/Doubleday.

Carrier, M., G. Massey, and L. Ruetsche, eds. (2000). *Science at Century's End: Philosophical Questions on the Progress and Limits of Science.* Pittsburgh: University of Pittsburgh Press.

Carter, R. (1999). *Mapping the Mind.* Berkeley: University of California Press.

Chalmers, D. "The Puzzle of Conscious Experience. " *Scientific American* (December 1995) 62–68.

Chaudhuri, H., and F. Spiegelberg, eds. (1960). *The Integral Philosophy of Sri Aurobindo: A Commemorative Symposium.* London: George Allen & Unwin.

Childre, D., and H. Martin (1999). *The HeartMath Solution.* New York: HarperCollins.

Chodron, P. (1991). *The Wisdom of No Escape.* Boston: Shambhala Publications.

Clarke, C. J. S. (1996). *Reality through the Looking Glass: Science and Awareness in the Postmodern World.* Edinburgh, UK: Floris Books.

Clarke, J. J. (1997). *Oriental Enlightenment: The Encounter between Asian and Western Thought.* London: Routledge.

Collinge, W. (1998). *Subtle Energy: Awakening To the Unseen Forces in Our Lives.* New York: Warner Books.

Combs, A. (1995). *The Radiance of Being: Complexity, Chaos, and the Evolution of Consciousness.* St. Paul, MN: Paragon House.

Cooper, R. (1996). *The Evolving Mind: Buddhism, Biology, & Consciousness.* Birmingham, UK: Windhorse Publications.

Cornelissen, M. (2000). "The Integration of Psychological Knowledge from the Spiritual Traditions into the Psychology Curriculum. " *Consciousness and Experiential Psychology* 4, at http://www. infinityfoundation. com/mandala/i_es/i_es_corne_curriculum. htm

———. (2002). "Integrality. " A talk given at the Cultural Integration Fellowship. San Francisco, April 6, 2002, at http://www. saccs. org. in/TEXTS/Others/Matthijs/CIF-2002-Integrality. html

———. [ed]. (2001). *Consciousness and Its Transformation: Papers presented at the Second International Conference on Integral Psychology.* Pondicherry, India: Sri Aurobindo International Centre of Education.

S. Cranston and C. Williams. (1984). *Reincarnation: A New Horizon in Science, Religion, and Society.* New York: Julian Press.

Crick, F. (1994). *The Astonishing Hypothesis: The Scientific Search for the Soul.* New York: Charles Scribner's Sons.

Csikszentmihalyi, M. (1993). *The Evolving Self: A Psychology for the Third Millenium.* New York: HarperCollins.

Dalal, A. S. (1991). *Psychology, Mental Health, and Yoga: Essays on Sri Aurobindo's Psychological Thought: Implications of Yoga for Mental Health.* Pondicherry, India: Sri Aurobindo Ashram Press.

Damasio, A. (1994). *Descartes' Error: Emotions, Reason, and the Human Brain.* New York: HarperCollins.

———. (1999). *The Feeling of What Happens: Body and Emotion in the Making of Consciousness.* San Diego: Harcourt.

———. (2003). *Looking for Spinoza: Joy, Sorrow, and the Feeling Brain.* Orlando: Harcourt.

Damiani, A. (1990). *Looking into Mind: How to Recognize Who You Are and How You Know.* Burdett, NY: Larson Publications.

Davidson, J. (1991). *Natural Creation & The Formative Mind.* Longmead, UK: Element Books.

DeCharms, C. (1998). *Two Views of Mind: Abhidharma and Brain Science.* Ithaca, NY: Snow Lion Publications.

Dembksi, W, (1998). *The Design Inference: Eliminating Chance through Small Probabilities.* Cambridge, UK: Cambridge University Press.

Denzin, N. K., and Y. S. Lincoln eds. (1994). *Handbook of Qualitative Research.* Thousand Oaks, CA: Sage Publications.

Depraz, N., F. J. Varela, and P. Vermersch. (1984). *On Becoming Aware: A Pragmatics of Experiencing.* Amsterdam: John Benjamin.

Dienstfrey, H. (1991). *Where the Mind Meets the Body: Type A, The Relaxation Response, Psychoneuroimmunology, Biofeedback, Neuropeptides, Hypnosis,*

Imagery—and the Search for the Mind's Effects on Physical Health. New York: HarperCollins.

Diwakar, R. R. (1988). *Mahayogi: Life, Sadhana, and Teachings of Sri Aurobindo.* Bombay, India: Bharatiya Vidya Bhavan.

Dixey, R. (1994). "Mind, Matter and Metaphysics: Can We Create a Total Science?" In W. Harman and J. Clark, eds., *New Metaphysical Foundations of Modern Science.* Sausalito, CA: Institute of Noetic Sciences.

Donald, M. (2001). *A Mind So Rare.* New York: W. W. Norton.

Dossey, L. (1982). *Space, Time & Medicine.* Boston: Shambhala Publications.

———. (2001). *Healing beyond the Body: Medicine and the Infinite Reach of the Mind.* Boston: Shambhala.

Durgananda, S. (2002). *The Heart of Meditation: Pathways To a Deeper Experience.* South Fallsburg, NY: Syda Foundation.

Edleglass, G. Maier, H. Gebert, and J. Davy. (1992). *Matter and Mind: Imaginative Participation in Science.* Hudson, NY: Lindisfarne Press.

Ehrlich, Paul R. (2000). *Human Natures: Genes, Cultures, and the Human Prospect.* New York: Penguin Books.

Elgin, D. (1993). *Awakening Earth: Exploring the Evolution of Human Culture and Consciousness.* New York: William Morrow.

———. (2000). *Promise Ahead: A Vision of Hope and Action for Humanity's Future.* New York: HarperCollins.

Feuerstein, G. (1987). *Structures of Consciousness: The Genius of Jean Gebser: An Introduction and Critique.* Lower Lake, CA: Integral Publishing.

Fichtelius, K. E. and S. Sjolander. (1972). *Smarter Than Man? Intelligence in Whales, Dolphins, and Humans.* New York: Sutton Books.

Fleischman, P. R. (1999). *Karma and Chaos: New and Collected Essays on Vipassana Meditation.* Seattle: Vipassana Research Publications.

Fodor, J. A. "The Big Idea: Can There be a Science of Mind." *Times Literary Supplement* (July 1992) 5–7.

Forman, R. (2004). *Grassroots Spirituality: What It Is; Why It Is Here; Where It Is Going.* Exeter, UK: Imprint Academic.

Frawley, D. (1992). *From the River of Heaven: Hindu and Vedic Knowledge for the Modern Age.* Delhi, India: Motilal Banarsidass Publishers.

Gandhi, K. (1991). *Social Philosophy of Sri Aurobindo and the New Age.* Pondicherry, India: Sri Aurobindo Ashram Publication Department.

Gardner, H. (1991). *The Unschooled Mind: How Children Think & How Schools Should Teach.* New York: Basic Books.

———. (2000). *The Disciplined Mind: Beyond Facts and Standard Tests, The K-12 Education that Every Child Deserves.* New York: Penguin Books.

Gardner, J. N. (2003). *Biocosm: The New Scientific Theory of Evolution: Intelligent Life Is the Architect of the Universe.* Makawao, HI: Inner Ocean Publishing.

Garfield, P. (1974). *Creative Dreaming.* New York: Ballantine Books.

Gebser, Jean (1985.) *The Ever-Present Origin.* Trans. Noel Barstad. Athens: Ohio University Press.

Giorgi, A, ed. (1985). *Phenomenology and Psychological Research.* Pittsburgh: Duquesne University Press.

Glass, M. (2001). *Yuga: An Anatomy of Our Fate.* Hillsdale, NY: Sophia Perennis.

Godwin, R. W. (2004). *One Cosmos under God: The Unification of Matter, Life, Mind & Spirit.* St. Paul, MN: Paragon House.

Goerner, S. J. (1999). *After the Clockwork Universe: The Emerging Science and Culture of Integral Society.* Edinburgh, UK: Floris Books.

Goleman, D. (1988). *The Meditative Mind: The Varieties of Meditative Experience.* Los Angeles: Jeremy Tarcher.

———., and J. Gurin. (1993). *Mind Body Medicine: How to Use Your Mind for Better Health.* Yonkers, NY: Consumer Reports Books.

Goswami, A. (2000). *The Visionary Window: A Quantum Physicist's Guide To Enlightenment.* Wheaton, IL: Theosophical Publishing House.

Govinda, L. A. (1991). *Buddhist Reflections.* York Beach, ME: Samuel Weiser.

———. (1970). *The Way of the White Clouds: A Buddhist Pilgrim in Tibet.* Berkeley, CA: Shambhala Publications.

———. (1976). *Creative Meditation and Multi-Dimensional Consciousness.* Wheaton, IL: The Theosophical Publishing House.

Grasse, R. (1996). *The Waking Dream: Unlocking the Symbolic Language of Our Lives.* Wheaton, IL: Theosophical Publishing House.

Greenberg, L. S., L. N. Rice, and R. Elliot. (1993). *Facilitating Emotional Change: The Moment-By-Moment Process*. New York: Guilford.

Gregory, R. L. (1966). *Eye and Brain: The Psychology of Seeing*. New York: McGraw-Hill.

Griffin, D. R. (1997). *Parapsychology, Philosophy, and Spirituality: A Postmodern Exploration*. Albany: State University of New York Press.

———., ed. (1988). *The Reenchantment of Science: Postmodern Proposals*. Albany, NY: State University of New York Press.

———. (1992). *Animal Minds: Beyond Cognition To Consciousness*. Chicago: University of Chicago Press.

Hafen, B. Q., K. J. Karren, K. J. Frandsen, and N. L. Smith. (1996). *Mind/Body Health: The Effects of Attitudes, Emotions, and Relationships*. Needham Heights, MA: Allyn & Bacon.

Hagen, S. (1995). *How the World Can Be the Way It Is: An Inquiry for the New Millenium into Science, Philosophy, and Perception*. Wheaton, IL: Theosophical Publishing House.

Hall, E. T. (1976). *Beyond Culture*. New York: Doubleday.

———. (1983). *The Dance of Life: The Other Dimension of Time*. New York: Anchor Books/Doubleday.

Harman, W. (1998). *Global Mind Change*. San Francisco: Berrett Koehler Publishers.

Harman, W. W., and E. Sahtouris. (1998). *Biology Revisioned*. Berkeley, CA: North Atlantic Books.

Harter, S. (1999). *The Construction of the Self: A Developmental Perspective*. New York: Guilford Press.

Hartmann, Thom. (2004). *The Last Hours of Ancient Sunlight: The Fate of the World and What We Can Do Before It's Too Late*. New York: Three Rivers Press.

Hayward, J. "A rDzogs-chen Buddhist Interpretation of the Sense of Self." *Journal of Consciousness Studies* 5, nos. 5–6 (1998) 611–26.

Hayward, J. W. (1984). *Perceiving Ordinary Magic: Science & Intuitive Wisdom*. Boulder, CO: New Science Library.

———. (1997). *Letters To Vanessa: On Love, Science, and Awareness in an Enchanted World*. Boston: Shambhala Publications.

Hedges, C. (2002). *War Is a Force that Gives Us Meaning*. New York: Anchor Books/Doubleday.

Hitchcock, J. (1999). *Healing Our Worldview: The Unity of Science and Spirituality*. West Chester, PA: Chrysalis Books.

Hobson, J. A. (1999). *Consciousness*. New York: Scientific American Library.

Hoffman, D. (2002). *Visual Intelligence: How We Create What We See*. New York: W. W. Norton.

Hunt, M. (1993). *The Story of Psychology*. New York: Anchor Books/Doubleday.

Hunt, S. A. (2002). *The Future of Peace: On the Front Lines with the World's Great Peacemakers*. San Francisco: HarperSanFrancisco.

Hunt, V. V. (1989). *Infinite Mind: Science of the Human Vibrations of Consciousness*. Malibu, CA: Malibu Publishing.

Iyengar, K. R. S. (1985). *Sri Aurobindo: A Biography and History*. Pondicherry, India: Sri Aurobindo International Centre of Education.

Jewett, R., and J. S. Lawrence. (2003). *Captain America and the Crusade Against Evil: The Dilemma of Zealous Nationalism*. Grand Rapids, MI: William B. Eerdmans.

Johnson, C. (2000). *Blowback: The Costs and Consequences of American Empire*. New York: Henry Holt.

Johnson, R. C. (1953). *The Imprisoned Splendor*. Wheaton, IL: Theosophical Publishing House.

John-Steiner, V. (1985). *Notebooks of the Mind: Explorations of Thinking*. New York: Harper & Row.

Jones, K. (1989). *The Social Face of Buddhism: An Approach To Political and Social Activism*. London: Wisdom Publications.

Jordan-Bychkov, T. G. (1982). *Human Mosaic: A Thematic Introduction To Cultural Geography*. New York: Longman.

Joseph, R. (1996). *Neuropsychiatry, Neuropsychology, and Clinical Neuroscience: Emotion, Evolution, Cognition, Language, Memory, Brain Damage, and Abnormal Behavior*. Baltimore: Williams & Wilkins.

Joshi, K. (1989). *Sri Aurobindo and the Mother*. New Delhi, India: The Mother's Institute of Research, in association with Motilal Banarsidass Publishers.

Kabat-Zinn, J. (1990). *Full Catastrophe Living: Using the Wisdom of Your Body and Mind to Face Stress, Pain, and Illness.* New York: Dell Publishing.

Kagan, J. (1989). *Unstable Ideas: Temperament, Cognition, and Self.* Cambridge: Harvard University Press.

Kaplan, R. D. (2005). *Imperial Grunts: The American Military on the Ground.* New York: Random House.

Kapleau, P. (1989). *Three Pillars of Zen.* New York: Anchor Books/Doubleday.

Karagulla, S., and D. van Gelder Kunz. (1989). *The Chakras and the Human Energy Fields.* Wheaton, IL: Theosophical Publishing House.

Kegan, R. (1982). *The Evolving Self: Problem and Process in Human Development.* Cambridge: Harvard University Press.

Kihlstrom, J. F. (1996). "Perception without Awareness of What Is Perceived, Learning without Awareness of What Is Learned. " In Velmans, ed., *The Science of Consciousness: Psychological, Neuropsychological, and Clinical Reviews.* London: Routledge.

Kiran, A. (1995). *Science, Materialism, Mysticism.* Waterford, CT: Integral Life Foundation.

Korten, D. C. (1999). *The Post-Corporate World: Life after Capitalism.* San Francisco: Berret-Koehler Publishers and West Hartford, CT: Kumarian Press.

———. (2001). *When Corporations Rule the World.* San Francisco: Berret-Koehler Publishers and Bloomfield, CT: Kumarian Press.

Kramer, G. (1999). *Meditating Together, Speaking from Silence: Experiencing Dharma in Dialogue.* Portland, OR: Metta Foundation.

Kranich, E. M. (1999). *Thinking beyond Darwin: The Idea of the Type as a Key To Vertebrate Evolution.* Hudson, NY: Lindisfarne Books.

Kunz, D. van Gelder. (1991). *The Personal Aura.* Wheaton, IL: Theosophical Publishing House.

LaBerge, S. (1985). *Lucid Dreaming: The Power of Being Awake & Aware in Your Dreams.* Los Angeles: Jeremy P. Tarcher.

Lancaster, B. (1991). *Mind, Brain, and Human Potential: The Quest for an Understanding of Self.* Longmead, UK: Element Books.

E. Laszlo, ed. (1991) *The New Evolutionary Paradigm: The World Futures General Evolution Studies.* vol. 2. New York: Gordon and Breach Science Publishers.

———. (2003). *The Connectivity Hypothesis: Foundations of an Integral Science of Quantum, Cosmos, Life, and Consciousness*. Albany: State University of New York Press.

———. (2004). *Science and the Akashic Field: An Integral Theory of Everything*. Rochester, VT: Inner Traditions.

Leahey, T. H. (2001). *A History of Modern Psychology*. Upper Saddle River, NJ: Prentice Hall.

———. , and R. J. Harris. (1980). *Learning and Cognition*. Upper Saddle River, NJ: Prentice Hall.

LeDoux, J. (1998). *The Emotional Brain: The Mysterious Underpinnings of Emotional Life*. New York: Touchstone.

Lemkow, A. F. (1990). *The Wholeness Principle: Dynamics of Unity within Science, Religion & Society*. Wheaton, IL: Theosophical Publishing House.

Leshan, L., and Margenau. (1982). *Einstein's Space & Van Gogh's Sky: Physical Reality and Beyond*. New York: Macmillan.

Lewis, M. (1997). *Altering Fate: Why the Past Does Not Predict the Future*. New York: Guilford Press.

Libet, B. (1999). "Do We Have Free Will?" In Libet et al. eds. (1999) *The Volitional Brain: Towards a Neuroscience of Free Will*. Thorverton, UK: Imprint Academic.

Loy, D. R. (2003). *The Great Awakening: A Buddhist Social Theory*. Boston: Wisdom Publications.

Loye, D. (1983). *An Arrow through Chaos: How We See into the Future*. Rochester, VT: Park Street Press.

———. (1984). *The Sphinx and the Rainbow: Brain, Mind, and Future Vision*. New York: Bantam Books.

Maharshi, R. (1972). *The Spiritual Teaching of Ramana Maharshi*. Berkeley, CA: Shambala Publications.

Maitra, S. K. (1956). *The Meeting of the East and the West in Sri Aurobindo's Philosophy*. Pondicherry, India: Sri Aurobindo Ashram Press.

McCrone, J. (2001). *Going Inside: A Tour Round a Moment of Consciousness*. New York: Fromm International.

McDermott, R. ed. (1973). *The Essential Aurobindo*. New York: Schocken Books.

McDonald, K. (1984). *How to Meditate: A Practical Guide.* Boston: Wisdom Publications.

McLaughlin, C., and G. Davidson. (1994). *Spiritual Politics: Changing the World from the Inside Out.* New York: Ballantine Books.

McLeod, K. (2001). *Wake Up To Your Life: Discovering the Buddhist Path of Attention.* San Francisco: HarperSanFrancisco.

McNeill, B., and C. Guion, C. eds. (1991). *Noetic Sciences Collection, 1980– 1990: Ten Years of Consciousness Research.* Sausalito, CA: Institute of Noetic Sciences.

McTaggart, L. (2002). *The Field: The Quest for the Secret Force of the Universe.* New York: HarperCollins.

Meeker-Lowry, S. (1988). *Economics as If the Earth Really Mattered: A Catalyst Guide To Socially Conscious Investing.* Philadelphia: New Society Publishers.

Mehmet, O. (1999). *Healing from the Heart: A Leading Surgeon Combines Eastern and Western Traditions to Create the Medicine of the Future.* New York: Penguin Putnam.

Melzack, R. "Phantom Limbs, the Self, and the Brain." *Canadian Psychology* 30 (1989) 1–16.

Midgley, M. (2001). *Science and Poetry.* London: Routledge.

———. "Being Scientific about Our Selves." *Journal of Consciousness Studies* 6 April (1999) 85–98.

Miller, M. E. and S. R. Cook-Greuter, eds. (1994). *Transcendence and Mature Thought in Adulthood: The Further Reaches of Adult Development.* Lanham, MD: Rowman & Littlefield.

Mishra, K. (1993). *Kashmir Saivism: The Central Philosophy of Tantrism.* Portland, OR: Rudra Press.

Mishra, R. S. (1987). *Fundamentals of Yoga: A Handbook of Theory, Practice, and Application.* New York: Harmony Books.

Mohrhoff, U. (1999). "The Physics of Interactionism." In Libet et al., eds. (1999) *The Volitional Brain: Towards a Neuroscience of Free Will.*

Morgan, J. (2002). *Born with a Bang, Book One: The Universe Tells Our Cosmic Story.* Nevada City, CA: Dawn Publications.

Mukherjee, J. K. (1990). *From Man Human To Man Divine.* Pondicherry, India: Sri Aurobindo International Centre of Education.

Murphy, M., and S. Donovan, (1997). *The Physical and Psychological Effects of Meditation: A Review of Contemporary Research with a Comprehensive Bibliography, 1931–1996*. Sausalito, CA: Institute of Noetic Sciences.

Narby, J. (2005). *Intelligence in Nature: An Inquiry into Knowledge*. New York: Jeremy P. Tarcher/Penguin.

Needleman, Jacob. (2002). *The American Soul: Rediscovering the Wisdom of the Founders*. New York: Jeremy P. Tarcher/Putnam.

Newberg, A., E. D'Aquili, and V. Rause. (2001). *Why God Won't Go Away: Brain Science & the Biology of Belief*. New York: Ballantine Books.

Nihilananda, S. trans. (1988). *The Gospel of Ramakrishna*. New York: Ramakrishna-Vivekananda Center.

Norretranders, T. (1998). *The User Illusion: Cutting Consciousness Down to Size*. New York: Penguin Group.

Nuernberger, P. (1981). *Freedom from Stress: A Holistic Approach*. Honesdale, PA: Himalayan Institute.

Ornstein, R. (1991). *The Evolution of Consciousness: Of Darwin, Freud, and Cranial Fire—The Origins of the Way We Think*. New York: Prentice Hall.

———. (1993). *The Roots of the Self: Unraveling the Mystery of Who We Are*. San Francisco: HarperSanFrancisco

———., and L. Carstensen. (1988). *Psychology: The Study of Human Experience*. San Diego: Harcourt Brace Jovanovich.

Palmo, T. (1998). *Cave in the Snow: Tenzin Palmo's Quest for Enlightenment*. London: Bloomsbury Publishing.

Pandit, M. P. (1988). *Upanishads: Gateways of Knowledge*. Wilmot, WI: Lotus Light Publications.

Parke, R. D., P. A. Ornstein, J . J. Rieser, and C. Zahn-Waxler, eds. (1995). *A Century of Developmental Psychology*. Washington, DC: American Psychological Association.

Pearsall, P. (1998). *The Heart's Code: Tapping the Wisdom and Power of Our Heart Energy: The New Findings about Cellular Memories and Their Role in the Mind/Body/Spirit Connection*. New York: Broadway Books.

Peat, F. D. (1987). *Synchronicity: The Bridge Between Matter and Mind*. Toronto: Bantam Books.

Pelletier, K. R. (1978). *Toward a Science of Consciousness*. New York: Dell Publishing.

Perlas, N. (2000). *Shaping Globalization: Civil Society, Cultural Power, and Threefolding*. Quezon City, Philippines: Center for Alternative Development Initiatives.

Podvoll, E. M. (1990). *The Seduction of Madness: Revolutionary Insights into the World of Psychosis and a Compassionate Approach To Recovery at Home*. New York: HarperCollins.

Prem, K. P., and M. Ashush. (1969). *Man, the Measure of All Things: In the Stanzas of Dzyan*. Wheaton, IL: Theosophical Publishing House.

Prem, S. K. (1976). *Initiation into Yoga: An Introduction To the Spiritual Life*. Wheaton, IL: Theosophical Publishing House.

———. (1982). *The Yoga of the Kathopanishad*. Ahmenabad, India: New Order Book Company.

———. (1988). *The Yoga of the Bhagavat Gita*. Longmead, UK: Element Books.

———. (1976). *Initiation into Yoga: An Introduction To the Spiritual Life*. Wheaton, IL: Theosophical Publishing House.

Radin, D. (1997). *The Conscious Universe: The Scientific Truth of Psychic Phenomena*. San Francisco: HarperEdge.

Randall, J. L. (1977). *Parapsychology and the Nature of Life*. New York: Harper Colophon Books.

Ratey, J. J. (2001). *A User's Guide To the Brain: Perception, Attention, and the Four Theatres of the Brain*. New York: Vintage Books.

Ray, P., and A. Anderson. (2000). *The Cultural Creatives: How 550 Million People are Changing the World*. New York: Harmony Books.

Reddy, K. (2003). *History of India: A New Approach*. New Delhi, India: Standard Publishers.

Rishabhchand. (1959). *The Integral Yoga of Sri Aurobindo*. Pondicherry, India: All India Press.

Robinson, D. N. (1986). *An Intellectual History of Psychology*. Madison: University of Wisconsin Press.

Rogers, Carl R. (1980). *A Way of Being*. Boston: Houghton Mifflin.

Rosch, E. "How to Catch James's Mystic Germ: Religious Experience, Buddhist Meditation and Psychology. " *Journal of Consciousness Studies* 9, nos. 9–10 (September/October 2002) 37–56.

Roy, D. K. (1992). *Yogi Sri Krishnaprem.* Bombay, India: Bharatiya Vidya Bhavan.

Russell, P. (1998). *Waking Up in Time: Finding Inner Peace in Times of Accelerating Change.* Novato, CA: Origin Press, Inc.

Sacks O. (1996). *An Anthropologist on Mars: Seven Paradoxical Tales.* New York: Vintage Books.

———. "Speed: Alterations of Time and Movement." *New Yorker* (August 23, 2004) 60–69.

Salmon, D. (1992). *Virtuous Reality: Music as an Aid in the Induction of Lucid Dreams—An Experiential Approach.* Unpublished manuscript.

———. (1999). *Attentional Control and the Deconstruction of the Schemas Underlying the Perception of Pain.* Unpublished manuscript.

Sastry, T. V. K. (1981). *Collected Works of T. V. Kapali Sastry, Volume Three: The Book of Lights-3.* Pondicherry, India: Dipti Publications.

Satprem. (1993). *Sri Aurobindo or The Adventure of Consciousness.* Mount Vernon, WA: Institute for Evolutionary Research.

Schlesinger, A. "Forgetting Reinhold Niebuhr." *New York Times*, September 18, 2005.

Schroeder, G. L. (1997). *The Science of God: The Convergence of Scientific and Biblical Wisdom.* New York: Broadway Books.

———. (2002). *The Hidden Face of God: Science Reveals the Ultimate Truth.* New York: Touchstone.

Schumacher, E. F. (1973). *Small Is Beautiful: Economics as If People Mattered.* New York: Harper & Row.

Schwartz, G. E. (1984). "Psychobiology of health: A New Synthesis. " In Hammonds, B. L. and C. J. Scheirer, eds., *Psychology and Health: Master Lecturers.* Washington, DC: American Psychological Association.

Schwartz, J. (2002). *The Mind and the Brain: Neuroplasticity and the Power of Mental Force.* San Francisco: HarperCollins.

Schwartz, J. M. (1999). "A Role for Volition and Attention in the Generation of New Brain Circuitry: Towards a Neurobiology of Mental Force. " In Libet et al. eds. (1999) *The Volitional Brain: Towards a Neuroscience of Free Will.*

Sen, I. (1986). *Integral Psychology: The Psychology System of Sri Aurobindo.* Pondicherry, India: Sri Aurobindo International Centre of Education.

Senge, P. (1994). *The Fifth Discipline*. New York: Currency/Doubleday.

Sheldrake, R. (1994). *The Rebirth of Nature: The Greening of Science and God*. Rochester, VT: Park Street Press.

———. (2003). *The Sense of Being Stared At and Other Unexplained Powers of the Human Mind*. New York: Crown Publishers.

Siegel, D. J. (1999). *The Developing Mind: How Relationships and the Brain Interact to Shape Who We Are*. New York: Guilford Press.

Silver, B. L. (1998). *The Ascent of Science*. New York: Oxford University Press.

Skinner, B. F. (1971). *Beyond Freedom and Dignity*. New York: Alfred A. Knopf.

Sloan, D. (1983). *Insight-Imagination: The Emancipation of Thought and the Modern World*. Westport, CT: Greenwood Publishing Group.

Smith, H. (1989). *Beyond the Post-Modern Mind*. New York: Crossroads Publishing.

Smith, L. ed. (1990). *Intelligence Came First: Life and Mind in the Field of Cosmic Consciousness*. Wheaton, IL: Theosophical Publishing House.

Sorokin, P. A. (1992). *The Crisis of Our Age*. Oxford, UK: Oneworld Publications.

Stapp, H. (1993). *Mind, Matter, and Quantum Mechanics*. Berlin: Springer-Verlag.

———. (1999). "Attention, Intention, and Will in Quantum Physics." In Libet, et al., eds. (1999) *The Volitional Brain: Towards a Neuroscience of Free Will*.

Stricker, G., and J. R. Gold, eds. (1993). *Comprehensive Handbook of Psychotherapy Integration*. New York: Plenum Press.

Swimme, B., and T. Berry. (1992). *The Universe Story: From the Primordial Flaring Forth to the Ecozoic Era: A Celebration of the Unfolding of the Cosmos*. San Francisco: HarperSanFrancisco.

Tagore, R. (1931). *The Religion of Man*. Boston: Beacon Press.

Taimi, I. K. (1974). *Man, God and the Universe*. Wheaton, IL: The Theosophical Publishing House.

Targ, R. (2004). *Limitless Mind: A Guide To Remote Viewing and Transformation of Consciousness*. Novato, CA: New World Library.

———. and J. Katra. (1998) *Miracles of Mind: Exploring Nonlocal Consciousness and Spiritual Healing*. Novato, CA: New World Library.

Tarnas, R. (1993). *The Passion of the Western Mind: Understanding the Ideas that Have Shaped Our World View.* New York: Ballantine Books.

Tart, C. T. (1989). *Open Mind, Discriminating Mind: Reflections on Human Possibilities.* San Francisco: Harper & Row.

Taylor, E. (1999). *Shadow Culture: Psychology and Spirituality in America.* Washington, D.C: Counterpoint.

————. "Desperately Seeking Spirituality." *Psychology Today* 27 (November 1, 1994).

————. "William James and Depth Psychology." *Journal of Consciousness Studies* 9, nos. 9–10 (September/October 2002) 11–36.

Taylor, G. R. (1981). *The Natural History of the Mind.* Harmondsworth, UK: Penguin Books.

Thomas, L. (1975). *The Lives of a Cell.* New York: Bantam Books.

Thompson, R. L. (1981). *Mechanistic and Nonmechanistic Science: An Investigation into the Nature of Consciousness and Form.* Los Angeles: Bhaktivedanta Book Trust.

Thurman, R. (1994). *The Tibetan Book of the Dead: Liberation through Understanding in the Between.* New York: Bantam Books.

————. (1998). *Inner Revolution: Life, Liberty, and the Pursuit of Real Happiness.* New York: Riverhead Books.

Tolle, E. (1999). *The Power of Now: A Guide to Spiritual Enlightenment.* Novato, CA: New World Library.

————. (2005). *A New Earth: Awakening To Your Life's Purpose.* New York: Dutton.

Underhill, E. (1915). *Practical Mysticism.* New York: E. P. Dutton.

Van Vrekham, G. (2001). *Overman: The Intermediary Between the Human & the Supramental Being.* New Delhi, India: Rupa & Co.

Varela, F., and J. Shear, eds. (1999). *The View From Within: First-Person Approaches To the Study of Consciousness.* Thorverton, UK: Imprint Academic.

Varela, F. J., E. Thompson, and E. Rosch, (1991). *The Embodied Mind: Cognitive Science and Human Experience.* Cambridge, MA: MIT Press.

Varghese, R. A. (2003). *The Wonder of the World: A Journey from Modern Science To the Mind of God.* Fountain Hills, AZ: Tyr Publishing.

Vaughan-Lee, L. (1993). *The Bond with the Beloved: The Mystical Relationship of the Lover and the Beloved.* Inverness, CA: Golden Sufi Center.

———. (1998). *The Face Before I Was Born: A Spiritual Biography.* Inverness, CA: Golden Sufi Center.

———. (2003). *Light of Oneness.* Inverness, CA: Golden Sufi Center.

Velmans, M. (2000). *Understanding Consciousness.* London, Routledge.

———. ed. (1996). *The Science of Consciousness: Pyschological, Neurophysiological, and Clinical Reviews.* London: Routledge.

Vrinte, J. (1996). *The Quest for the Inner Man: Transpersonal Psychology and Integral Sadhana.* Pondicherry, India: Sri Mira Trust.

Wallace, B. A. (1992). *A Passage from Solitude: Training the Mind in a Life Embracing the World.* Ithaca, NY: Snow Lion Publications.

———. (1993). *Tibetan Buddhism from the Ground Up: Practical Approach for Modern Life.* Boston: Wisdom Publications.

———. (1996). *Choosing Reality: A Buddhist View of Physics and the Mind.* Ithaca, NY: Snow Lion Books.

———. (1998). *The Bridge of Quiescence: Experiencing Tibetan Buddhist Meditation.* Chicago: Open Court.

———. (1999). *Boundless Heart: The Cultivation of the Four Immeasurables.* Ithaca, NY: Snow Lion Publications.

———. (2000). *The Taboo of Subjectivity: Toward a New Science of Consciousness.* Oxford, UK: Oxford University Press.

Wan-Ho, M. (1998). *The Rainbow and the Worm: The Physics of Organisms.* Singapore: World Scientific.

Watson, E. L. G. (1992). *The Mystery of Practical Life.* Hudson, NY: Lindisfarne Press.

Watson, G., S. Batchelor and G. Claxton. (2000). *The Psychology of Awakening: Buddhism, Science, and Our Day-To-Day Lives.* York Beach, ME: Samuel Weiser.

Watson, L. (1988). *Beyond Supernature: A New Natural History of the Supernatural.* Toronto: Bantam Books.

Weisman, A. (1998). *Gaviotas: A Village to Reinvent the World.* White River Junction, VT: Chelsea Green Publishing.

Wesson, R. (1989). *Cosmos and Metacosmos.* La Salle, IL: Open Court.

Whitehead, A. N. (1955). *Adventures of Ideas.* New York: New American Library of World Literature.

Wood, E. (1949). *Concentration: An Approach To Meditation.* Wheaton, IL: Theosophical Publishing House.

————. (1947). *Mind and Memory Training.* Adyar, India: Theosophical Publishing House.

Woodhouse, M. B. (1996). *Paradigm Wars: Worldviews for a New Age.* Berkeley, CA: Frog, Ltd.

Wright, R. (2000). *Nonzero: The Logic of Human Destiny.* New York: Pantheon Books.

Wyller, A. A. (1996). *The Creating Consciousness: Science as the Language of God.* Denver: MacMurray & Beck.

INDEX

CONTENTS OF CD

TEXT: JAN MASLOW AND DON SALMON   MUSIC: DON SALMON

We put together this CD to help you read *Yoga Psychology and the Transformation of Consciousness* in a more contemplative way. It may be helpful to listen to the CD once through before you begin reading the book. This will give you an overview of the major themes, and help you to read the book in a more contemplative way. As you are reading the book, it may also be helpful to pause from time to time to listen again to one or more tracks on the CD, and then try to maintain that meditative feeling as you resume reading.

When you listen to the CD, sit quietly with your back straight but relaxed, and your eyes closed. The meditative effect will be enhanced by listening through headphones.

The more often you practice some kind of meditation exercises—the ones we provide here or others—the deeper your experience and understanding of yoga psychology will become. Track 4, a guided meditation with music, is included to help you practice the same meditation techniques learned on Tracks 2 and 3. You can use Track 4 to develop and maintain a meditation practice if you don't already have one.

Our thanks to Harry O'Brien of Atlanta Recording Studio for his expertise, grace, and good humor during long hours of mixing and recording the CD.

For information on our yoga psychology website, see www.paragonhouse.com.